CRASH COURSE

Cell Biology
and Genetics

Other Titles in the Crash Course Series

There are 23 books in the Crash Course series in two ranges: Basic Science and Clinical. Each book follows the same format, with concise text, clear illustrations and helpful learning features including access to online USMLE test questions.

Basic Science titles
Pathology
Nervous System
Renal and Urinary Systems
Gastrointestinal System
Respiratory System
Endocrine and Reproductive Systems
Metabolism and Nutrition
Pharmacology
Immunology
Musculoskeletal System
Cardiovascular System
Cell Biology and Genetics
Anatomy

Clinical titles
Surgery
Cardiology
History and Examination
Internal Medicine
Neurology
Gastroenterology
OBGYN

Forthcoming:
Psychiatry
Imaging
Pediatrics

Cell Biology and Genetics

Neil E. Lamb, PhD
Director of Education
Department of Human Genetics
Emory University School of Medicine
Atlanta, Georgia

UK edition authors
Ania L. Manson
Emma Jones
Anna Morris

UK series editor
Daniel Horton-Szar

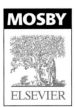

ELSEVIER

1600 John F. Kennedy Blvd.
Suite 1800
Philadelphia, PA 19103-2899

CRASH COURSE: CELL BIOLOGY AND GENETICS

Copyright 2007 by Mosby, Inc., an affiliate of Elsevier, Inc.

ISBN-13: 978-0-323-04494-3
ISBN-10: 0-323-04494-8

Adapted from Crash Course Cell Biology and Genetics by Ania L Manson, Emma Jones, and Anna Morris, ISBN: 0-7234-3248-1. Copyright © Elsevier Science Limited 2002, 1998. All rights reserved.

The rights of Ania L Manson, Emma Jones, and Anna Morris to be identified as the authors of this work have been asserted by them in accordance with the Copyright, Designs and Patents Act, 1988.

Library of Congress Cataloging-in-Publication Data

Lamb, Neil E.
   Crash course cell biology and genetics / Neil E. Lamb.—1st American ed.
     p. cm.
   ISBN 0-323-04494-8
   1. Cytology.   2. Genetics.   I. Title.
   QH581.2.L36 2007

   571.6–dc22

2006044879

Acquisitions Editor: Alex Stibbe
Project Development Manager: Stan Ward
Publishing Services Manager: David Saltzberg
Designer: Andy Chapman
Cover Design: Antbits Illustration
Illustration Manager: Mick Ruddy

Printed in China

Last digit is the print number:
9 8 7 6 5 4 3 2 1

Preface

Genetics and cell biology are fundamental components of medical education. A solid understanding of the fundamentals of cell structure and function, coupled with a background in the genetic contributions to simple and complex disorders, is a necessity for today's practicing physician.

The publication of the human genome sequence has accelerated the speed with which genetic information is incorporated into medical practice; this rate will only increase in years to come. The genetic impact on health and disease will be felt across all branches of medicine.

Historically, with an abundance of jargon and some very complex concepts, many students have approached this topic with anxiety and trepidation. It is the aim of this book to relieve the reader of those anxious thoughts and to present the fundamentals in clear, concise, and relevant terms. The first American edition builds upon the excellent content provided by the previous UK editions to highlight the key concepts underlying the genetic influence on disease and well-being.

It is our hope that you find this book an important reference, one that you continue to pull off the shelf, even after successfully passing your exams and completing your medical training.

Neil E. Lamb

Acknowledgments

I begin by thanking the authors of the previous editions of *Crash Course: Cell Biology and Genetics*—Ania L. Manson, Emma Jones, and Anna Morris. The excellent foundation they provided made this most recent revision a pleasure to undertake. I also wish to thank my fellow faculty in the Department of Human Genetics at Emory University for their support, assistance, and willingness to answer my many queries. Lastly, I want to acknowledge my family (both immediate and extended), especially my wife Cynthia, for the support they provided during (and, perhaps, even in spite of) the many hours I spent preparing this book.

Dedication

To my family:

My parents—David and Mary Lamb—for providing me with the best of genetic and environmental starts in life.

My wife Cynthia for her steadfast love and friendship, as well as the willingness to patiently overlook some of my genetically influenced quirks.

And my children—Preston, Olivia, and Emma Grace—for the untold blessings I have received by being part of their lives. I never knew watching one's genetic contributions unfold in the next generation could be so much fun.

Contents

Preface v
Acknowledgments vii
Dedication ix

Part I: Principles of Cell Biology and
Molecular Genetics 1

1. General Organization of the Cell 3
   Definitions 3
   Prokaryotes and eukaryotes 3
   Structure and function of eukaryotic
      organelles 5
   Cell diversity in multicellular organisms . . . 10

2. Proteins and Enzymes 13
   Amino acids 13
   Proteins 18
   Enzymes 23

3. The Cell Membrane 31
   Structure of the cell membrane 31
   Transport across the cell membrane 36
   Membrane potential 41
   Receptors 45

4. The Working Cell 53
   Cytoskeleton and cell motility 53
   Lysosomes 58
   Cell surface and cell adhesion 61

5. The Molecular Basis of Genetics 73
   Organization of the cell nucleus 73
   Cell cycle 74
   Mitosis and meiosis 77
   Nucleic acids 80
   DNA packaging and repair 84
   DNA replication 87

Transcription and RNA synthesis 94
Translation and protein synthesis 99
Control of gene expression and protein
   synthesis 104
Posttranslational modification
   of proteins 107
Structure of genes 109
Genetics of bacteria and viruses 110

Part II: Medical Genetics 119

6. Molecular Genetics as Applied
   to Medicine 121
   Basic techniques of molecular
      genetics 121
   The Human Genome Project 130
   Cloning and characterizing human
      disease genes 132
   Gene therapy 136

7. Genetic Disease 139
   Single gene disorders 139
   Chromosomal disorders 159
   Polygenic inheritance and
      multifactorial disorders 165
   Genetics of cancer 168

8. Principles of Medical Genetics 177
   Population genetics and screening 177
   Risk assessment and genetic
      counseling 184
   Genetic consultation and
      history taking 188
   Common presentations of
      genetic disease 190

Index 199

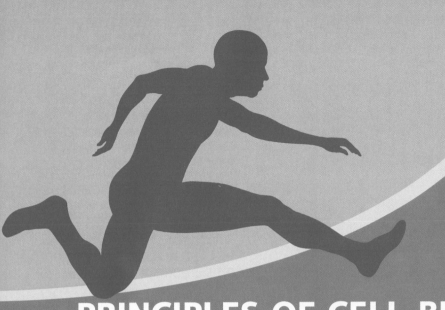

PRINCIPLES OF CELL BIOLOGY AND MOLECULAR GENETICS

1. General Organization of the Cell   3

2. Proteins and Enzymes   13

3. The Cell Membrane   31

4. The Working Cell   53

5. The Molecular Basis of Genetics   73

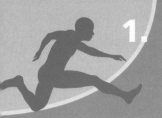

1. General Organization of the Cell

Definitions

Cell

The cell is the basic unit of life. If it is to survive, each cell must maintain an internal environment that supports its essential biochemical reactions, despite changes in the external environment. Therefore, a selectively permeable plasma membrane surrounding a concentrated aqueous solution of chemicals is a feature of all cells.

Organism

An organism is a system capable of self-replication and self-repair, which may be unicellular or multicellular. Unicellular organisms consist of a solitary cell able independently to perform all the functions of life. Multicellular organisms contain several different cell types that are specialized to perform specific functions.

Prokaryotes and eukaryotes

Prokaryotes are the simplest unicellular organisms. It is thought that by a process of mutation and natural selection all living organisms evolved from a common prokaryotic ancestor (Fig. 1.1).

The basic molecular machinery of life has been conserved in all species. The enzymes that perform common reactions such as glycolysis in bacterial and human cells show significant homology at both the DNA and protein level.

The prokaryotic cell

All microorganisms lacking a membrane-bound nucleus (i.e., the various types of bacteria) are classified in the prokaryote superkingdom. The

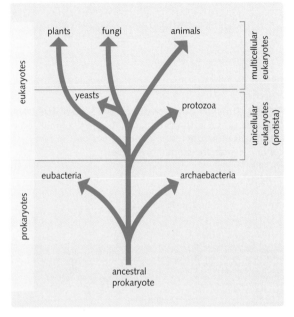

Fig. 1.1 Evolutionary relationships between organisms. Prokaryotes are thought to represent the most primitive life form, with eukaryotic unicellular and multicellular organisms evolving from an ancestral prokaryotic cell by a process involving mutation followed by natural selection. (Adapted from *Molecular Biology of the Cell*, 3rd edn, by B. Alberts *et al.*, Garland Publishing Co., 1994, with permission of Routledge, Inc., part of The Taylor & Francis Group.)

typical prokaryotic cell (Fig. 1.2) shows the following features:
- A single cytoplasmic compartment containing all the cellular components.
- Cell division by binary fission.

In order for the prokaryotic cell to survive, molecules required for energy and biosynthesis must diffuse into the cell and waste products must diffuse out of the cell across the plasma membrane. The rate of diffusion is related to membrane surface area.

When the diameter of a cell increases:
- The cell volume expands to the cube of the linear increase.
- The surface area only expands to the square of the linear increase.

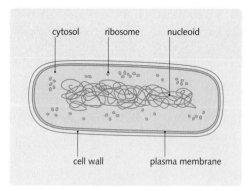

cytosol   ribosome   nucleoid

cell wall   plasma membrane

Fig. 1.2 Structure of a typical prokaryotic cell. The DNA molecule is free in the cytoplasm. Bacteria contain some subcellular structures such as ribosomes but do not contain membrane-bound organelles.

Thus, small cells have a larger surface area to volume ratio than large cells. Prokaryotic cells rely on simple diffusion for the delivery of nutrients to the center of the cell. Therefore, if prokaryotes expand above a certain size, the rate of diffusion of nutrients across the plasma membrane will not be sufficient to sustain the increased needs of its larger cell volume. Hence, prokaryotic cells are small.

The eukaryotic cell

All organisms consisting of cells with a membrane-bound nucleus are classified in the eukaryote superkingdom. The Animalia, Plantae, Protista, and Fungi kingdoms all belong within this group. The typical eukaryotic cell (Fig. 1.3) shows the following features:

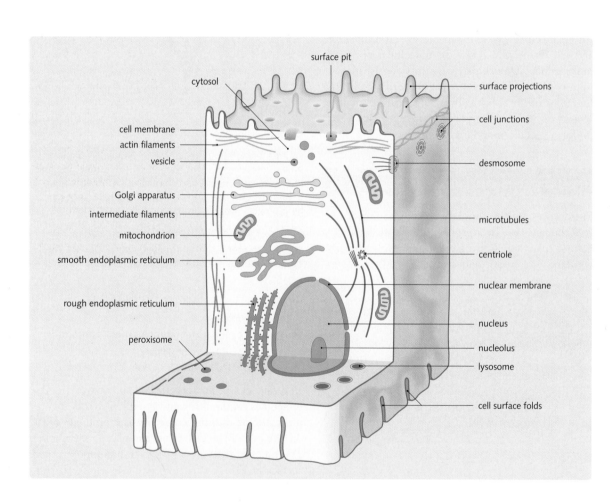

surface pit

cytosol

surface projections

cell membrane

cell junctions

actin filaments

vesicle

desmosome

Golgi apparatus

intermediate filaments

mitochondrion

microtubules

smooth endoplasmic reticulum

centriole

nuclear membrane

rough endoplasmic reticulum

nucleus

peroxisome

nucleolus

lysosome

cell surface folds

Fig. 1.3 Structure of a typical eukaryotic cell. Genetic material is contained within the nuclear membrane. Membrane-bound organelles serve as compartments for specific cellular functions, permitting greater cellular specialization and diversity. Cytoskeletal components maintain cell shape and facilitate dynamic functions such as endocytosis. (Adapted from Stevens and Lowe, 1997.)

- A complex series of inner membranes that separate the cell into distinct compartments which perform specific functions.
- Cell division by mitosis.
- Specialized organelles such as centrioles, mitotic spindles, mitochondria, and microtubules.

Unlike prokaryotes, eukaryotic cells are capable of endocytosis (see Chapter 4). By this means, patches of the plasma membrane pinch off to form membrane-bound vesicles that deliver nutrients from the external environment to compartments deep within the cell. Endocytosis thus liberates eukaryotic cells from the constraints of simple diffusion, allowing them to sustain a relatively small surface area to volume ratio. Eukaryotic cells are, therefore, on average, much larger than prokaryotic cells (Fig. 1.4). In the typical animal cell, the various specialized organelles occupy about half the total cell volume.

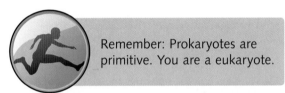

Remember: Prokaryotes are primitive. You are a eukaryote.

Structure and function of eukaryotic organelles

The whole cell is surrounded by the plasma membrane, which forms a dynamic interface between the cytosol and the environment. Eukaryotic cells have a complex ultrastructure comprising membranous and nonmembranous organelles. These structures serve specific functions within the cell.

Membranous organelles

Membranous organelles are enclosed within a phospholipid bilayer, and they maintain discrete biochemical environments that contain characteristic sets of enzymes.

Plasma membrane

The plasma membrane is a selectively permeable barrier that surrounds cell cytoplasm (Fig. 1.5). Nonpolar (lipid-soluble) molecules diffuse across the lipid bilayer by passive transport. Proteins embedded within the bilayer are responsible for transport of polar molecules between the cell and extracellular fluid by facilitated diffusion and active transport (see Chapter 3). The ability of the cell to regulate transport protein activity is fundamental to many biological processes, such as muscle contraction generation and conduction of nerve cell action potentials.

Many of the proteins and lipids on the outer surface of the cell membrane have oligosaccharides covalently attached to them. This "glycocalyx" coat:

- Produces a negative charge, which separates cells within a multicellular layer.
- Acts as a receptor surface that is sensitive to chemical and other changes in the environment.

Prokaryotic compared with eukaryotic cells	
Prokaryotic cells	**Eukaryotic cells**
Includes bacteria and blue–green algae	Four major groups: protista, fungi, plants, and animals
No true nucleus	True nucleus
DNA circular and free	DNA linear and within nucleus
No membrane-bound organelles	Internal compartmentalization with organelles, hence division of labor (specialization)
Simple binary reproduction	Mitotic reproduction (and meiotic)
No development of tissues	Tissue and organ systems common
Multicellular types rare	Independent unicellular organism or part of multicellular organism
Size: 1–10 µm	Size: 10–100 µm

Fig. 1.4 Basic features of prokaryotic and eukaryotic cells.

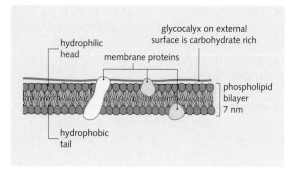

Fig. 1.5 Structure of the plasma membrane. Proteins that penetrate one or both layers interrupt the structural continuity of the phospholipid bilayer. The glycocalyx forms an outer coat to the cell.

- Carries chemical signals enabling other cells (e.g., cells of the immune system) to recognize it.

In certain cell types, such as epithelia, the plasma membrane may show specializations that enhance cell function:

- The intercellular surfaces are linked together by cell junctions to form a continuous sheet of cells (see Chapter 4).
- The basal surface is linked to extracellular matrix by hemidesmosomes.
- Luminal surfaces may incorporate cilia (motile structures, e.g., lining the fallopian tubes and trachea), microvilli (increase surface area, e.g., in small intestine), or stereocilia (extra long microvilli, e.g., in epididymis).

Nucleus

The nucleus (Fig. 1.6):

- Sequesters and replicates DNA.
- Transcribes and splices RNA.
- Allows facilitated selective exchange of molecules such as RNA, e.g., transfer RNA (tRNA), with the cytoplasm.

DNA replication occurs when the genetic code is copied exactly before cell division. In RNA transcription and splicing, genes are copied and adapted to form complementary strands of

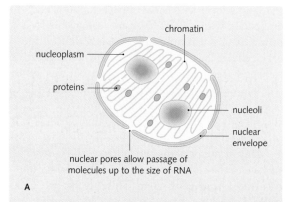

A

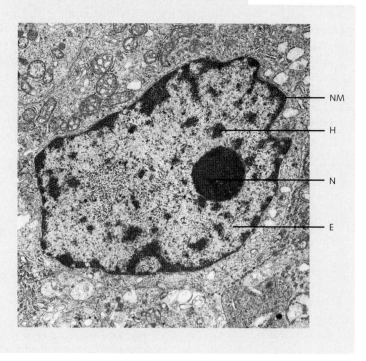

B

Fig. 1.6 (A) Structure of the nucleus. (B) Electron micrograph showing the double nuclear membrane (NM), nucleolus (N), heterochromatin (H), which is dense staining, and euchromatin (E), which is light staining. (Courtesy of Dr. Trevor Gray.)

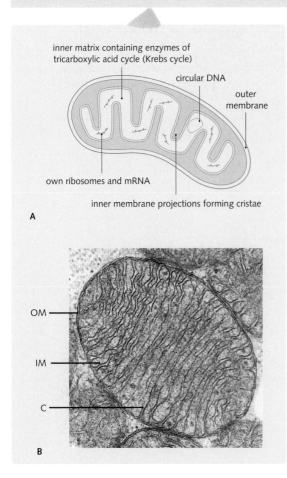

inner matrix containing enzymes of tricarboxylic acid cycle (Krebs cycle)

circular DNA

outer membrane

own ribosomes and mRNA

inner membrane projections forming cristae

A

OM

IM

C

B

Fig. 1.7 (A) Structure of a mitochondrion. (B) Electron micrograph showing outer membrane (OM), inner membrane (IM), and cristae (C). (Courtesy of Dr. Trevor Gray.)

messenger RNA (mRNA), which can be translated into protein.

Chromosomes are long strands of DNA that carry the genetic code. In eukaryotes, DNA is complexed with histone and nonhistone proteins to form chromatin. Histones are DNA-binding proteins that are important for DNA packaging. Other DNA-associated proteins function as enzymes for replication and transcription. Nucleoli are dense-staining areas within the nucleus where ribosomal RNA (rRNA) is made.

Mitochondria

The structure of a mitochondrion is illustrated in Fig. 1.7. Mitochondria perform aerobic respiration, and they are self-replicating. They have their own DNA, and they are thought to originate from primitive bacteria.

Rough (granular) endoplasmic reticulum

Rough endoplasmic reticulum (RER) is a labyrinth of membranous sacs, called cisternae, to which ribosomes are attached giving a "rough" appearance on electron microscopy. Enzymes are attached to cisternae membranes or contained within the lumen (Fig. 1.8). Ribosome clusters occur free in the cytoplasm or attached to the outer surface of the cisternae. They make polypeptides, which are then in turn:

- Inserted into the membrane.
- Released into the lumen of the cisternae.
- Transported to the Golgi complex or elsewhere.

Proteins made within RER are kept within vesicles or secreted. Cells that make large quantities of secretory protein have large amounts of RER (e.g., pancreatic acinar cells, plasma cells).

Free ribosomes synthesize proteins for immediate use in the cytoplasm.

Smooth (agranular) endoplasmic reticulum

Smooth endoplasmic reticulum (SER) is a labyrinth of cisternae with many enzymes attached to its surface or found within its cisternae. SER:

- Makes steroid hormones (e.g., in the ovary).
- Detoxifies body fluids (e.g., in the liver).

Golgi apparatus

The Golgi apparatus (Fig. 1.9) is a system of membranous flattened sacs involved in modifying (e.g., addition of carbohydrate), sorting, and packaging macromolecules for secretion or delivery to other organelles. Cells that produce many secretory products have well-developed Golgi apparatus (e.g., hepatocytes).

Lysosomes

Lysosomes are primary components of intracellular digestion (see Chapter 4). Cells specializing in phagocytosis (e.g., macrophages) have many lysosomes which:

- Are vesicular bodies containing granular amorphous material and about 60 types of hydrolytic enzymes.
- Vary in size from 50 nm to over 1 mm.
- Digest material with hydrolases that are active at acid pH.

Peroxisomes

Peroxisomes are vesicular bodies that are smaller than lysosomes, and contain specific enzymes. They

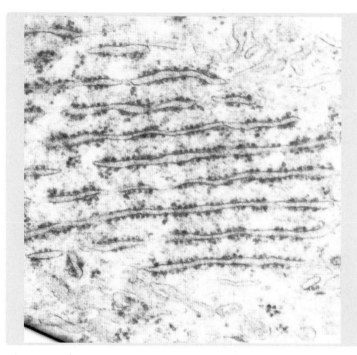

Fig. 1.8 Electron micrograph of rough endoplasmic reticulum (RER). The membranous tubules that make up the ER are studded with ribosomes giving a rough appearance. (Courtesy of Dr. Trevor Gray.)

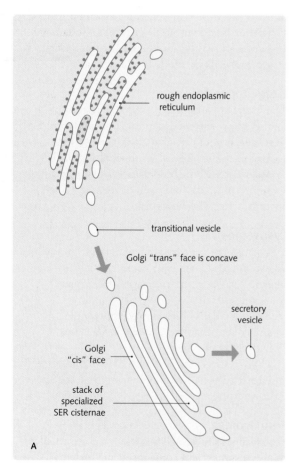

rough endoplasmic reticulum

transitional vesicle

Golgi "trans" face is concave

secretory vesicle

Golgi "cis" face

stack of specialized SER cisternae

A

Fig. 1.9 (A) Structure of the Golgi apparatus.

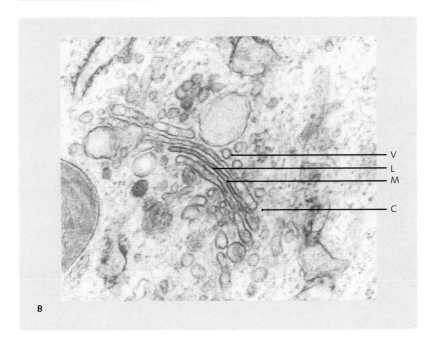

B

Fig. 1.9—cont'd (B) Electron micrograph with parallel stacks of membrane (M) delineating Golgi lumen (L) from the cytosol (C). Transport vesicles (V) can be seen on their way from endoplasmic reticulum. (Courtesy of Dr. Trevor Gray.)

perform oxidation and detoxify hydrogen peroxide, which is a product of many metabolic reactions in the cell.

Nonmembranous organelles
The cytoskeleton

The cytoskeleton is the internal framework of the cell, consisting of filaments and tubules. Cytoskeletal structures maintain and change cell shape by rearrangement of the cytoskeletal elements. They are thus essential for endocytosis, cell division, ameboid movements, and contraction of muscle cells. There are several classes of cytoskeletal structural components:

- Microfilaments formed from actin.
- Microtubules formed from tubulin.
- Intermediate filaments formed from intermediate filament proteins such as keratin.

These structures may be cross-linked by other proteins into networks or specialized organelles, the most common of which are:

- Centrioles—these usually occur in pairs and they are the site of spindle assembly in cell division. Each centriole is a short cylinder comprised of nine groups of three fused microtubules arranged around a central cavity.
- Cilia—used by some cells to transport substances (e.g., fallopian cells move ova

toward the uterus). Cilia self-assembly is seeded at basal bodies on the cell surface, which are identical in structure to centrioles. Microtubules are arranged in a "9 + 2" arrangement consisting of nine microtubule doublets surrounding two single microtubules (Fig. 1.10). Dynein side arms extend between adjacent doublets and hydrolyze ATP to generate a sliding force between them. This action underlies ciliary beating.

- Flagella—very long cilia used for propulsion by spermatozoa (NB prokaryotic and eukaryotic flagellae have different molecular structures).
- Microvilli—nonmotile extensions of plasma membrane supported by actin, which increase the surface area of the cell (e.g., the small intestine brush-border).

Kartagener syndrome is an inherited disorder characterized by bronchiectasis, sinusitis, and dextrocardia. It is associated with ultrastructural defects in dynein or microtubule proteins leading to ciliary dyskinesia.

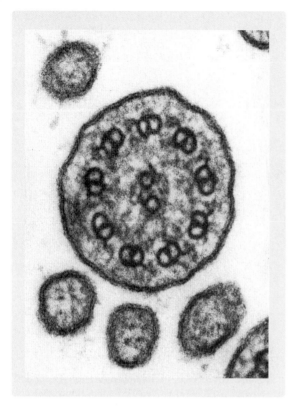

Fig. 1.10 Structure of a cilium. Electron micrograph of transverse section through a cilium, showing the characteristic 9 + 2 structure of the microtubules. (Courtesy of Dr. Trevor Gray.)

Cell diversity in multicellular organisms

Cell specialization

It is thought that multicellular organisms evolved because specialized cells acting together can combine to form a single organism that is able to exploit ecological niches not available to any of its component cells acting alone.

Similar types of specialized cells combine together to form tissues, of which there are four main types each adapted to a specific function (Fig 1.11). By definition, specialized cells show structural features that enable them to perform their designated function. In order to cooperate and coordinate their activities in the multicellular animal:

- Cells are bound together by adhesions between their plasma membranes and the extracellular matrix (see Chapter 4).
- Cells interact and communicate with one another (see Chapter 3).

Differentiation

Over 200 types of cell are identifiable in human tissue, differing in terms of their structure, function, and chemical metabolism. All cell types are derived from a single cell (the zygote) following conception. The zygote is described as being totipotent since it is ultimately able to differentiate into all the cell types that make up the adult organism. There is no loss of genetic material from somatic cells during human development (red blood cells are an exception), so different cell types arise as a result of differences in gene expression.

During development, cells differentiate as successive cascades of proteins are expressed that regulate the DNA in each cell, restricting transcription from specific sections of the genome. The developmental signals that initiate differentiation in a human cell come from the cells that surround it. However, even when removed from its normal environment the differentiated cell and its progeny will retain many of its functional characteristics. This concept is termed cell memory because the DNA modifications restricting transcription ("epigenetic" changes) persist and are transmitted to daughter cells.

Gene expression in multicellular eukaryotes

The Human Genome Project estimates there are between 25,000 and 30,000 protein-coding genes in the haploid human genome (see Chapter 6). The expression of these genes may be spatially or temporally regulated:

- "Housekeeping genes" are expressed in all cell types because they code for proteins necessary for eukaryotic cell survival (e.g., TCA cycle genes).
- The expression of some genes is confined to differentiated cells with a specific function (e.g., insulin in pancreatic beta cells).
- Some genes are expressed for only a short period during a specific stage of development (e.g., PAX genes are expressed early in neural development).

Cell specialization in tissues		
Tissue structure	**Function**	**Specialized cell types**
Epithelial tissue Consists of continuous sheets of cells that are bound together by tight junctions	Epithelial tissue lines inner and outer surfaces of the body to form a selectively permeable barrier Epithelial surfaces may be specialized for: • absorption • substance movement • secretion	Absorptive cells—the luminal plasma membrane is folded into microvilli to increase the surface area (e.g., intestinal villi) Ciliated cells—the luminal plasma membrane is coated with cilia that beat in synchrony (e.g., tracheal mucociliary escalator) Secretory cells—the RER and Golgi apparatus are highly developed (e.g., chief cells in the stomach)
Muscle tissue Consists of groups of cells containing fibrillar proteins arranged in an organized manner in the cytoplasm and linked by intermolecular bonds Skeletal and cardiac muscle appear striated	Muscle functions to produce movement. Contraction results from the rearrangement of internal bonds between fibrillar proteins Muscle tissue is specialized to allow: • voluntary movement of the skeleton • involuntary movement of substances through the viscera • continuous synchronous contraction of the heart	Skeletal muscle cells—each muscle fiber is an enormous multinucleated cell that extends the full length of the muscle (nuclei are located at the cell periphery). Thus, excitation results in simultaneous contraction of the full length of muscle in a longitudinal direction Visceral (smooth) muscle cells—cells are relatively small with tapered ends and only a single nucleus. The cells are arranged in layers at right angles to one another to facilitate peristalsis Cardiac muscle cells—cells are Y shaped with one nucleus that is centrally located. The longitudinal branches of adjacent cells join at intercalated discs. This structure allows for the rapid spread of contractile stimuli from one cell to another
Connective tissue Consists of cells and extracellular material. The extracellular material is secreted by the cells and determines the physical properties of the tissue. It is composed of ground substance, fibers (collagen and elastin). and structural glycoproteins	Connective tissue provides structural and metabolic support for other tissues and organs Loose connective tissue acts as biological packing material Dense connective tissue provides tough physical support. For example, it forms the skeleton, the dermis, and organ capsules	Fibroblasts—synthesize and maintain extracellular material. They are active in wound healing where specialized contractile fibroblasts (myofibroblasts) bring about shrinkage of scar tissue Adipocytes—store and maintain fat. They are found in clumps in loose connective tissue and form the main cell type in adipose tissue. Fat stored in adipocytes forms a large droplet that occupies most of the cytoplasm Chondroblasts and chodrocytes—produce and maintain cartilage Osteoblasts, osteocytes, and osteoclasts—specialized cells that produce, maintain, and break down bone, respectively
Nervous tissue Peripheral nervous tissue is composed of neurons and Schwann cells Central nervous tissue consists of neurons and neuroglial cells (oligodendrocytes, astrocytes, microglia, and ependymal cells). It is divided macroscopically into gray and white matter. White matter consists of tracts of myelinated nerves. Gray matter contains neuronal cell bodies	Nervous tissue detects changes in the internal and external environments. By transmitting and processing this information it coordinates the activities of the multicellular organism to produce an appropriate response Nervous tissue is specialized for: • sensing environmental change • conducting information • integrating and analyzing information	Sensory receptors—there are numerous cell types specialized for detecting environmental change, for example, Pacinian corpuscles (mechanoreceptor that detects skin pressure) Neurons—these are specialized for receiving and transmitting information. Therefore, they synthesize neurotransmitters and neurotransmitter receptors. Multiple dendrites allow communication with many neighboring cells and function as sites of information input. The axon may be extremely long, and it facilitates transmission of information to distant sites. Terminal boutons arise at the end of the axon and communicate with other nerve cells or the effector organ Schwann cells/oligodendrocytes—specialist cells that wrap around the neuronal axon to form the myelin sheath and provide structural and metabolic support

Fig. 1.11 Cell specialization in epithelial, connective, nervous, and muscle tissue.

Some large sections of the genome, such as the centromeres or the inactive X chromosome, are not transcriptionally active in mammalian cells. In certain cytological preparations these regions stain differently to parts of the chromosome that are transcribed (see Fig. 1.6):

- Heterochromatin consists of the dark staining, late-replicating sections of the genome, which are transcriptionally inactive.
- Euchromatin consists of the lighter staining, early-replicating sections of the genome, which are transcriptionally active.

- Draw and label a typical prokaryotic and a typical eukaryotic cell.
- Explain why eukaryotic cells are larger than prokaryotic cells.
- Outline the differences between prokaryotes and eukaryotes—name at least six.
- Describe epithelial cell membrane specializations.
- List four membranous organelles and describe their structure and function.
- List the three components of the cytoskeleton.
- Outline the structure and function of cilia.
- Describe two types of specialized cell and explain how the structure of each reflects its function.
- Explain cell differentiation and cell memory.
- Define heterochromatin and euchromatin.

2. Proteins and Enzymes

Amino acids

Amino acids are the subunits of proteins, and they all have the same basic structure (Fig. 2.1):
- A central carbon atom (the α carbon).
- An amino (NH_2) group at the α carbon.
- A carboxyl group (COOH).
- A side group (R).

There are 20 naturally occurring amino acids, which differ in their side group, the simplest being hydrogen (H) in the amino acid glycine. D and L stereoisomer forms exist for all except glycine, as the α carbon is asymmetrical in all but this amino acid (Fig. 2.2). Only the L form is found in humans.

Amino acids form proteins by joining together through peptide bonds that result from the condensation of the amino group of one amino acid with the carboxyl group of the next (Fig. 2.3).

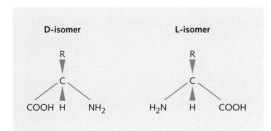

nonionized form   ionized form

Fig. 2.1 Structure of an amino acid. R is the side group. In solution at pH 7 the amino acid exists in its ionized form. The charges on the amino and carboxyl groups disappear when they form peptide bonds.

D-isomer   **L-isomer**

R   R
| |
C   C
COOH H   NH₂   H₂N   H   COOH

Fig. 2.2 D and L isomers of amino acid. The stereoisomers are mirror images of one another.

There may be a few to several thousand amino acid residues in a polypeptide, the sequence being determined by the base sequence in DNA. By convention, the free amino group is considered the start of a polypeptide sequence and the free carboxyl group its end.

Essential and nonessential amino acids

There are 10 essential and 10 nonessential amino acids in human biochemistry:
- Nonessential amino acids can be synthesized in the human body, so they are not required in the diet.
- Essential amino acids cannot be synthesized by the body—either not at all or not at a sufficient rate to meet requirements—they must be supplied by dietary protein.

One essential amino acid is required only during growth (arginine), but the others are required throughout life (see *Crash Course, Metabolism and Nutrition* for further details).

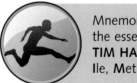

Mnemonic for remembering the essential amino acids: **PVT TIM HALL** (Phe, Val, Thr, Trp, Ile, Met, His, Arg, Leu, Lys).

Structure of amino acids

The amino acids can be classified by the nature of their R group or side chain (Fig. 2.4).

Properties of amino acids

The three-dimensional structure of a protein and therefore its behavior are determined by the characteristics and interactions of the side chains in its amino acid sequence.

Size and structure

Larger, bulky side chains impede bending of the polypeptide chain, while ring structures prevent it forming the turns required to make α-helices

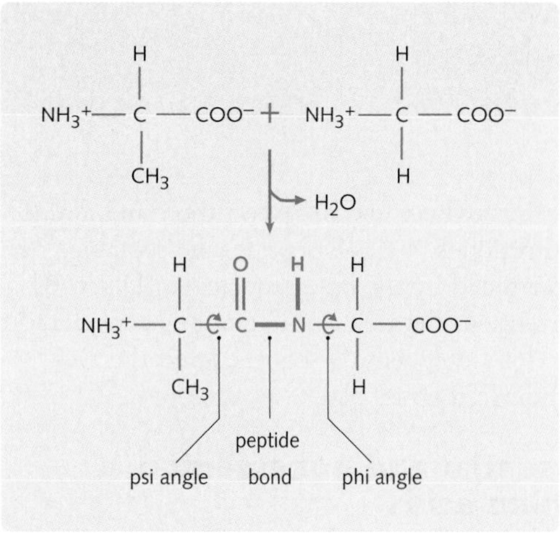

Fig. 2.3 Condensation of amino acids into protein. The C–N bond is the peptide bond. This has a partial double bond character, so the atoms highlighted remain in the same plane. Psi and phi angles are rotational angles about the indicated bonds. (Adapted from Stevens and Lowe, 1997.)

(these effects are called steric hindrance). Small or hydrophobic amino acids favor α-helical secondary structure.

Cross-linkages

Links between amino acid residues occur through hydrogen bonds, disulfide bridges, hydrophobic bonds, and ionic bonds, all of which act to stabilize the protein in its characteristic conformation.

- Hydrogen bonds occur between carbonyl (C=O) and imino (N–H) groups.
- Disulfide bridges are covalent bonds between thiol (–SH) groups of cysteine residues.
- Noncovalent hydrophobic bonds form between two hydrophobic residues.
- Electrovalent (ionic) bonds occur between a negative group of one amino acid residue and a positive group of another amino acid residue.

Solubility

In aqueous solution, colloidal proteins such as cytoplasmic enzymes are globular with polar R groups, which attract water, arranged on the outside and nonpolar groups arranged on the inside.

Covalent modification

Specific side groups can be modified by the addition of a chemical group in post-translational

modification reactions (see Chapter 5). Such modification alters the conformation of the protein, which may influence its activity. For example, tyrosine residues are phosphorylated by tyrosine kinases. This property is exploited in cell–cell signaling and in the regulation of enzyme activity (see Chapter 3).

Ionization properties of amino acids

Amino acids with nonpolar R groups form amphions at neutral pH because the carboxyl group donates a hydrogen to the amino group, producing a molecule that has both a positively and a negatively charged group (see Fig. 2.1). This molecule is called a zwitterion, and its overall electrical charge is neutral. Amphions such as amino acids have the ability to act as both donors and acceptors of protons:

- At very low (acidic) pH both the amino group and the carboxyl group are protonated and the molecule (cation) has an overall positive charge.
- At very high (alkaline) pH both the amino group and the carboxyl group are deprotonated and the molecule (anion) has an overall negative charge.
- Between these extremes the protonation of the amino and carboxyl groups and the overall charge of the molecule vary with pH (Fig. 2.5).
- The pH at which the net charge on the molecule is neutral, such that the molecule would not move in an electric field, is called the "isoelectric point."

The Henderson–Hasselbalch equation

Depending on the pH, both the amino and the carboxyl groups of an amino acid may act as weak acids. A weak acid (HA) is one that only partially dissociates to its anion (A^-) and a proton (H^+). The value of the dissociation constant (K_a) for a weak acid indicates its tendency to dissociate. Rearranging the formula for the dissociation constant gives the Henderson–Hasselbalch equation (Fig. 2.6):

$$pH = pK_a + \log [A^-]/[HA]$$

This equation permits the calculation of:

- The pH of a conjugate acid–base pair, given the pK_a and the molar ratio of the pair.
- The value of pK_a for a weak acid given the pH of a solution of known molar ratio.

Classification of amino acids by side-group type

Name	Symbol	Stereochemical formula	Side-group type
Aliphatic side chains			
Glycine	Gly (G)	$H-CH-COO^-$ $\quad\quad\mid$ $\quad NH_3^+$	Small
Alanine	Ala (A)	$CH_3-CH-COO^-$ $\quad\quad\quad\mid$ $\quad\quad NH_3^+$	Hydrophobic +
Valine	Val (V)	CH_3 $\quad\mid$ $CH-CH-COO^-$ $\quad\mid\quad\mid$ $CH_3\quad NH_3^+$	Hydrophobic ++
Leucine	Leu (L)	CH_3 $\quad\mid$ $CH-CH_2-CH-COO^-$ $\quad\mid\quad\quad\quad\mid$ $CH_3\quad\quad\quad NH_3^+$	Hydrophobic +++
Isoleucine	Ile (I)	CH_3 $\quad\mid$ CH_2 $\quad\mid$ $CH-CH-COO^-$ $\quad\mid\quad\mid$ $CH_3\quad NH_3^+$	Hydrophobic +++
Aromatic rings			
Phenylalanine	Phe (F)	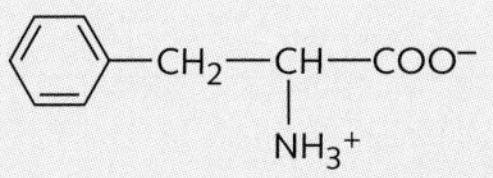 $\bigcirc-CH_2-CH-COO^-$ $\quad\quad\quad\quad\mid$ $\quad\quad\quad NH_3^+$	Hydrophobic ++++
Tyrosine	Tyr (Y)	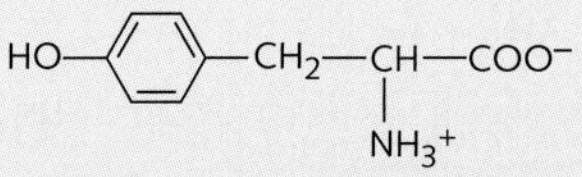 $HO-\bigcirc-CH_2-CH-COO^-$ $\quad\quad\quad\quad\quad\mid$ $\quad\quad\quad\quad NH_3^+$	Hydrophobic (polar)
Tryptophan	Trp (W)	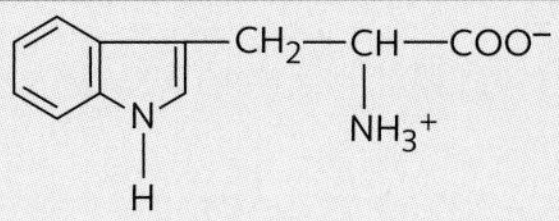 $CH_2-CH-COO^-$ $\quad\quad\quad\mid$ $\quad\quad NH_3^+$ (indole ring)	Hydrophobic
Imino acids			
Proline	Pro (P)	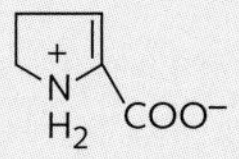 (pyrrolidine ring) N_+ $H_2\quad COO^-$	Closed ring
Acidic groups or amides			
Aspartic acid	Asp (D)	$^-OOC-CH_2-CH-COO^-$ $\quad\quad\quad\quad\quad\mid$ $\quad\quad\quad\quad NH_3^+$	Weak acid, pK 4 negative charge

Fig. 2.4 Classification of amino acids by side-group type.

Name	Symbol	Stereochemical formula	Side-group type
Acidic groups or amides (*cont.*)			
Asparagine	Asn (N)	$H_2N-\underset{\parallel O}{C}-CH_2-\underset{NH_3^+}{CH}-COO^-$	Polar
Glutamic acid	Glu (E)	$^-OOC-CH_2-CH_2-\underset{NH_3^+}{CH}-COO^-$	pK 4 negative charge
Glutamine	Gln (Q)	$H_2N-\underset{\parallel O}{C}-CH_2-CH_2-\underset{NH_3^+}{CH}-COO^-$	Polar
Basic groups			
Arginine	Arg (R)	$H-\underset{\underset{NH_2^+}{\overset{\parallel}{C}-NH_2}}{N}-CH_2 \quad CH_2-\underset{NH_3^+}{CH}-COO^-$	Weak base, pK 12 positive charge
Lysine	Lys (K)	$\underset{NH_3^+}{CH_2}-CH_2-CH_2-CH_2-\underset{NH_3^+}{CH}-COO^-$	pK 10 positive charge
Histidine	His (H)	$\underset{\underset{CH}{HN\;\;NH^+}}{CH=C}-CH_2-\underset{NH_3^+}{COO^-}$	pK 6 positive charge
Hydroxylic groups			
Serine	Ser (S)	$\underset{OH}{CH_2}-\underset{NH_3^+}{CH}-COO^-$	Polar
Threonine	Thr (T)	$CH_3-\underset{OH}{CH}-\underset{NH_3^+}{CH}-COO^-$	Polar
Sulfur groups			
Cysteine	Cys (C)	$NH_3^+-\underset{\underset{COO^-}{\overset{H}{\mid}}}{CH}-CH_2-SH$	
Methionine	Met (M)	$NH_3^+-\underset{\underset{COO^-}{\overset{H}{\mid}}}{CH_2}-CH_2-S-CH_3$	

Fig. 2.4—cont'd.

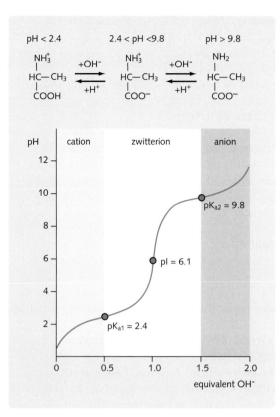

Fig. 2.5 Titration of glycine. The ionic species that predominates in each region is shown above the graph. pI is the isoelectric point (at which there is no net charge on the molecule). (Adapted from Baynes and Dominiczak, 1999.)

By the Henderson–Hasselbalch equation, when [A⁻] equals [HA], pH equals pK_a, i.e., the pK_a of a weak acid is the pH at which it is half dissociated.

Amino acids as buffers

A buffer consists of a weak acid and its conjugate base. Buffers cause a solution to resist changes in pH when acid or base is added. In amino acids, the amino and the carboxyl groups may both act as buffers. At a pH of 9.8 the amino group of glycine functions as a buffer (see Fig. 2.5).

- At pH 9.8 glycine is in equilibrium between the anion and the zwitterion.
- If protons are added they are removed from solution as they combine with the anion to produce the zwitterion.
- If alkali is added protons dissociate from the zwitterion to produce the anion and a water molecule.

The dissociation constant for a weak acid is:

$$K_a = \frac{[H^+][A^-]}{[HA]} = [H^+] - \frac{[A^-]}{[HA]}$$

Take the log of each of the terms in this equation.

$$\log K_a = \log [H^+] + \log \frac{[A^-]}{[HA]}$$

Rearrange thus:

$$- \log [H^+] = - \log K_a + \log \frac{[A^-]}{[HA]}$$

Substitute pH for $- \log [H^+]$ and pK_a for $- \log K_a$.

$$pH = pK_a + \log \frac{[A-]}{[HA]}$$

Fig. 2.6 Derivation of the Henderson–Hasselbalch equation.

Since at the pK_a of the amino group (9.8) there is an equal concentration of the weak acid (the zwitterion) and its conjugate base (the anion) it functions best as a buffer at this pH. A similar situation arises at pH 2.4 for the carbonyl group, though in this case the cation is the weak acid and the zwitterion its conjugate base. When glycine is titrated with an alkali (see Fig. 2.5):

- Two pK_a values are observed at pH 2.4 (carboxyl group) and at pH 9.8 (amino group).
- The addition of alkali produces very little change in pH within one pH unit of each pK_a.
- The addition of alkali produces a large change in pH at the isoelectric point.
- The isoelectric point lies midway between pK_{a1} and pK_{a2}.

Amino acids with ionizable side chains have a third pK_a corresponding to the pH range in which the proton on the side chain dissociates.

The glycine titration curve is a common short answer question. Make sure you can draw and explain it.

17

Proteins

Functions of proteins

Proteins serve a variety of diverse functions in the human body (Fig. 2.7). Protein isoforms have almost identical biologic activity, but they differ in amino acid sequence. For example:

- Myosin expressed in heart tissue.
- Myosin expressed in fast muscle fibers.

Protein conformation is defined by the sequence of its amino acid residues, which is critical to its function (Fig. 2.8).

Organization of proteins

Primary structure

Primary structure is specified by the linear sequence of amino acid residues linked via peptide bonds. The amino acid sequence is determined by the base sequence in DNA (see Chapter 5).

Secondary structure

Most proteins contain local regions of the polypeptide chain folded into α-helices and β-pleated sheets. These structures are particularly common because they are formed from hydrogen bonding interactions between peptide bonds (Fig. 2.9). They are favored by:

- Hydrogen bonding.
- Repulsion of side groups.
- Limited flexibility of the polypeptide chain.

Tertiary structure

Folding occurs to form the unique three-dimensional shape of a polypeptide chain (Fig. 2.10). It is determined by interactions between side groups of the amino acid residues, including disulfide bridges and electrostatic/hydrophobic interactions.

Quaternary structure

Two or more polypeptide chains (subunits) associate to form dimers, tetramers, or oligomers (Fig. 2.11). The subunits are held together by the same types of bond that stabilize tertiary structure.

Forces that shape proteins

Peptide bond

The peptide bond is formed between two amino acids by condensation (see Fig. 2.3). This is a strong covalent bond, which is resistant to heat, pH extremes, and detergent, with a bond energy of 380 kJ/mol, and length 0.132 nm or 1.32Å. The peptide group is planar as it has a partial double-bond character. However, free rotation occurs around the other bonds, giving different phi and psi angles (see Fig. 2.3) that allow considerable flexibility in the polypeptide chain. Consequences of the peptide bond are as follows:

- The polypeptide chain has considerable, though restricted, flexibility.
- The partial charge present at the oxygen and nitrogen of the bond enables attraction between

Functions of proteins	
Protein function	Examples
Structural	Collagen in skin, keratin in hair
Metabolism	Enzymes (e.g., lysozyme, pepsin, amylase)
Signal transduction	Cytoplasmic kinases
Defense	Antibodies
Movement	Actin and myosin in muscle contraction
Transport	Hemoglobin carries oxygen, transferrin carries iron
Communication	Hormones, receptors, and adhesion molecules (e.g., insulin, β-adrenergic receptor, steroid receptor, integrins)
Recognition	Major histocompatibility complex proteins
Storage	Ferritin stores iron in the liver

Fig. 2.7 Functions of proteins.

Proteins and ligands	
Protein	Ligand
Enzymes	Substrate
Myosin	Actin and other proteins
Antibodies	Antigen
Receptors	Hormones, neurotransmitters, counterreceptors

Fig. 2.8 Proteins and ligands.

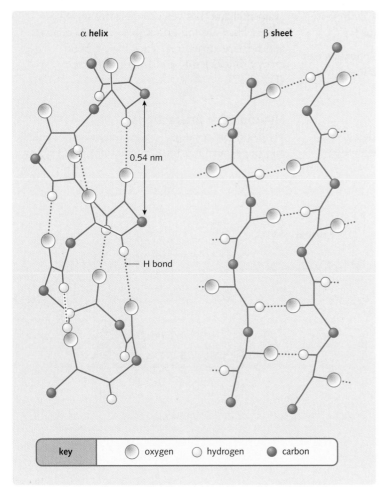

Fig. 2.9 Secondary structure of a protein. In both the α-helix and β-pleated sheet, regions of secondary structure are stabilized by hydrogen bonds (H bonds) between the C=O and N–H groups of the peptide bonds in the protein.

α helix   β sheet

0.54 nm

H bond

| key | oxygen | hydrogen | carbon |

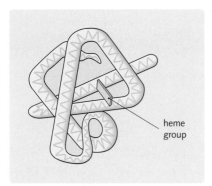

Fig. 2.10 Tertiary structure of a protein. One complete protein chain (β-chain of hemoglobin) is illustrated here.

heme group

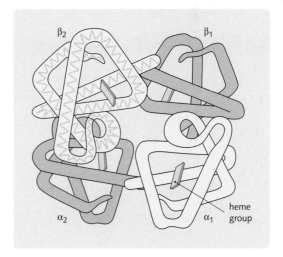

β₂   β₁

α₂   α₁

heme group

Fig. 2.11 Quaternary structure of a protein. Four separate chains of hemoglobin are assembled into an oligomeric protein.

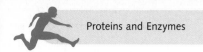

two peptide bonds, forming a weak hydrogen bond with a bond energy of 5 kJ/mol.

Many biologically active proteins will spontaneously fold into one conformation that is stabilized by a variety of intramolecular bonds.

Hydrogen bonds
Hydrogen bonds occur between peptide bond atoms and polar side groups where a hydrogen

atom is shared between two electronegative atoms; they are important in forming secondary and tertiary structures. They have a bond energy of 20 kJ/mol and length of 0.3 nm (Fig. 2.12).

Hydrophobic interactions
Hydrophobic residues (e.g., valine, alanine, leucine, and phenylalanine) form interactions, rather than

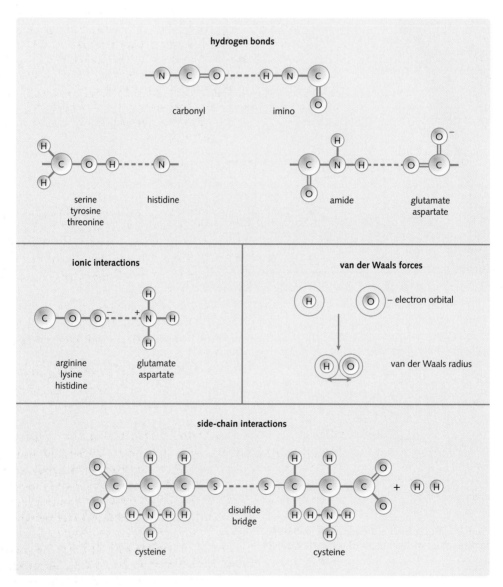

Fig. 2.12 Forces shaping proteins. Proteins are stabilized by chemical bonds that may depend on interactions between the carbonyl and imino groups in the polypeptide chain (e.g., some hydrogen bonds) or on specific side-chain interactions (e.g., disulfide bridges).

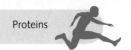

true bonds, where they cluster close together. Bond energy comes from the displacement of water.

Ionic interactions

Ionic interactions result from strong attractions between positive and negative atoms. These bonds are important in tertiary structure and have a bond energy of 335 kJ/mol and length of 0.25 nm (see Fig. 2.12).

van der Waals forces

van der Waals forces (dipole-induced dipole) are weak attractions between two atoms as the electron orbitals approach each other (see Fig. 2.12). The bond energy is very weak, being 0.8 kJ/mol, and the length is 0.35 nm. Collectively, these bonds "add" to significant energy in the tertiary structure of large polypeptides.

Side-chain interactions

Side-chain interactions form bonds, the most important being between the thiol groups of two cysteine residues, forming a covalent bond of 210 kJ/mol called a disulfide bridge (see Fig. 2.12). Disulfide bridges are important in tertiary structures and in the secondary structure of elastin. This reaction is not favored intracellularly, so disulfide bridges are normally found in exported proteins, for example:

- The digestive enzyme ribonuclease has four disulfide bonds.
- The peptide hormone insulin has three disulfide bonds.

Protein folding

The correct "folded shape" of a protein is determined by the amino acid sequence. Chaperone proteins bind to the polypeptide chain, assist in folding to the correct conformation, and then detach. Groups far away in the primary sequence may be brought close together in the final three-dimensional structure. Large proteins are composed of several domains linked by flexible regions of polypeptide. Domains have specific tertiary structure associated with a particular function, which may be conserved between proteins. For example, all known NAD-dependent dehydrogenase enzymes share a conserved NAD-binding domain.

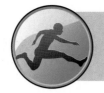

Protein structure and folding are often asked about in essay questions.

Structures within proteins

α-helix

The α-helix is a right-handed helix (L form) with a backbone of peptide linkages, from which side chains radiate outwards. Small or hydrophobic amino acid residues favor α-helix formation, so glycine or proline are usually found at the α-helix bends. The structure is stabilized by hydrogen bonds between every first and fourth amino acid, each hydrogen bond being relatively weak, but as all are parallel and "intrachain" they provide reinforcement. The helix has:

- 0.15 nm rise.
- 0.54 nm pitch.
- 3.6 residues per turn.

The structure is a rigid rod-like cylinder that is very stable, with side groups pointing out and, therefore, free to interact with other α-helices (see Fig. 2.9). α-Helices make up 90–100% of fibrous proteins and 10–60% of globular proteins. For example:

- α-Keratin, a fibrous protein that is a component of skin, consists of long rod-like coils made from two identical α-helices wound around one another.
- Myoglobin, the globular protein that binds oxygen in muscle, has eight α-helical segments, and it is 75% α-helix in total.

β-pleated sheet

β-pleated sheets are extended chains formed from two or more pleated polypeptides joined by hydrogen bonds. In a parallel sheet the terminal amino acids are at the same end, whereas in the more common antiparallel sheet, terminal amino acids are at opposite ends, so forming a more stable structure (see Fig. 2.9). The sheet is a rigid nonelastic "platform," which is commonly found in fibrous proteins, for example:

- β-Keratins in claws, scales, feathers, and beaks are made of antiparallel strands.
- Silk is made of regular β-sheets.

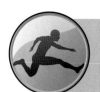

Prion diseases, which include BSE, may be genetic or infective. It has been proposed that disease-causing prion proteins interact with a normal cellular version of the same protein to produce a conformational change. Whereas cellular prion protein is normally rich in β-sheets, infective prion proteins are predominantly α-helix.

Zinc fingers

Zinc fingers are a common motif in DNA-binding proteins such as transcription factors. The "zinc finger domain" is a folded amino acid projection surrounding a central zinc atom (Fig. 2.13). Zinc finger proteins recognize and bind to specific DNA regulatory sequences and, therefore, influence transcription.

Collagen helix

Collagen is a fibrous protein that is a major component of connective tissue. It is composed of three polypeptide chains wound around one another and linked by hydrogen bonds. Every turn of the triple helix contains three amino acid residues such that every third amino acid lies between the other two chains at the center of the structure. Glycine is the only side chain small enough to fit in this position, so every third amino acid on each polypeptide chain is glycine.

Stability of proteins

Denaturation is the loss of the three-dimensional structure of a protein due to breaking of structural bonds. It is usually associated with loss of biological activity (Fig. 2.14). Any treatment that disrupts chemical bonding (e.g., heat, pH extremes, detergents, oxidation, and physical effects such as shaking) may cause denaturation. Therefore, most proteins only function within narrow environmental limits. If the denaturing conditions are not extreme, most proteins return to their active states when returned to optimal conditions.

Complex structures

Individual polypeptides may not be biologically active themselves, but they may serve as subunits in the formation of larger, active complexes.

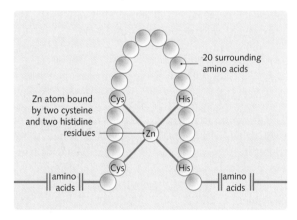

Fig. 2.13 Zinc finger domain. The bonds between the four amino acids and zinc stabilize a loop of polypeptide into a finger-like structure.

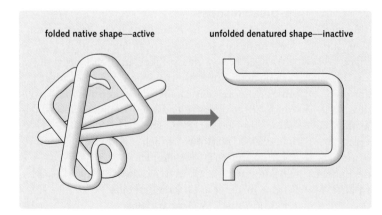

folded native shape—active   unfolded denatured shape—inactive

Fig. 2.14 Denaturation of protein. The function of most proteins is dependent on their shape. Therefore, treatment with agents such as heat or solvents, which disrupt the chemical bonds that stabilize proteins, may inactivate them.

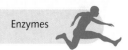

- The pyruvate dehydrogenase complex contains multiple subunits. In addition to the three enzymes that catalyze the overall reaction the complex includes subunits that regenerate cofactors and subunits that regulate its activity. This arrangement improves the efficiency of the overall reaction.
- Hemoglobin A is a tetramer composed of two α-subunits and two β-subunits, each associated with a prosthetic heme group (Fig. 2.15). Crucial to hemoglobin's function is its ability to bind oxygen when pO_2 is high and release it when it is low. When oxygen joins the first heme group it causes a change in the bonding affinity of the second heme group via conformational changes in the globin chains. This enables the second heme to combine more rapidly with an oxygen molecule, which in turn alters the third heme. This is an example of positive cooperativity, and it explains the sigmoidal hemoglobin saturation curve.

Some proteins are dependent on their interaction with other, nonprotein, molecules:

- Prosthetic group is the term given to the portion of a complex protein that is not polypeptide, for example the heme group in hemoglobin or the zinc atom in zinc finger proteins. Prosthetic groups frequently form an integral part of the active site.
- Coenzymes are organic molecules that must be associated with a given enzyme for it to function. They bind to the enzyme, undergo chemical change, and are ultimately released as the reaction is completed. For example, alcohol dehydrogenase requires the presence of the coenzyme NAD.
- Polypeptides may be glycosylated to form glycoproteins, which are important in cell–cell recognition.

Enzymes

Properties of enzymes

Enzymes are biologic catalysts. Without them, metabolic reactions would proceed too slowly for life. Enzymes have the following properties:

- They bind specific ligands (substrates) at active sites and catalyze their conversion to products.
- They greatly alter the speed of a reaction.
- They remain in the same chemical state at the end of the reaction as at the beginning, so can be reused.
- They catalyze the forward and the reverse reaction.
- They show great specificity. Some enzymes may only recognize one stereoisomer.

An enzyme's name is normally the name of the substrate with the suffix -ase added, the substrate being the substance on which the enzyme acts. Isoenzymes catalyze the same reaction, but they have different primary structures and may work under different optimum conditions, for example:

- Lactate dehydrogenase has heart and muscle isoforms.
- Creatine kinase has brain and muscle isoforms.

Classification of enzymes

All known enzymes can be classified into one of six groups defined by the International Union of Biochemistry (Fig. 2.16).

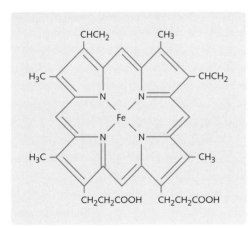

Fig. 2.15 Structure of heme b. Hemes consist of a porphyrin ring coordinated with an atom of iron.

Mnemonic for remembering the six classes of enzyme: **O**ver **T**he **HILL** (**O**xidoreductases, **T**ransferases, **H**ydrolases, **I**somerases, **L**igases, **L**yases). Enzymes get reactants over the activation energy "hill."

23

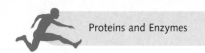

Classification of enzymes		
Enzyme class	**Reaction**	**Example**
Oxidoreductases Oxidize or reduce substrates a) dehydrogenases dehydrogenases transfer hydrogen to coenzymes: b) oxidases oxidases transfer hydrogen to oxygen molecules:	Substrate + coenzyme $\longrightarrow$ oxidized substrate + reduced coenzyme $AH_2 + 2NAD^+ \longrightarrow A^+ + 2NADH$ Substrate $\longrightarrow$ oxidized substrate $AH_2 + {}^1/_2 O_2 \longrightarrow A + H_2O$	Alcohol dehydrogenase catalyzes: $CH_3CH_2OH + NAD^\oplus \longrightarrow CH_3\!-\!\overset{\overset{\textstyle H}{\vert}}{C}\!=\!O + NADH + H^\oplus$ ethanol $\qquad\qquad\qquad$ acetaldehyde Cytochrome oxidase catalyzes: Cyt.H_2(reduced cytochrome) + ${}^1/_2 O_2 \longrightarrow$ Cyt + H_2O (cytochrome)
Transferases Transferases move molecules from one substrate to another:	$AB+C \longrightarrow A + BC$	Glucokinase catalyzes: D-Glucose + ATP $\longrightarrow$ D-Glucose-6-phosphate + ADP
Hydrolases Hydrolases form two products from a single substrate by hydrolysis, coupling the hydrogen atom from water to one component and the hydroxyl group to another:	$AB + H_2O \longrightarrow AH + BOH$	Carboxypeptidase A catalyzes: C-terminal of polypeptide $\qquad$ polypeptide $\quad$ C-terminal $\qquad\qquad\qquad\qquad\qquad$ shortened $\qquad$ residue
Isomerases isomerases change the isomeric configuration of a molecule, so transfer atoms from one part of the molecule to another:	$ABC \longrightarrow ACB$	Malate isomerase catalyzes: $\quad$ malate $\qquad\qquad$ fumarate
Lyases lyases break down C — C bonds. Two simpler products are formed as with hydrolases but water is not involved:	$AB \longrightarrow A + B$	Pyruvate decarboxylase catalyzes: $^\ominus OOC\!-\!\overset{\overset{\textstyle O}{\|}}{C}\!-\!CH_3 + H^\oplus \longrightarrow CO_2 + \overset{\overset{\textstyle O}{\|}}{\underset{\underset{\textstyle H}{/}}{C}}\!-\!CH_3$ $\quad$ pyruvate $\qquad\qquad\qquad$ acetaldehyde
Ligases ligases form new bonds, with energy provided by ATP:	$A + B + ATP \longrightarrow AB + ADP + P$	Pyruvate carboxylase catalyzes: $^\ominus OOC\!-\!\overset{\overset{\textstyle O}{\|}}{C}\!-\!CH_3 + CO_2 + ATP \longrightarrow {}^\ominus OOC\!-\!\overset{\overset{\textstyle O}{\|}}{C}\!-\!CH_2\!-\!COO^\ominus + ATP + P$ $\quad$ pyruvate $\qquad\qquad\qquad\qquad\qquad$ oxaloacetate

Fig. 2.16 Classification of enzymes.

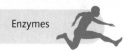

Mechanism of enzyme action
Catalysts
In any chemical reaction, when a reactant is converted to a product, highly unstable intermediates are produced as chemical bonds are broken and reformed. These intermediates have higher free energy than the reactant, and so they are not favored energetically (Fig. 2.17).
- The difference in free energy between the reactant and the unstable intermediate is the activation energy.
- Reactants must have in excess of the required activation energy.

The energy level of individual reactants in a population follows a normal distribution. If activation energy is high, only a few molecules will have sufficient energy to react at any one time and the reaction will be slow.

A catalyst speeds up chemical reaction but is itself unchanged by it. Catalysts bind transition molecules and stabilize them, so reducing the activation energy for the reaction. Therefore, in a catalyzed reaction, more molecules will have the required activation energy and the reaction rate will increase. However, since they accelerate the reaction in both directions the position of the equilibrium is unchanged. A catalyzed reaction has the following features relative to a noncatalyzed reaction:
- The rate of the reaction is increased.
- The overall change in free energy between reactants and products is the same.
- The position of the equilibrium is the same.

Increasing the temperature of reactants increases their mean energy level. For a reaction catalyzed by an inorganic catalyst, rate increases directly proportionally to temperature. However, enzyme-catalyzed reactions show maximum activity at 37°C, but much reduced reaction rates at higher temperatures. This is because enzyme activity depends on the active site, and outside physiologic parameters the bonds that maintain its structure are disrupted.

Active sites
The active site is the region to which substrate molecules bind. Enzyme specificity occurs because the shape of the active site is such that only substrates with a complementary structure can bind. This has been likened to the fitting of a key into its lock. However, rather than viewing the active site as a rigid structure the "induced fit" model (Fig. 2.18) proposes that:
- The substrate binds to a substrate-binding domain, which induces a conformational change at the active site.

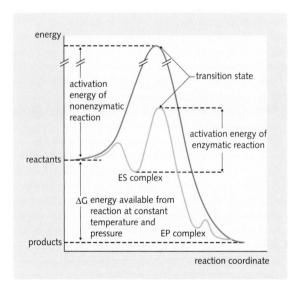

Fig. 2.17 Reaction profile for catalyzed and noncatalyzed reactions. Activation energy is less for the catalyzed reaction. (ES complex, enzyme–substrate complex; EP complex, enzyme–product complex.) (Adapted from Baynes and Dominiczak, 1999.)

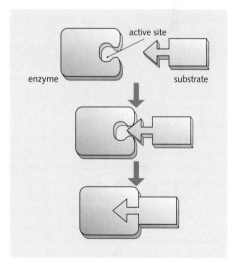

Fig. 2.18 The "induced fit" hypothesis explains how the binding of the substrate to the enzyme changes the conformation of the active site.

25

- The conformational change in the active site reveals functional groups.
- As the product dissociates the enzyme returns to its original conformation and so can bind more substrate.

Structure of enzymes

X-ray crystallography has provided an insight into how enzymes work at the molecular level. Lactate dehydrogenase (LDH) is an oxidoreductase, which catalyzes the following reaction:

Pyruvate + NADH + H$^+$ → Lactate + NAD$^+$

The reduction of pyruvate to form lactate depends on the presence of the cofactor NADH as well as pyruvate, i.e., LDH is a bisubstrate enzyme. NADH binds to the enzyme first producing a conformational change that permits the binding of lactate to the active site by induced fit. The conformational change brings the bound substrate into close proximity to the nicotinamide ring (the part of the coenzyme that is oxidized) to facilitate the transfer of hydrogen (Fig. 2.19).

LDH is a tetramer consisting of four identical subunits (Fig. 2.20), each one containing a nicotinic acid binding domain:

- The NAD binding domain has a βαβ turn conserved in all known NAD-dependent dehydrogenases (Fig. 2.21).
- NAD binding domains are composed of four α-helices and six strands of parallel β-sheets.
- One-half of the domain binds the nicotinamide unit of NAD, the other its adenosine moiety.

Regulation of enzyme activity

The coordinated regulation of enzyme activity allows the organism to adapt to environmental change. In multistep metabolic pathways, the slowest enzyme determines the rate at which the final product is produced. The activity of such "rate-determining" enzymes is regulated so that metabolism is coordinated and energy is not wasted. Five mechanisms are involved:

- Transcription from the enzyme coding gene may be regulated (see Chapter 5).
- Enzymes may be irreversibly activated or deactivated by proteolytic cleavage.

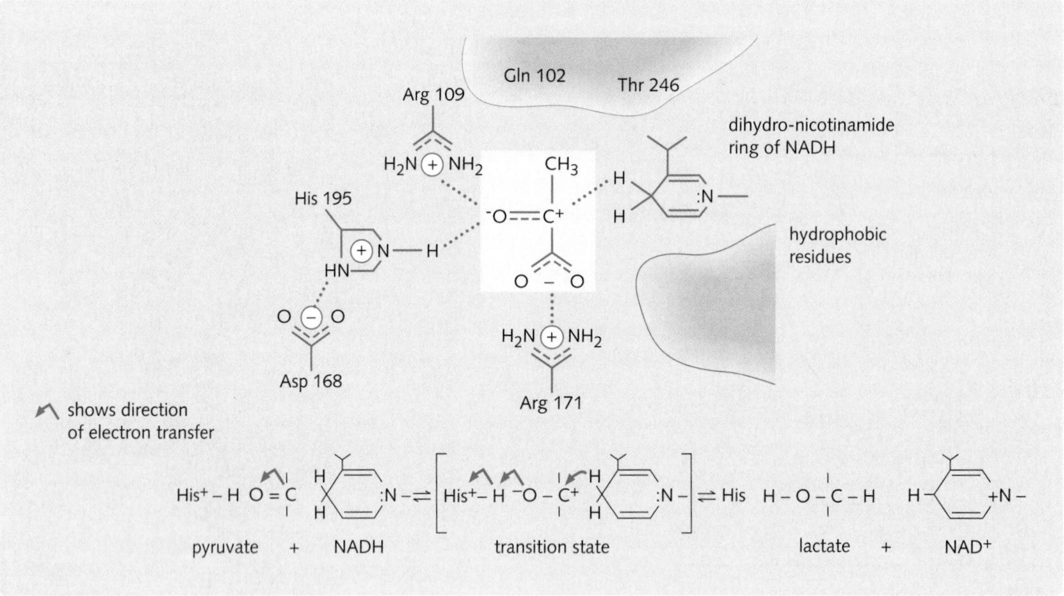

Fig. 2.19 Enzyme–substrate–coenzyme complex of lactate dehydrogenase. The adenine moiety of NADH is bound to the enzyme in a hydrophobic crevice, whereas its dihydro-nicotinamide moiety, which functions as the proton donor, is bound so that the reactive part of the ring is in a polar environment. Binding of the coenzyme induces a conformational change that allows pyruvate to bind to the substrate binding domain by virtue of hydrogen and electrostatic bonds. The conformation of the active site is such that when the substrate molecules are bound pyruvate is aligned to react with NADH as shown.

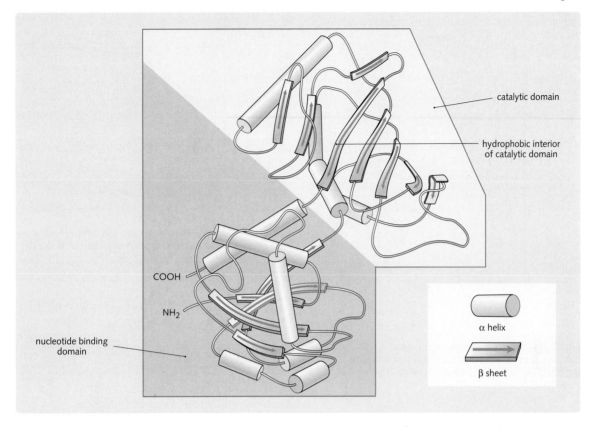

Fig. 2.20 Structure of lactate dehydrogenase. The α-helix and β-pleated sheets form two globular binding domains.

- Enzymes may be reversibly activated and deactivated by covalent modifications such as phosphorylation.
- Enzymes may be subject to allosteric modification. This occurs when the binding of a small molecule to a site distant from the active site alters the conformation of the enzyme and, therefore, its activity.
- The rate of degradation of the enzyme may be regulated.

Enzyme kinetics

Enzyme kinetics is the study of the rate of change of reactants and products. Enzyme assays use biosensors, oxygen electrodes, chromogenic substances, and other methods to measure the progress of reactions.

Reaction rates

By plotting the amount of product formed against time, the initial velocity of the reaction can be estimated (Fig. 2.22A). The initial velocity (V) equals the reaction rate. Reaction rate varies according to enzyme and substrate concentration. Increasing enzyme concentration increases the reaction linearly, so follows first-order kinetics (Fig. 2.22B).

Increasing substrate concentration increases the reaction rate in an asymptotic, nonlinear, fashion; as the enzyme becomes saturated the reaction rate reaches a limit—this is a Michaelis–Menten graph (Fig. 2.23). For simple enzymes the curve is a rectangular hyperbola. At low substrate concentrations the graph is linear (rate is proportional to [substrate]), so follows first-order kinetics. At high substrate concentrations a plateau is reached, so follows zero-order kinetics. The Michaelis–Menten equation relates the reaction rate to the substrate concentration:

$$E + S \underset{K_2}{\overset{K_1}{\rightleftharpoons}} ES \underset{K_4}{\overset{K_3}{\rightleftharpoons}} E + P$$

K_1, K_2, etc., are individual rate constants. K_4 is insignificant so is ignored.

27

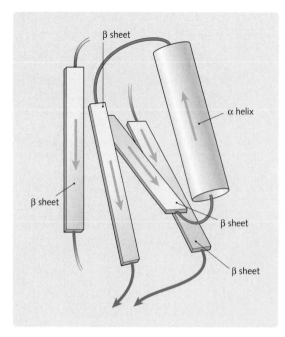

Fig. 2.21 Core structure of the nucleotide cofactor binding domain. All NAD- or NAPH-dependent dehydrogenases have a similar binding domain.

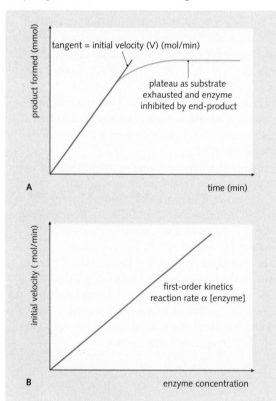

Fig. 2.22 (A) Calculation of initial velocity. (B) Effect of enzyme concentration on reaction rate.

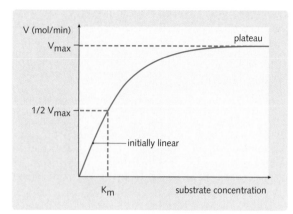

Fig. 2.23 Michaelis–Menten graph showing effect of increasing substrate concentration against reaction rate. (K_m, Michaelis constant; V, initial velocity; V_{max}, maximum velocity.)

The Michaelis constant (K_m) is the rate of breakdown of the enzyme–substrate complex:

$$K_m = \frac{K_2 + K_3}{K_1}$$

The maximum velocity (V_{max}) is reached under saturating conditions when the substrate concentration is high:

$$V_{max} = K_3[ES]$$

where K_3 is rate of enzyme and product formation and [ES] is enzyme–product complex concentration. The velocity (V) of a Michaelis–Menten reaction is therefore:

$$V = \frac{V_{max}[S]}{K_m[S]}$$

- V_{max} and K_m are constants for each different enzyme.
- For most enzymes, K_m is the substrate concentration at which the reaction rate is half of V_{max}.
- K_m is a measure of the affinity of the enzyme for its substrate, with a low K_m (low enzyme–substrate complex breakdown) corresponding to high affinity (tight binding) and vice versa.
- V_{max} and K_m are difficult to estimate from a Michaelis–Menten graph, so an alternative graph representation is used, the Lineweaver–Burk graph (Fig. 2.24).

Inhibitors

Enzyme inhibitors are substances that lower enzyme activity. False inhibitors include denaturing

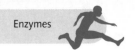

treatments and irreversible inhibitors (e.g., organophosphorus compounds). True inhibitors can be:

- Competitive.
- Noncompetitive.
- Allosteric.

Competitive inhibitors resemble the substrate, and they compete for the active site (Fig. 2.25A). The K_m is increased, so affinity of the enzyme is decreased; for example, azidothymidine (AZT) used to treat HIV infection resembles deoxythymidine, so it is a competitive inhibitor of HIV reverse transcriptase.

Noncompetitive inhibitors (e.g., heavy metals such as lead) do not resemble the substrate, so they do not compete for the binding site. They bind to the enzyme and abolish its catalytic activity, although substrate may still bind (Fig. 2.25B). V_{max} is decreased as there is less catalytically active enzyme, but K_m is unchanged as affinity of the enzyme is not altered.

Allosteric inhibitors do not bind to the active site; instead, they bind to a different allosteric site elsewhere on the enzyme. Binding causes a conformational change, which can alter V_{max} and/or K_m; for example, phosphofructokinase I (PFK I) is allosterically inhibited by high concentrations of ATP and by citrate (Fig. 2.26).

Clinical significance of genetic variation of enzyme function

Genetic variation of enzyme function can have clinical consequences:

- The cholinesterase enzyme may be functionally altered if there is a mutation in its gene located on chromosome 3. This enzyme normally metabolizes suxamethonium, a short-acting induction agent used in anesthesia. A mutant form fails to act on the drug, resulting in prolonged paralysis and apnea.
- The glucose-6-phosphate dehydrogenase enzyme is encoded on the X chromosome, and it protects erythrocytes from oxidative damage. Variations in this enzyme can cause a hemolytic anemia.

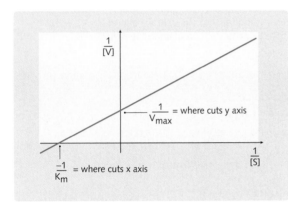

Fig. 2.24 Lineweaver–Burk plot. (K_m, Michaelis constant; S, substrate; V, velocity; V_{max}, maximum velocity.)

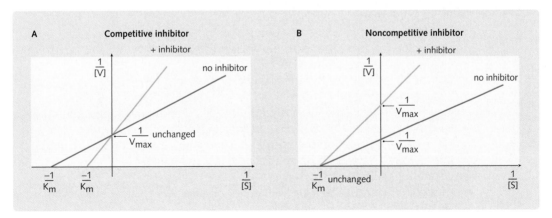

Fig. 2.25 (A) Competitive inhibition of enzyme. The inhibitor increases K_m. V_{max} is unchanged. (B) Noncompetitive inhibition of enzyme. The inhibitor decreases V_{max}. K_m remains unchanged. (K_m, Michaelis constant; S, substrate; V, initial velocity; V_{max}, maximum velocity.)

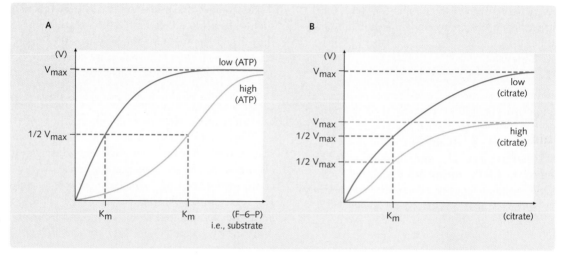

Fig. 2.26 Allosteric inhibition of phosphofructokinase 1, which adds a second phosphate group to fructose-6-phosphate. (A) ATP increases K_m (decreases affinity), but it does not alter V_{max}. (B) Citrate decreases V_{max}, but it does not alter K_m. (K_m, Michaelis constant; S, substrate; V, initial velocity; V_{max}, maximum velocity.)

- Explain the difference between an essential and a nonessential amino acid, and give three examples of each.
- Describe the classification of amino acids, and give an example for each group.
- List three characteristics of amino acid side chains, and discuss how they influence protein structure.
- Draw the titration curve for glycine, and indicate which ionic species predominates in each region.
- Define and mark on the glycine titration curve the pK_a for the amino and carboxyl groups and the isoelectric point.
- Discuss the characteristics of peptide bonds and their formation.
- Define what is meant by primary, secondary, tertiary, and quaternary protein structure.
- Describe the role of three different types of chemical bonds in maintaining three-dimensional protein structure.
- What is a protein domain?
- Outline how the structure of hemoglobin reflects its function.
- Define the following: catalyst, enzyme, substrate, coenzyme, and isoenzyme.
- List four properties of enzymes.
- List the six groups used in the classification of enzymes.
- Draw a diagram of the reaction profile of a catalyzed and noncatalyzed reaction, and explain why catalyzed reactions reach equilibrium more quickly.
- Discuss the relationship between enzyme activity and temperature.
- Describe the interaction between the enzyme active site and its substrate.
- List four ways in which enzyme activity can be regulated.
- Define K_m and V_{max}.
- Describe a typical Michaelis–Menten graph and Lineweaver–Burk graph.
- What are the effects of each class of inhibitor on enzyme kinetics?

3. The Cell Membrane

Structure of the cell membrane

Fluid mosaic model

Singer and Nicholson first suggested the fluid mosaic model in 1972. They proposed that biologic membranes consist of a phospholipid bilayer with proteins embedded in it (Fig. 3.1). It has been verified by freeze fracture and freeze etching electron microscopy, which have shown the distribution of proteins within the 6–10 nm-wide membrane.

The phospholipid molecules that are the major component of the bilayer are amphipathic; i.e., they have hydrophobic and hydrophilic regions (Fig. 3.2). The phospholipid molecules form a stable bilayer in aqueous solutions as a result of:

- Hydrophilic interactions of polar head groups with the extracellular and intracellular aqueous environments.
- Hydrophobic interactions of the hydrophobic fatty acid molecules in the bilayer interior.

The proteins embedded in the membrane may be peripheral or integral:

- Peripheral proteins are associated with one leaf of the lipid bilayer.
- Integral proteins usually span the lipid bilayer.

The membrane is a dynamic structure, and many proteins are able to move freely through it in a manner that has been likened to "icebergs floating in a sea of phospholipids."

The fluid mosaic model is a common topic in exams; remember to draw a diagram including peripheral and integral proteins, even for short-answer questions. Mention that the membrane is dynamic, and in essay questions discuss the movement of phospholipids and proteins within it.

Components of the biologic membrane

Lipids

A lipid is a molecule that is soluble in an organic solvent (e.g., chloroform), but only sparingly soluble in water. Triglycerides, which are hydrophobic, consist of three fatty acids attached to a glycerol backbone by ester linkages.

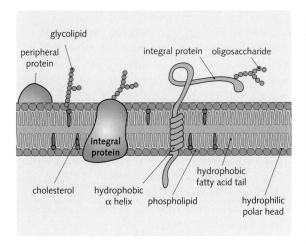

Fig. 3.1 Fluid mosaic model of the cell membrane.

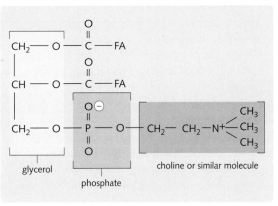

Fig. 3.2 Structure of a phospholipid. The shaded areas correspond to the hydrophilic parts of the molecule. (FA, fatty acid.)

Phospholipids

The hydrophilic moiety in a phospholipid arises because one of the fatty acid chains is replaced by an amine-containing polar group linked to glycerol (at C3) by a phosphodiester bond (see Fig. 3.2). There are four major phospholipids in the plasma membrane (Fig. 3.3):

- Phosphatidylethanolamine.
- Phosphatidylserine.
- Phosphatidylcholine.
- Sphingomyelin—this molecule is not a true phospholipid (Fig. 3.3).

Phospholipids are arranged asymmetrically, with the first two occurring in the inner layer of the membrane, and the second two in its outer layer. Since they aggregate into a continuous sheet impervious to ions, the molecules must pack very closely. Most lipids pack as cylinders or slightly truncated cones, although lysophospholipids, which have one fatty acid missing, are shaped like cones (Fig. 3.4). The presence of a double bond in a fatty acid side chain introduces a kink. This disrupts van der Waals forces and so reduces the ability of the molecule to fit tightly with its neighbors, therefore, increasing membrane fluidity.

Cholesterol

Cholesterol is a lipid molecule that consists of four hydrophobic rings and a hydrophilic hydroxyl group (Fig. 3.5). It orientates in the membrane such that the rings lie parallel to the hydrophobic fatty acids groups, with the hydroxyl group forming a hydrogen bond with the carboxyl group on an adjacent phospholipid. The result is that:

- At physiologic temperature cholesterol restricts the movement of the fatty acid chains and, therefore, reduces membrane fluidity.
- At low temperatures it inhibits phospholipid packing, which increases membrane fluidity.

Membrane proteins
Integral proteins

Integral proteins span the membrane, and they have intracellular and extracellular domains:

- The membrane-spanning domains are rich in hydrophobic amino acid residues and traverse the membrane as α-helical loops.
- The cytosolic and extracellular domains are rich in polar amino acid residues.
- Extracellular domains may be glycosylated.

Monotopic integral proteins traverse the membrane once, while bitopic and polytopic proteins pass through the membrane twice and many times, respectively.

Peripheral proteins

Peripheral proteins are associated with either the cytoplasmic or extracellular leaf of the lipid bilayer. They may be attached to the membrane by:

- Electrostatic attachment to integral proteins.
- Covalent attachment to nonprotein components of the cytoplasmic layer.
- Covalent attachment to phospholipids via an oligosaccharide linker in the extracellular layer.

Examples of membrane proteins, their function, and their means of attachment to the membrane are included in Fig. 3.6.

Isolation of membrane proteins

Peripheral membrane proteins can be dissociated from the membrane by mild procedures that leave the membrane intact, for example, changing the pH of the solution may interfere with electrostatic binding. Dissociation of integral membrane proteins poses a problem, as both the cell membrane and protein are hydrophobic. Detergents that disrupt the membrane and compete for nonpolar interactions may isolate such proteins (Fig. 3.7), though strong detergents may denature the protein.

Properties of biologic membranes
Fluidity

The transition temperature occurs when the membrane transforms from a rigid gel-like structure to a relatively disordered, fluid state (Fig. 3.8). In its fluid state, proteins embedded in the membrane are free to interact. The membrane is heterogeneous, and ordered regions alternate with more fluid ones.

Fluidity is determined by factors that influence the interactions of phospholipids (Fig. 3.9):

- Temperature—membranes are more fluid at high temperatures when phospholipid molecules have more kinetic energy.
- Saturation of fatty acid chains—membranes are more fluid if they have a high proportion of unsaturated fatty acids.
- Cholesterol—the effects of cholesterol depend on temperature.

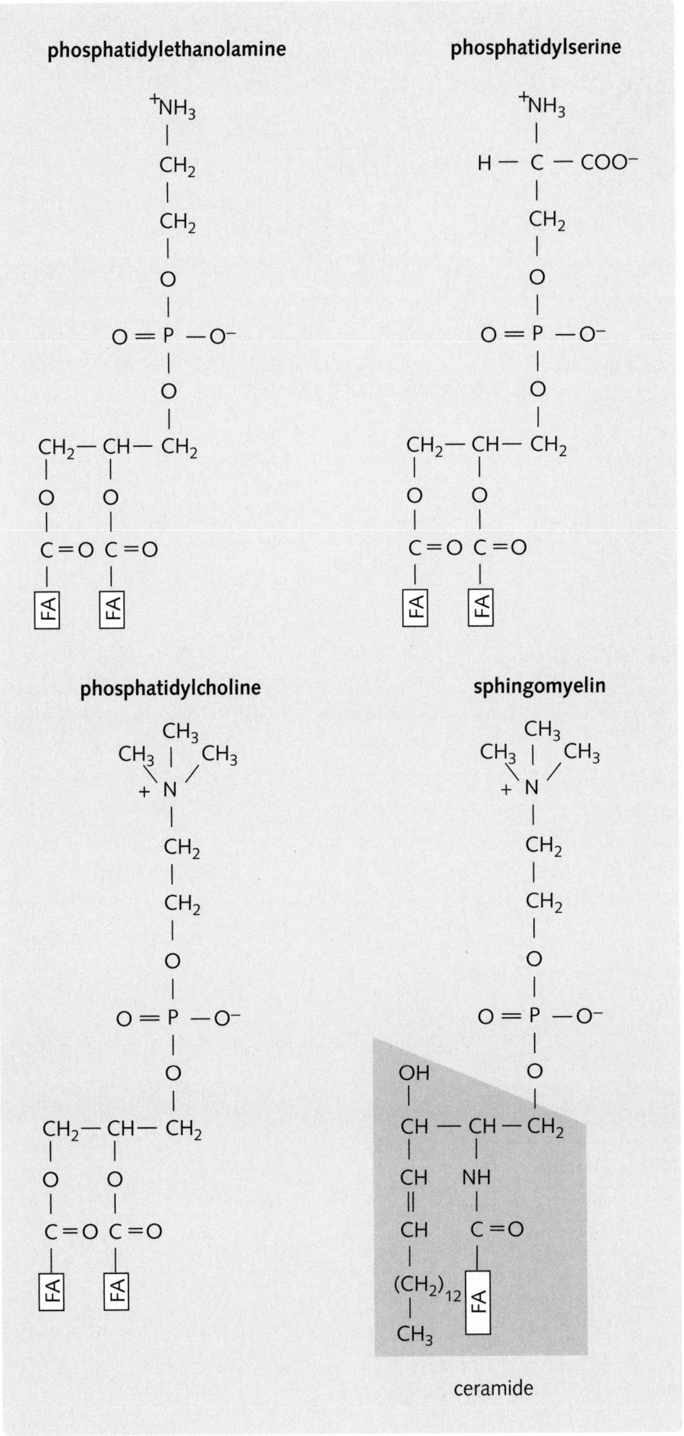

phosphatidylethanolamine

$^+NH_3$
|
CH_2
|
CH_2
|
O
|
$O = P — O^-$
|
O
|
$CH_2 — CH — CH_2$
| |
O O
| |
$C = O$ $C = O$
| |
FA   FA

phosphatidylserine

$^+NH_3$
|
$H — C — COO^-$
|
CH_2
|
O
|
$O = P — O^-$
|
O
|
$CH_2 — CH — CH_2$
| |
O O
| |
$C = O$ $C = O$
| |
FA   FA

phosphatidylcholine

CH_3
CH_3 | CH_3
$+$ N
|
CH_2
|
CH_2
|
O
|
$O = P — O^-$
|
O
|
$CH_2 — CH — CH_2$
| |
O O
| |
$C = O$ $C = O$
| |
FA   FA

sphingomyelin

CH_3
CH_3 | CH_3
$+$ N
|
CH_2
|
CH_2
|
O
|
$O = P — O^-$
|
O
|
OH
|
$CH — CH — CH_2$
|
CH NH
‖ |
CH $C = O$
| |
$(CH_2)_{12}$ FA
|
CH_3

ceramide

Fig. 3.3 The three major phospholipids, phosphatidylethanolamine, phosphatidylserine, and phosphatidylcholine, differ with respect to their polar head groups. Sphingomyelin is a sphingolipid as opposed to a phospholipid, and it consists of a choline group attached via a phosphate molecule to a ceramide group. (FA, fatty acid.)

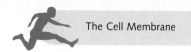

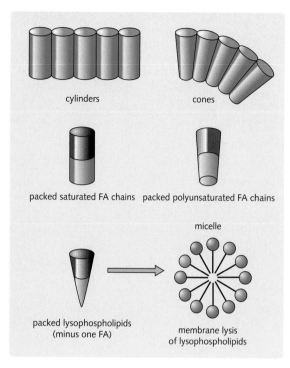

packed saturated FA chains   packed polyunsaturated FA chains

micelle

packed lysophospholipids
(minus one FA)

membrane lysis
of lysophospholipids

Fig. 3.4 Packing of phospholipids. The nature of the fatty acid side chains influences their packing. Lysophospholipids, which lack one fatty acid, form micelles preferentially. However, the favored structure for phospholipids with two fatty acid chains in aqueous solution is a lipid bilayer because they are too bulky to form micelles. (FA, fatty acid.)

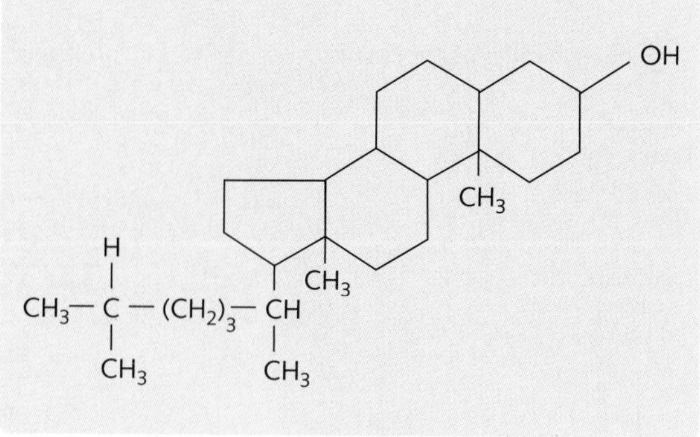

$$CH_3 - \underset{\underset{CH_3}{|}}{\overset{\overset{H}{|}}{C}} - (CH_2)_3 - \underset{\underset{CH_3}{|}}{CH}$$

Fig. 3.5 Structure of cholesterol.

Examples of membrane proteins			
Protein	**Type**	**Bonding with membrane**	**Function**
Cadherin	Monotopic integral	Hydrophobic with phospholipids	Mediates cell–cell adhesion
CFTR	Polytopic integral	Hydrophobic with phospholipids	Gated chloride channel in epithelial tissue
Ankyrin	Peripheral	Electrostatic with the anion exchange protein on the cytoplasmic surface of the lipid bilayer	Maintains erythrocyte structure by forming a link between spectrin and the anion exchange protein (band 3)
Ras	Peripheral	Covalent attachment to the cytoplasmic layer of the lipid bilayer	GTP-binding protein that relays signals from the cell surface to the nucleus

Fig. 3.6 Examples of membrane proteins and their functions. (CFTR, cystic fibrosis transmembrane regulator

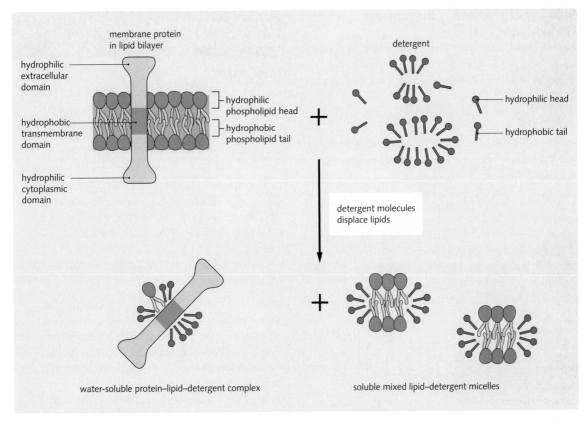

Fig. 3.7 Solubilizing membrane proteins with detergent. The detergent competes with phospholipids to form hydrophobic interactions with proteins and so displaces them from the membrane. (Adapted from *Molecular Biology of the Cell*, 3rd edn, by B. Alberts *et al.*, Garland Publishing Co., 1994, with permission of Routledge, Inc., part of The Taylor & Francis Group.)

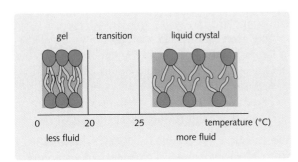

Fig. 3.8 Membrane transition from gel to liquid crystal.

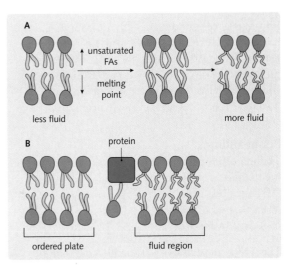

Fig. 3.9 Factors affecting membrane fluidity. (A) Increasing the concentration of unsaturated fatty acids (FAs) decreases the melting point of the membrane and so increases fluidity. (B) Uneven distribution of membrane lipids affects the fluidity.

35

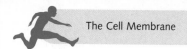

Mobility of membrane components
Phospholipids

Phospholipid molecules show four different modes of movement to varying degrees:

- Intrachain movements, such as flexing of fatty acid chains.
- Axial rotation of the molecules in the plane of the bilayer.
- Lateral diffusion within the plane of the bilayer.
- Movement from one half of the bilayer to the other ("flip-flop").

Lateral diffusion of phospholipids occurs readily, resulting in a fluid two-dimensional membrane. Flip-flop is rare in the absence of the enzyme "flippase," enabling asymmetry of phospholipid composition between membrane layers. Membrane asymmetry is functionally important and, for example, phosphatidylserine is concentrated on the cytoplasmic side where it may interact with protein kinase C.

Proteins

Proteins show three types of movement:

- Lateral movement, though this may be restricted by interactions with the cytoskeleton or covalent attachment to lipid molecules.
- Axial rotational movements in the plane of the membrane.
- Conformational changes.

Flip-flop is thermodynamically unfavorable, since it would require hydrophilic protein moieties to rotate through the bilayer and it is, therefore, rare. Protein directionality is important for function, and it ensures, for example, that hormone receptors are correctly orientated.

Permeability

There are three main forms of transport across the membrane:

- Passive diffusion.
- Facilitated diffusion.
- Active transport.

Though permeable to lipid-soluble compounds, lipid bilayers are impermeable to ionic and polar substances, and these require dedicated channels to cross the membrane. Although polar, water is membrane permeable because it is a very small molecule.

Transport across the cell membrane

Concepts

Concentrations are measured in moles and the dissociation of ions is not taken into account.

$$1 \text{ mole} = 6.02 \times 10^{23} \text{ molecules (of any kind)}$$
$$= \text{Avogadro's constant (the number of atoms in exactly 12 g of carbon 12)}$$

For example:

- A molar solution of $NaCl$ contains one mole of Na atoms and one mole of Cl atoms in 1 L.
- A molar solution of sucrose contains one mole of sucrose in 1 L.
- A molar solution of $CaCl_2$ contains one mole of Ca^{2+} and two moles of Cl in 1 L.

Diffusion is the movement of particles from a region of high concentration to a region of low concentration until they are evenly distributed. Osmosis is the movement of solvent molecules (usually water) across a semipermeable membrane from a region of high solvent concentration to a region of low solvent concentration. The osmotic pressure is the pressure required to prevent the net movement of pure water into an aqueous solution across a semipermeable membrane. In osmotic pressure the dissociation of ions is important.

$$1 \text{ osmole} = 10^{23} \text{ osmotically active particles}$$

For example:

- One osmol/L of $NaCl$ contains 0.5 moles of the ion Na^+ and 0.5 moles of the ion of Cl^-.
- One osmol/L of sucrose contains one mole of sucrose.
- Three osmol/L of $CaCl_2$ contains one mole of the ion Ca^{2+} and two moles of the ion Cl^-.

The osmolarity of plasma is critical, as changes affect plasma volume, cell volume, and water and ion homeostasis.

The term "tonicity" relates to the behavior of cells immersed in a solution:

- Isotonic extracellular solutions have the same osmotic pressure as the inside of the cell, so osmosis does not occur and the cell remains the same size.
- Hypotonic solutions are less concentrated, so water will pass into the cell and it will swell.
- Hypertonic solutions are more concentrated, so water will pass out of the cell and it will shrink.

Distribution of ions across the cell membrane		
Component	Outside	Inside
K$^+$ (mmol/L)	4.5	140 (varies with cell type)
Na$^+$ (mmol/L)	140	10
Ca^{2+} total (mmol/L)	3	1
Ca^{2+} free (μmol/L)	1	0.1
Cl$^-$ (mmol/L)	110	3
HCO$_3^-$ (mmol/L)	24	10
pH	7.35	7
Amino acids, proteins	10	120

Fig. 3.10 Distribution of ions across the cell membrane.

Normal plasma osmolarity is approximately 0.3 osmol/L (i.e., 300 mosmol/L). K$^+$, Na$^+$, and Cl$^-$ are fully dissociated, whereas Ca^{2+}, Mg^{2+}, and H$^+$ are only partially dissociated in living systems. Dissociation is affected by pH, temperature, and binding of ions to compounds (e.g., Ca^{2+} binding to myosin during muscle contraction).

Distribution of ions across the cell membrane

Life's essential chemical reactions can only occur within narrow physiologic parameters, so the cell must regulate the entry and exit of intracellular molecules. Some biological processes, such as muscle contraction, depend upon an electrochemical gradient across the cell membrane. The distribution of ions across the cell membrane is shown in Fig. 3.10. Distribution is influenced by:
• The semipermeable membrane concept.
• Electrochemical gradient.
• Pumps.

Semipermeable membrane concept
Polar molecules cannot diffuse through the lipid bilayer, and they rely on the proteins embedded in the membrane for transport. These proteins are generally specific for particular molecules. The cell regulates the activity of membrane transport proteins such that only certain molecules can get through at any one time. It is, therefore, semipermeable.

Electrochemical gradient
It is thermodynamically favorable for ions to move from areas of high concentration to low concentration and for positively charged ions to move to negatively charged environments.

Pumps
Pumps are used to maintain energetically unfavorable concentration gradients. For example, the cell is able to maintain an energetically unfavorable sodium gradient because it expends energy in the form of ATP to drive sodium out of the cell.

Transport across the membrane
If the transport of a molecule can occur spontaneously, it is termed passive transport or diffusion. If the transport process requires energy, it is active transport (Fig. 3.11).

Passive diffusion
Passive diffusion is the free movement of molecules across a membrane down a concentration gradient. Small nonpolar molecules (e.g., O$_2$ and CO$_2$) and uncharged polar molecules (e.g., urea) may diffuse directly through the lipid bilayer by this means. No energy is required and diffusion continues until equilibrium is reached. Saturation does not occur because no binding sites are involved. Diffusion rate is directly proportional to the ion gradient, hydrostatic pressure, and electrical potential, and it can be summarized by Fick's law of diffusion:

Rate of diffusion = D × A × Δ conc

Where D = diffusion constant, A = membrane area, and Δ conc = concentration gradient.

Facilitated diffusion
Charged molecules cannot diffuse directly through the lipid bilayer; they depend on specific proteins. The transport of molecules by a protein receptor down a concentration gradient is called facilitated diffusion, which is a form of passive transport that continues until equilibrium. Proteins mediating facilitated diffusion may be channels or carrier proteins. Transport with carrier proteins shows Michaelis–Menten kinetics (Fig. 3.12):
• Substrate specificity or selectivity, affinity for a particular ligand (measured as K$_L$).
• Saturability of ligand binding (B$_{max}$).

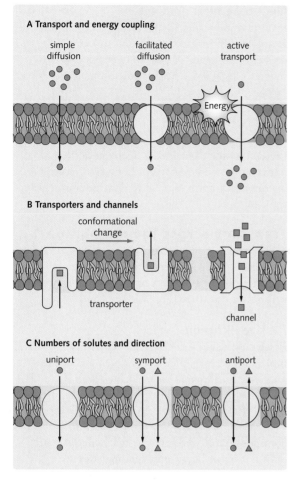

A Transport and energy coupling

simple diffusion	facilitated diffusion	active transport

Energy

B Transporters and channels

conformational change

transporter

channel

C Numbers of solutes and direction

uniport	symport	antiport

Fig. 3.11 A summary of solute movement across membranes. (Adapted from Baynes and Dominiczak, 1999.)

- Transferability (T_{max}) the maximum rate of molecule transfer across the membrane.
- Inhibition (e.g., transport of glucose into erythrocytes).

The rate of movement of ions through a membrane via channels depends on the concentration gradient, the speed with which the ion moves through the channel (a constant) and the number of open channels. It is, therefore, analogous to passive diffusion, with the number of open channels being equivalent to the surface area. Channels may be gated such that the cell controls when they are open. Irrespective of the electrochemical gradient, an ion cannot cross the membrane if there are no open channels.

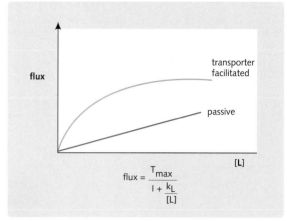

flux

transporter facilitated

passive

[L]

$$flux = \frac{T_{max}}{1 + \frac{k_L}{[L]}}$$

Fig. 3.12 Kinetics of facilitated diffusion. Passive diffusion is slower than transporter facilitated diffusion and its rate is directly proportional to substrate concentration. Transporter facilitated diffusion behaves like an enzyme and becomes saturated. (T_{max}, maximum transport rate; k_L, affinity for ligand; [L], concentration of ligand.)

Active transport

Active transport couples the movement of molecules against an unfavorable electrochemical gradient to a thermodynamically favorable reaction:

- Primary active transport is coupled directly to the hydrolysis of ATP.
- Secondary active transport is coupled indirectly to the hydrolysis of ATP.

Primary active transport

Sodium and potassium are examples of ions that are transported across the cell by primary active transport by the Na^+/K^+ dependent ATPase (also called "the sodium pump"). This transporter pumps three Na^+ ions outward and two K^+ ions inward, against their respective concentration gradients, for every molecule of ATP hydrolyzed. The Na^+/K^+-dependent ATPase is found in all cells, and it may consume half of the cell's ATP.

Secondary active transport

The action of the Na^+/K^+ ATPase establishes K^+ and Na^+ concentration gradients across the membrane. Movement of Na^+ into the cell, down its electrochemical gradient, is thermodynamically favored, and in secondary transport this is coupled to the movement of a second ion against a gradient. The Na^+ electrochemical gradient may drive the transport of ions in either direction across the membrane (Fig. 3.13):

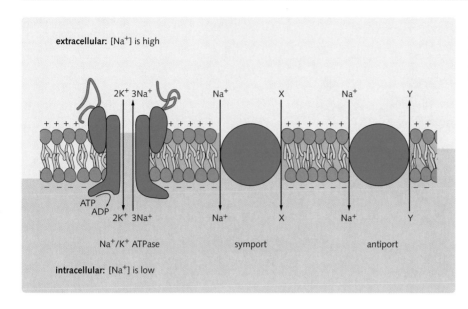

Fig. 3.13 Secondary active transport. The action of the Na⁺/K⁺ ATPase results in a sodium concentration gradient across the membrane. This potential energy may be used to drive molecules into the cell via symports or out of the cell via antiports.

- Symports transport both ions in the same direction.
- Antiports transport the ions in opposite directions.

Summary of types of transport

In summary:
- Passive diffusion is through the plasma membrane, and it does not expend energy.
- Facilitated diffusion requires specific proteins but energy is not expended.
- Active transport requires specific proteins and energy expenditure.

Transport mechanisms

Membrane transport proteins may be channels or carriers (see Fig. 3.11). Most transport proteins are reversible, and depending on the prevailing conditions may transport ions into or out of the cell.

Ion channels

Ion channels are proteins that span the membrane and have central water-filled pores. The pores are specific, allowing either cations or anions through. Transport speed is greater than 10^6 ions/s, and it is always down a concentration gradient. Potassium channels are the most common type. One type is perpetually open, with the leakage of potassium through these channels being critical to the membrane potential. Defects or damage can cause muscular dysfunction (e.g., periodic paralysis).

Many channels are gated, and open and close under specific conditions.

Cystic fibrosis is a recessive disease characterized by airway disease, pancreatic insufficiency, and male infertility. It is caused by mutations in the gene encoding CFTR (cystic fibrosis transmembrane regulator). CFTR is a gated channel that permits passive chloride movement across the apical membrane of some epithelial cell types.

Carrier proteins

Carrier proteins bind specific ligands (the transported molecule) and undergo conformational change during transport. They transport polar and ionic molecules by active transport and facilitated diffusion. Transport is hundreds of times slower than via ion channels. Carrier proteins can become saturated, limiting the rate of transport. Uniports transport single molecules across the membrane (see Fig. 3.11). Coupled transporters transfer molecules across the membrane with simultaneous transfer of

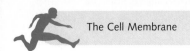

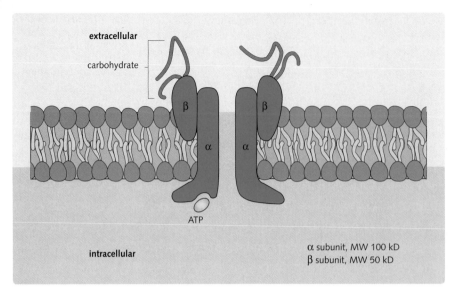

Fig. 3.14 Structure of the sodium pump.

α subunit, MW 100 kD
β subunit, MW 50 kD

another molecule (symports and antiports). Different cells have different carrier cell populations, and so they have different permeabilities.

Glucose transporter

Most cells transfer glucose by facilitated diffusion through uniports, as the concentration of glucose is greater outside the cell. In the intestine and kidney some cells absorb glucose from low extracellular concentrations, which is achieved by secondary active transport via symports cotransporting sodium.

Active transporters

Active transporters are carrier proteins that are linked to a source of energy, such as ATP or an ionic gradient.

Sodium pump

The sodium pump is an example of an active transporter. It is a heterodimer or oligomer consisting of α-subunits and glycosylated β-subunits (Fig. 3.14).

The glycosylated subunit is important for the assembly and localization of the pump. The α-subunit is the catalytic unit, and it has binding sites for sodium and ATP on its intracellular surface and potassium on its extracellular surface. Binding of sodium causes phosphorylation of the cytoplasmic side and a conformational change, which transfers the sodium outside the cell.

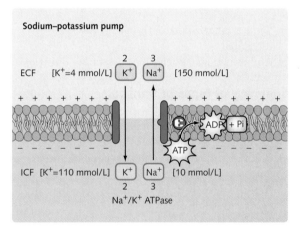

Sodium–potassium pump

ECF [K^+=4 mmol/L] K^+ Na^+ [150 mmol/L]

ICF [K^+=110 mmol/L] K^+ Na^+ [10 mmol/L]

Na^+/K^+ ATPase

Fig. 3.15 The Na^+/K^+ ATPase. The hydrolysis of one molecule of ATP is associated with the transport of three sodium ions out of the cell and two potassium ions into the cell against their respective concentration gradients. (ECF, extracellular fluid; ICF, intracellular fluid.) (Adapted from Baynes and Dominiczak, 1999.)

Binding of potassium causes dephosphorylation, so the subunit returns to its original state, transferring the potassium inside the cell simultaneously (Fig. 3.15). The biochemical name for the sodium pump is the Na^+/K^+ ATPase. Its functions are as follows:

- Maintaining the intracellular sodium concentration at a low level.
- Maintaining a constant cell volume.

- Providing a sodium gradient as an energy source for cotransport. The gradient is exploited by many body processes, including the transporters that regulate intracellular pH and those that drive glucose into kidney cells.
- Generation of membrane potential.

Summary of types of transporter molecule

In summary (see Fig. 3.11):
- All transport molecules are proteins.
- Ion channels span the membrane, never require energy, and transport down gradient.
- Carrier proteins bind molecules, may be linked to an energy source, and can transport with or against a gradient.

Membrane potential

Definition

A membrane potential (E_m) is defined by the difference in electrical charge on each side of a membrane. It is very important in the functioning of excitable cells, especially nerve and muscle cells. These cells use the controlled opening of gated ion channels to cause a change in their membrane potential. There are three major types of gated channels in excitable cells:
- Voltage-gated channels (e.g., voltage-gated sodium channels used in action potential generation).
- Chemically gated channels (e.g., acetylcholine receptor channels in neuromuscular transmission).
- Mechanical receptors (e.g., touch receptor channels in sensory neurons).

Maintenance of membrane potential

Electrochemical potential difference of ions

When a solution is not at equilibrium, the movement of its ions is influenced by both chemical and electrical gradients. If these factors operate in different directions across a cell membrane, net ion flow will tend to be down whichever gradient is the steepest. The electrochemical potential difference ($\Delta\mu$) of an ion X^+ across a membrane separating compartments A and B can be calculated as follows:

$$\Delta\mu(X^+) = (RTln\ [X^+]_A/[X^+]_B + zF(E_A - E_B)$$

(Where $\Delta\mu$ is the electrochemical potential difference between A and B; R is the ideal gas constant; T is absolute temperature; $[X^+]_{A/B}$ is the concentration of X^+ in A and B; z is valency; F is Faraday's number; $E_A - E_B$ is the electric potential difference across the membrane.)

This equation includes the contributions of both the concentration difference and the electrical potential difference to the tendency for the ion to flow across the membrane. Since $\Delta\mu$ was defined as the electrochemical potential of the ion on side A minus that of the ion on side B:
- If $\Delta\mu$ is positive, ions move from A to B.
- If $\Delta\mu$ is negative, ions move from B to A.
- If $\Delta\mu$ is zero, there is no net movement of ions (the reaction is at equilibrium).

When a potential difference for an ion exists across a membrane there is a tendency for it to move down a chemical or electrical gradient. This potential energy can be harnessed, which is the basis of secondary active transport.

The Nernst equation

When a reaction is at equilibrium there is no net movement of ions across the cell membrane—i.e., the concentration gradient and the electrical gradient are balanced ($RTln[X^+]_A/[X^+]_B = zF(E_A - E_B)$). In this situation, the electrochemical potential difference equation above can be rearranged to give the Nernst equation (Fig. 3.16):

$$E_A - E_B = (60\,mV/z)\ (log\ ([X^+]_B/[X^+]_A))$$

When moving down a chemical gradient, an ion is moving from an area of high concentration to low concentration. Ion movement down an electrical gradient is dictated by charge. An ion crossing a membrane down an electrochemical gradient is responding to both chemical and electrical gradients.

The Nernst equation can be used to calculate:
- The electrical potential difference that must exist between two chambers for an ion to be in equilibrium across the membrane.

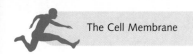

When no net movement of X^+ across a membrane occurs it is at equilibrium and the electropotential difference ($\Delta\mu$) for X^+ is zero, therefore:

$$RT\ln \frac{[X^+]_A}{[X^+]_B} + zF(E_A - E_B) = 0$$

Solving for $E_A - E_B$ gives:

$$E_A - E_B = \frac{-RT}{zF} \ln \frac{[X^+]_A}{[X^+]_B} = \frac{RT}{zF} \ln \frac{[X^+]_B}{[X^+]_A}$$

A convenient form of the equation is obtained by converting to a form that involves $\log_{10}$ ($\ln y = 2.303 \log y$). At 29°C the quantity 2.303 RT/F is equal to 60 mV:

$$E_A - E_B = \frac{60mV}{z} \log \frac{[X^+]_B}{[X^+]_A}$$

Fig. 3.16 Derivation of the Nernst equation. ($E_A - E_B$, the electric potential difference across the membrane; R, ideal gas constant; T, absolute temperature; $[X^+]_{A/B}$, concentration of X^+ in A and B; z, valency; F, Faraday's number.)

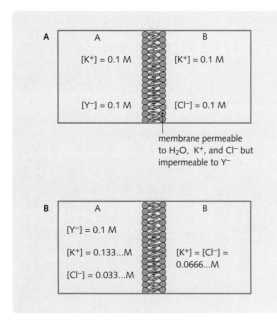

Fig. 3.17 Gibbs–Donnan equilibrium. (A) Ion concentrations at the start of the experiment. (B) Ion concentrations when Gibbs–Donnan equilibrium has been reached. (Adapted from Berne *et al.*, 1998.)

- The direction an ion will flow when the reaction is not in equilibrium, given an experimentally derived electrical potential difference.

The electrochemical potential difference when an ion is at equilibrium is called the equilibrium potential, e.g., $E_{Cl} = -70\,mV$.

Gibbs–Donnan equilibrium

In an experimental system

The Gibbs–Donnan equilibrium is the electrochemical equilibrium that develops when two solutions are separated by a membrane permeable to only some of the ions in solution. If an experimental system consists of two compartments containing equimolar solutions of KCl (compartment B) and KY (compartment A) is separated by a membrane permeable to K^+ and Cl^-, but impermeable to the Y^- anions, the permeant ions will redistribute as follows (Fig. 3.17):

- Cl^- moves down its concentration gradient from B to A.
- Electroneutrality is preserved, so K^+ follows, moving from B to A.
- Y^- cannot diffuse across the membrane, and it is trapped in compartment A.
- Electroneutrality is preserved, so K^+ remains trapped in compartment A.

Electroneutrality is preserved when ions cross the membrane because the movement of Cl^- sets up a local electrical potential that draws K^+ across the membrane. The movement of ions continues until the reaction is at equilibrium (Fig. 3.17B) at which point:

- The tendency for Cl^- to move down the concentration gradient from B to A is offset by its tendency to move down the electrical gradient from A to B.
- The tendency for K^+ to move down its concentration gradient from A to B is offset by its tendency to move down the electrical gradient from B to A.

At equilibrium, $\Delta\mu K^+$ and $\Delta\mu Cl^-$ both equal zero. This is the basis for the derivation of the Gibbs–Donnan equation, which states that the product of the concentrations of both permeant ions is the same in each compartment:

$$[K^+]_A[Cl^-]_A = [K^+]_B[Cl]_B$$

The Gibbs–Donnan equation holds for any univalent anion cation pair in equilibrium between two chambers. A system in Gibbs–Donnan equilibrium has a number of important features at equilibrium:

- The compartment containing the impermeant ion contains more osmotically active ions (Fig. 3.17B).
- The compartment containing the impermeant anion has a negative electropotential (NB a compartment containing an impermeant cation would have a positive electropotential).

In living cells

Living cells resemble the experimental Gibbs–Donnan equilibrium above in a number of respects:

- They contain impermeant ions in the form of proteins and nucleic acids.
- The membrane is permeable to K^+ and Cl^-, and these ions are abundant.

However, there are significant differences:

- The cell is sensitive to osmotic gradients.
- The cell membrane is not entirely impermeable to positively charged ions such as Na^+ and Ca^{2+}, and these leak into the cell down an electrochemical gradient.
- If allowed to accumulate, they would exert osmotic pressure and the cell would swell.
- Osmotic effects are avoided by actively transporting such ions out of the cell.
- Cell swelling is avoided because the Na^+/K^+ ATPase pumps three Na^+ ions out of the cell, while only two K^+ ions are pumped back in.

Resting membrane potential

The membrane potential (E_m) of a cell is proportional to the concentration gradient of the dominant ions (Na^+, K^+, and Cl^-) and the membrane permeability to each one. If an ion is freely permeable across the cell membrane, it will tend to force E_m toward its own equilibrium potential. Resting excitable cells are most permeable to K^+ so E_m reflects the balance between K^+ leaking out of the cell down its concentration gradient and being pulled in down the electrical gradient (i.e., E_K). This movement is not accompanied by the extrusion of an anion because the membrane is only permeable to Cl^-, which has an opposing concentration gradient. Thus, E_m is

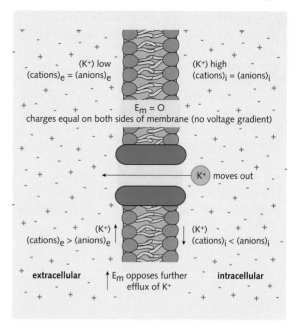

Fig. 3.18 Role of potassium in generating the cell membrane potential. (E_m, membrane potential; e, extracellular; i, intracellular.)

proportional to the concentration of K^+ on each side of the membrane (Fig. 3.18).

Resting E_m (−70 mV) is not quite equal to E_K (−90 mV) because the membrane is slightly permeable to other ions, such as Na^+. Sodium influx makes the membrane potential slightly more positive because E_{Na} is positive (+60 mV), reflecting its tendency to move into the cell down its electrochemical gradient. However, note that Na^+ is not at equilibrium across the resting cell membrane because it is not freely permeable to this ion.

The action of the Na^+/K^+ ATPase, being electrogenic, contributes a small amount to the membrane potential directly. However, the majority of the membrane potential arises from the indirect action of the pump and reflects the movement of K^+ and Na^+ down the concentration gradients that it has established.

The excitable cell may manipulate its resting potential to control activity:

- Depolarization means the E_m becomes less negative, so there is a decrease in the potential difference. A depolarized nerve cell is more likely to fire.
- Hyperpolarization means that the potential difference increases in magnitude, by increasing

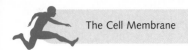

the relative negative charge inside the cell. A hyperpolarized nerve cell is less likely to fire.

Action potentials

An action potential is a rapid, transient, self-perpetuating electrical excitation of the membrane. It is initiated and proceeds as follows (Fig. 3.19):

- The trigger for initial depolarization varies between cell types, e.g., binding of acetylcholine to its receptor.
- If depolarization exceeds the threshold potential, voltage-gated sodium channels open.
- Na^+ flows into the cells down the electrochemical gradient and E_m tends toward E_{Na}.
- Na^+ channels remain open very briefly before changing conformation to a closed "inactivated state."
- The depolarization caused by proximal open Na^+ channels causes distal voltage-gated Na^+ channels to open, allowing further Na^+ in. In this way, a wave of depolarization spreads down the axon.
- Repolarization of the membrane occurs by the combined action of closure of the Na^+ channels and the opening of voltage-gated K^+ channels that permit K^+ efflux (these are activated by depolarization, but they are slower to respond than the Na^+ channels). The Na^+/K^+ ATPase plays a minimal role in the process.
- When the membrane repolarizes to its resting potential, the Na^+ channels undergo a further conformational change to a closed, but potentially activated, form.

Membrane potential is highly sensitive to the concentration of K^+. An increase in the extracellular concentration of K^+ (hyperkalemia) will partially depolarize excitable cells, bringing the resting potential closer to the threshold potential. Moreover, since K^+ efflux after an action potential is inhibited repolarization is impeded. Hypokalemia (a decrease in the extracellular concentration of K^+) will tend to hyperpolarize cells, making them less excitable. Both conditions affect cardiac cells, causing arrhythmias.

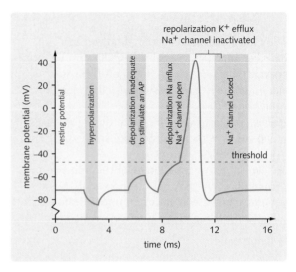

Fig. 3.19 Generation of an action potential.

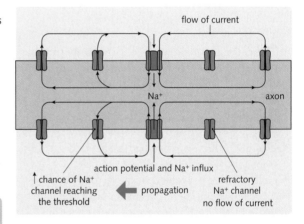

Fig. 3.20 Propagation of the action potential, illustrating the local circuit hypothesis.

The local circuit hypothesis states that propagation occurs where the current flows along the membrane, generating areas of local depolarization, which produces further depolarization in distal areas ahead (Fig. 3.20). Propagation is unidirectional, as regions that have just been excited are refractory because the Na^+ channels are in an inactivated state. The thousands of channels summate to create a current across the membrane that can be measured with a microelectrode.

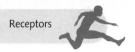

Receptors

Concepts of transmembrane signaling

Mechanisms to signal from extracellular to intracellular are necessary. It is essential that cells in a multicellular organism are able to communicate in order to coordinate their activities. Signal transduction has been shown to be a universal path through which cells are directed to divide, differentiate, migrate, degranulate, and many other activities. Such processes enable responses to be made to external factors governing cell activity. The pathway begins at cell surface receptors and ends in the nucleus with proteins that regulate gene expression. Since different cell types may respond differently to the same signal at the level of transcription, these processes facilitate the coordination of the whole organism's response to a stimulus.

Only certain lipid-soluble molecules can cross the cell membrane directly (e.g., steroid hormones); other molecules transfer their signal by binding to cell surface receptors. The signal transduction pathways are formed by interacting proteins, which can amplify, dampen, or process signals before passing them downstream. Each cell may be confronted with many different signals coming from its cellular neighbors, environment, substratum contact, and the presence of growth factors and hormones. The resulting signal pathways are integrated so that the cellular response is appropriate. When signal pathways malfunction, the cell may multiply uncontrollably, and this may result in malignancy.

Definitions

Important definitions include the following:
- A hormone is a molecule produced by an endocrine cell, which is released into the bloodstream and acts on specific receptors.
- Cell surface receptors are specific proteins that bind a signaling molecule and convert this binding into intracellular signals, which alter the cell's behavior.
- A ligand is a molecule such as a hormone that binds the receptor, and is termed the first messenger.
- The second-messenger system is a set of intracellular molecules that are activated by cell surface receptors and affect cell function, producing a physiological response, e.g., AMP, GMP, DAG, IP_3. Second-messenger systems produce a signal cascade that amplifies the initial signal and facilitates a variety of cellular responses, the details of which vary between cell types.

The three mechanisms of cell signaling to surface receptors are (Fig. 3.21):
- Endocrine.
- Paracrine.
- Autocrine.

Types of receptor

The presence or absence of a specific receptor on a cell governs the responsiveness of that cell to signaling molecules. There are a number of different types of receptor.

Ionotropic receptors

These receptors are linked to an ion channel and are made of multimeric proteins of about

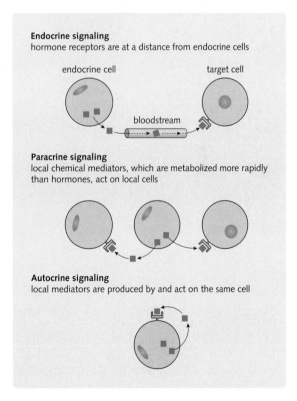

Fig. 3.21 The three mechanisms of cell signaling. A single signaling molecule may fall into more than one of these categories depending on where it is synthesized and released.

45

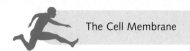

250,000 D. They are predominantly found in the nervous system, and their signaling is very fast (e.g., nicotinic acetylcholine receptor; Fig. 3.22).

Tyrosine kinase (TK) receptors

These are catalytic receptors that signal directly to the cell (Fig. 3.23). There are four classes and these are illustrated in Fig. 3.24. TK phosphorylates target proteins at tyrosine residues (Fig. 3.25). They often phosphorylate their own cytoplasmic tail in a process known as "autophosphorylation." Cytoplasmic proteins, which are often enzymes, bind to activated TK through a common domain, the SH2 domain.

Examples of TK receptors are:
- Epidermal growth factor (EGF) receptor—a type I TK receptor; its ligands are epidermal growth factor (EGF), transforming growth factor-alpha (TGF-α), and heparin-binding EGF, which all have a similar core structure. In inflammatory disease such as pancreatitis there may be upregulation of EGF receptors, which bind TGF-α that can lead to abnormal growth and possibly carcinoma.
- Insulin growth factor (IGF) I receptor—a type II TK receptor.
- Fibroblast growth factor (FGF) receptors—all type IV TK receptors. There are four FGF receptors, which bind the seven FGF ligands. FGF is important in angiogenesis, and abnormalities of FGF and the FGF receptor are seen in some carcinomas (e.g., pancreatic), facilitating both paracrine and autocrine mediated proliferation.

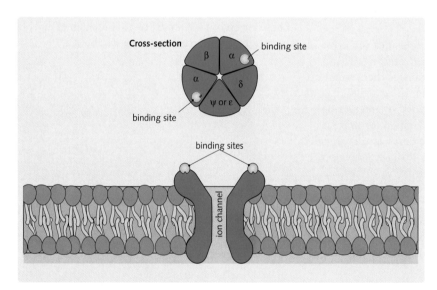

Fig. 3.22 Structure of the nicotinic acetylcholine receptor.

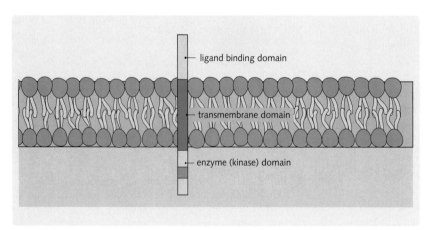

Fig. 3.23 Structure of the tyrosine kinase (TK) receptor.

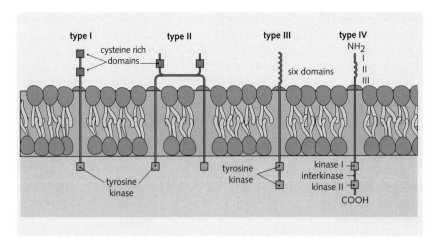

Fig. 3.24 The four classes of tyrosine kinase (TK) receptor. All these receptors have tyrosine kinase activity and SH2 binding domains on their cytoplasmic portions. The main differences between receptors are in their ligand binding domains.

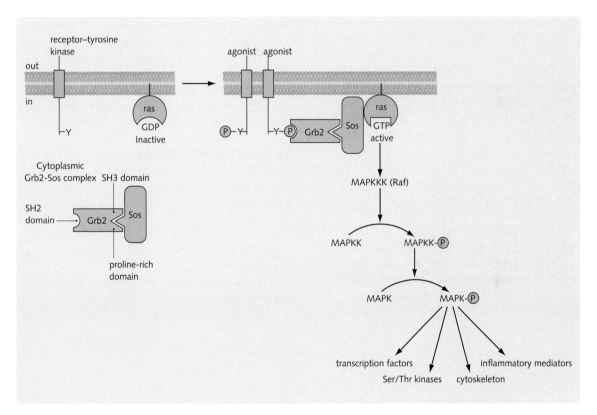

Fig. 3.25 Tyrosine kinase (TK) signal transduction, showing phosphorylation path of target proteins. The binding of its ligand (a growth factor) to the receptor–tyrosine kinase induces a conformational change that results in dimerization. Each monomer phosphorylates its partner on multiple tyrosine residues. Phosphorylation of the receptor initiates a cascade of reactions in which proteins including Ras and MAP kinase are progressively activated by phosphorylation. MAP kinase ultimately phosphorylates transcription factors and other protein kinases that are important for cell growth and differentiation. Mutations that increase the activity of proteins in this pathway are frequent in tumors. Such mutated genes are called oncogenes (the unmutated form is a proto-oncogene). (Y, tyrosine; MAPK, mitogen activated protein kinase; MAPKK, mitogen activated protein kinase kinase; etc.) (Adapted from Norman and Lodwick, 1999.)

47

Metabotropic receptors (G-protein coupled)

These receptors all have a common structural feature, a region that spans the membrane seven times (Fig. 3.26). Some receptors are composed of multiple subunits, and they are activated by dissociation of these subunits.

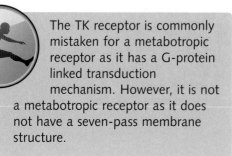

The TK receptor is commonly mistaken for a metabotropic receptor as it has a G-protein linked transduction mechanism. However, it is not a metabotropic receptor as it does not have a seven-pass membrane structure.

Metabotropic receptors activate G-proteins. G-proteins are a family of proteins that are bound to the inner plasma membrane and involved in the regulation of second-messenger activity. When activated, G-proteins bind and hydrolyze GTP, functioning like a binary switch (Fig. 3.27). The Ras protein (encoded by an oncogene) belongs to a subset of monomeric G-proteins that are homologous to the α-subunit of the more common trimeric version. Activated G-proteins subsequently activate intracellular second-messenger pathways. For example:

- Cyclic AMP (cAMP) (Fig. 3.28).
- Calcium (directly by opening of calcium channels in the plasma membrane, or indirectly by the inositol lipid pathways).
- Inositol lipid pathways (Fig. 3.29).

Different G-proteins activate different pathways. For example:

- G_s increases cAMP (see Fig. 3.28).
- G_i decreases cAMP.
- G_q activates the inositol lipid pathway.

An example of a metabotropic receptor is the β-adrenergic receptor.

Steroid receptors

These are not membrane bound receptors, but soluble cytoplasmic proteins (Fig. 3.30). Steroid receptors bind water-insoluble steroid, retinoid, and thyroid hormones, which pass through the lipid membrane easily, and which are metabolized more slowly when released into the bloodstream than are hydrophilic molecules.

Once activated, the receptors may or may not dimerize before binding specific nucleotide sequences on the DNA, so regulating the transcription of specific genes. The product of the gene may in turn regulate the transcription of further genes, termed the secondary response. The testosterone receptor is a steroid receptor.

Receptors and drugs

Many drugs produce their pharmacological effect by acting on cell surface receptors. The effect produced depends upon whether the drug acts as an agonist or antagonist:

- Agonists are molecules that activate receptors, and they may be pharmacologic or physiological agents.
- Antagonists are molecules that bind receptors and do not activate them. They block the

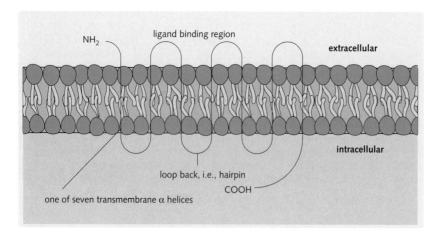

Fig. 3.26 Structure of a metabotropic receptor (e.g., a β-adrenergic receptor).

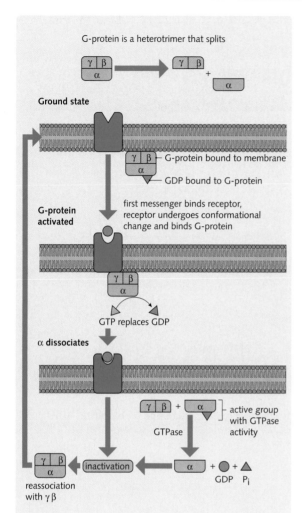

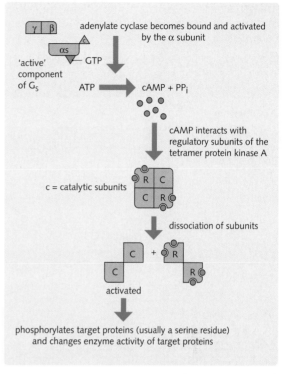

Fig. 3.27 Activation of G-proteins. The G-protein in its inactive state is a heterotrimer that has a GDP bound via its α-subunit. Interaction of the receptor with its ligand drives the exchange of GTP for GDP. This induces a conformational change in the α-subunit that results in its dissociation from both the receptor and the $\beta\gamma$-subunits. The dissociated subunits are free to interact with effectors that generate secondary messengers. Eventual hydrolysis of GTP by the α-subunit permits the regeneration of the inactive heterotrimer. (GDP, guanosine diphosphate; GTP, guanosine triphosphate; P_i, inorganic phosphate.)

Fig. 3.28 Adenylate cyclase pathway. Increased cAMP levels lead to numerous downstream actions, including the activation of protein kinase A. (cAMP, cyclic adenosine monophosphate; ATP, adenosine triphosphate; C, catalytic subunits; GTP, guanosine triphosphate; PP_i, pyrophosphate; R, regulatory subunits.)

receptor's ligand from binding, so preventing its action.

Reversible antagonists, also called competitive antagonists, compete with the ligand for the receptor. Competitive antagonism can be reduced by increasing the concentration of agonist. Irreversible antagonists cannot be removed from the receptor; thus they reduce the effective number of receptors, and increasing the agonist concentration has no effect.

The specificity of a drug reflects its ability to combine with one receptor type. The desired action of a drug is to combine with a specific receptor in the targeted tissue. Adverse effects may be caused by nonspecific binding to other receptor types, or by binding with the desired receptor, but in a different tissue.

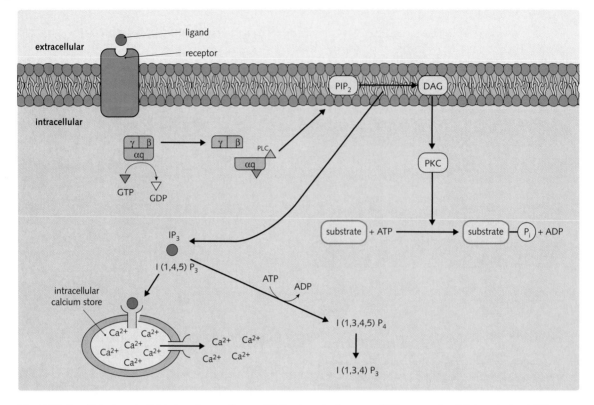

Fig. 3.29 Inositol phospholipid signaling pathway. (PLC, phospholipase c; GTP, guanosine triphosphate; ADP, guanosine monophosphate; PIP$_2$, phosphoinositol diphosphate; DAG, diacylglycerol; PKC, phosphokinase C; P$_i$, inorganic phosphate; IP$_3$, inositol triphosphate; Ca^{2+}, calcium ions.)

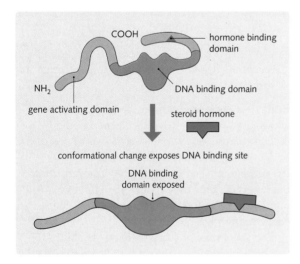

Fig. 3.30 Structure of a steroid receptor.

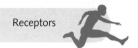

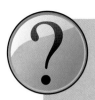

- Draw a labeled diagram of the fluid mosaic model of the plasma membrane.
- Discuss the chemical properties of phospholipids and their significance in the plasma membrane.
- Describe the two classes of membrane protein and the nature of their attachment to the plasma membrane.
- Outline the factors that influence membrane fluidity.
- List the modes of movement available to phospholipids and proteins in the plasma membrane.
- Define diffusion, osmosis, osmotic pressure, isotonic, hypotonic, and hypertonic.
- Describe the relative concentrations of K^+, Na^+, Cl^-, and Ca^{2+} across the resting cell membrane.
- Describe secondary active transport, and state how it differs from primary active transport.
- Compare and contrast active transport and facilitated diffusion.
- Outline the structure of the Na^+/K^+ ATPase, suggest what type of transport it mediates, and describe its function with reference to ionic gradients.
- With reference to the values in Fig. 3.10 use the Nernst equation to calculate E_K.
- Explain why, for an experimental system in Gibbs–Donnan equilibrium, the compartment containing the impermeable anion is hypertonic relative to its neighboring compartment.
- What is the major mechanism for the maintenance of the resting potential in cells?
- Discuss the ionic basis of the action potential.
- Suggest why excitable cells are sensitive to fluctuations in extracellular potassium concentrations.
- What are the salient features of endocrine, paracrine, and autocrine signaling.
- Define what a second messenger is, and list three. What is the advantage to the cell of having second messengers?
- Discuss tyrosine kinase mediated signal transduction. Briefly, suggest how mutations in the genes that code for the proteins in this pathway might be associated with cancer.
- Draw a diagram showing the activation–inactivation cycle of a G-protein.
- In general terms, discuss how drugs influence receptors.

4. The Working Cell

Cytoskeleton and cell motility

Concepts

In eukaryotic cells, the cytoskeleton is a system of proteins that supports the topography of the cell membrane and organizes the arrangement of the cytoplasmic components into defined areas. Cell shape is extremely important, and it may be fundamental to function, e.g., microvilli increase the surface area available for absorption in intestinal cells. The cytoskeleton is composed of three types of filaments: actin (or microfilaments), microtubules, and intermediate filaments. Its major functions are:

- Determining cell shape (mechanical).
- Organelle anchoring and polarity determination.
- Motility (and migration).
- Anchoring of the cell to external structures.
- Metabolic functions.
- Separating duplicated chromatids and homologous chromosomes into separate cells.

In general, actin filaments have a structural role or are associated with cell movement; microtubules appear to be important in organelle organization and intracellular transport; and intermediate filaments provide the cell with mechanical strength. The three types of filament are formed from the polymerization of different protein subunits:

- Actin filaments are polymers of G-actin.
- Microtubules are polymers of tubulin.
- Intermediate filaments are polymers of members of a family of fibrous proteins that includes lamin.

Actin and tubulin subunits have a pair of appropriately orientated, complementary binding sites that allow each subunit to bind two other monomers. In this way, long, helical structures are formed. Each subunit is asymmetrical and, therefore, the resulting filament is polarized. The filaments are dynamic, and they may be transient because while one end (the plus end) is capable of rapid growth the other (the minus end) tends to lose subunits if not stabilized. Actin and tubulin are highly conserved throughout evolution, and they are found in all eukaryotic cells. However, by interacting with a range of accessory proteins, actin fibers and microtubules are able to perform a variety of distinct functions.

In contrast to actin and tubulin, the subunits of intermediate filaments are symmetrical. These fibrous monomers wind together to form the ropelike intermediate filaments.

The functions of the cytoskeleton are a common topic for exam questions. For top marks in long-answer questions, give some examples and consider the role of actin-associated and microtubule-associated proteins.

Components of the cytoskeleton

Actin

A microfilament is composed of actin and is 6–7 nm wide. Actin filaments form a layer just beneath the plasma membrane called the cortex. The subunit, G-actin, is globular, and at least six kinds are known. The filament, F-actin, is formed by the polymerization of G-actin subunits (Fig. 4.1). The cell closely regulates polymerization and depolymerization of fibers. For example, extracellular signals may influence polymerization via cell surface receptors that act through G-proteins; this facilitates cell processes such as chemotaxis in neutrophils.

Actin is the product of different genes in muscle and nonmuscle cells. These isoforms may allow distinct protein interactions in accordance with the differing functions of the muscle and nonmuscle forms. Actin has a contractile function in muscle cells. In nonmuscle cells, actin:

- Maintains structure of microvilli.
- Is a component of a specialized region of the cell cortex, the terminal web, which lies beneath microvilli and desmosomes.

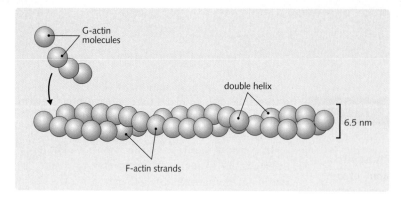

Fig. 4.1 Structure of a microfilament (actin). Actin filaments consist of a tight helix of uniformly oriented actin molecules. The filament is extended as globular actin polymerizes at the plus end. Because of its appearance when complexed with myosin, the minus end is also referred to as the "pointed end" and the plus end as the "barbed end."

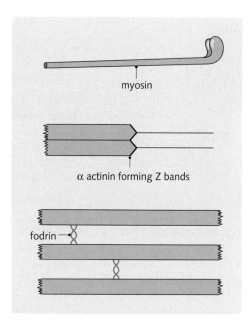

Fig. 4.2 Examples of actin-binding proteins.

- Facilitates movement of macrophages by gel–sol transition of the actin network.
- Facilitates movement of fibroblasts and nerve growth cones by controlled polymerization and rearrangement of actin filaments.

Various actin-binding proteins cause changes in the molecular forms of actin (Fig. 4.2), and they can be classified into groups according to their function:

- Severing proteins such as gelsolin will cleave actin filaments in the presence of calcium ions. This property allows the cell to break up the cell cortex when required to facilitate processes such as phagocytosis.

- Linking proteins that bind actin strands together. Actin may be bound into tight arrays of parallel strands by "bundling proteins" such as fimbrin and α-actinin. Alternatively, it may be arranged into a loose gel by "gel-forming proteins" such as filamin that bind crosswise intersections between strands.
- Myosin proteins are members of a protein family that move groups of oppositely oriented actin filaments past each other. This is the basis for contraction in muscle cells, but it is also important in nonmuscle cells, where a transient assembly of actin and myosin produces the contractile ring that separates the cells in cell division. Other accessory proteins such as troponin affect actin and myosin interactions.
- Attachment proteins mediate linking of actin filaments to the plasma membrane—this group includes fodrin, talin, and vinculin.

Intermediate filaments

Intermediate filaments are 8–11 nm wide (Fig. 4.3). They tend to be more stable than microfilaments and microtubules, and they do not dissociate into monomers under physiological conditions. Intermediate filaments are thought to be the major structural determinants in cells. There are many varieties:

- Cytokeratins—these are typically expressed in the epithelium. Ten cytokeratins are specific to "hard" tissues (e.g., nail and hair). Approximately 20 cytokeratins are found more generally in epithelia lining internal body cavities.
- Neurofilaments—these are found in neuron axons. They may account for the strength and rigidity of the axon.

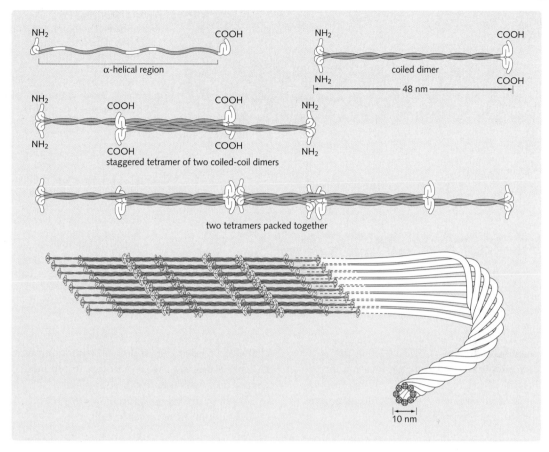

Fig. 4.3 Structure of an intermediate filament. Identical monomers bind in a parallel fashion to form dimers. Two dimers associate in antiparallel arrays to form tetramers, which wind together in groups of eight to produce the final rope-like intermediate filament. Since the association of the dimers in tetramers is antiparallel, intermediate filaments are not polarized. (Adapted from Norman and Lodwick, 1999.)

- Glial fibrillary acidic protein (GFAP)—this is found in glial cells surrounding neurons.
- Vimentin—this is expressed in mesenchymal cells such as fibroblasts, and in endothelial cells. These fibers often end at the nuclear membrane and desmosomes. They are closely associated with microtubules, and they form cages around lipid droplets in adipose tissue.
- Desmin—this is found predominantly in muscle cells. It forms an interconnecting network perpendicular to the long axis of the cell. Desmin fibers anchor and orientate the Z bands in myofibrils, thus generating the striated pattern.

Rapidly growing cells and myelin-producing glial cells do not have intermediate filaments. Cells usually contain only one type of intermediate filament.

Microtubules

Microtubules are hollow tubules and are 25 nm wide (Fig. 4.4). They extend from microtubule organizing centers, such as centrosomes, that stabilize the negative pole of the extending polymer. Tubulin is the dimeric structural subunit (α β dimer) that polymerizes to form microtubules. All cells have microtubules, except for mature erythrocytes, and they are particularly abundant in neurons.

There are many microtubule-associated proteins (MAPs), which have specific interactions with the tubulin, with different microtubules associating with different MAPs, e.g., Tau in the nerve axon. MAPs have specific interactions with tubulin:
- Some MAPs function as ATP-dependent molecular motors (e.g., dynein and kinesin). Such motors may carry a cargo, such as an

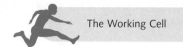

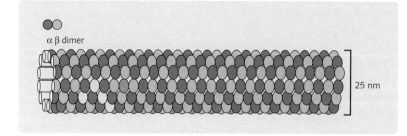

Fig. 4.4 Structure of a microtubule. There are normally 12–13 tubulin units per turn in the assembled microtubule. (Adapted from *Biology of the Cell*, 3rd edn, by B. Alberts *et al.*, Garland Publishing, 1994, with permission of Routledge, Inc., part of The Taylor & Francis Group.)

α β dimer

25 nm

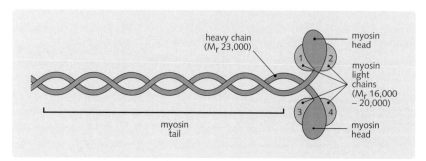

heavy chain (M_r 23,000)

myosin head

myosin light chains (M_r 16,000 – 20,000)

myosin head

myosin tail

Fig. 4.5 Structure of myosin. Myosin II, which is the form found in muscle cells, is composed of two heavy and four light chains. The α-helices of the two heavy chains wrap around one another to produce a dimer. (M_r, relative molecular mass.) (Adapted from Stevens and Lowe, 1997.)

organelle or transport vesicle, along the microtubule to its designated location in the cell.

- Some MAPs influence the polymerization of tubulin (e.g., centrioles).

Microtubules form cilia in the respiratory tract and the sperm flagella, both of which move via cycles of ATP-powered dynein arm linkage.

> The formation of microtubule spindles is essential for cell division. Nocodazole, taxol, and vinblastine are antimitotic cancer chemotherapy drugs that interfere with the exchange of tubulin subunits between the microtubules and the free tubulin pool.

Myosin

Myosin is an actin accessory protein that functions as a molecular motor. There are several isoforms of myosin, and muscle and nonmuscle forms have slightly divergent amino acid sequences. It is composed of two heavy chains and four light chains (Fig. 4.5). The two essential light chains have ATPase action, while the two regulatory light

chains determine the binding of calmodulin to myosin. Actin and myosin interact to produce contraction, which is regulated by:

- Troponin in skeletal muscle.
- Calmodulin in nonmuscle cells.

See *Crash Course, Musculoskeletal System* for further details.

Examples of cytoskeletal function
Erythrocyte cytoskeleton

Erythrocytes have a very rigid but malleable shape. The erythrocytic cytoskeleton is atypical, being present in only a thin strip below the cell membrane. The cell shape is maintained by spectrin, which links actin to ankyrin and band 4.1, which are in turn bound to integral proteins (Fig. 4.6). Patients with hereditary spherocytosis and elliptocytosis produce smaller amounts or defective spectrin, so their erythrocytes are less tractable, lose their biconcave shape, and become trapped in the circulation (see *Crash Course, Immune, Blood, and Lymphatic Systems*).

Cilia

Cilia are formed of a 9 + 2 arrangement of microtubules with a basal body. Dynein arms connect microtubule pairs, and the sliding mechanism enables the cilia to bend (see Chapter 1).

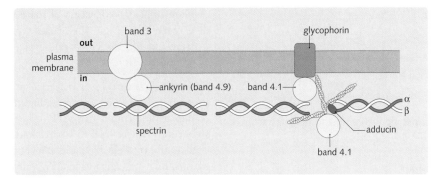

Fig. 4.6 The erythrocyte spectrin-based cytoskeleton. Spectrin is a dimer consisting of antiparallel α- and β-subunits. It is linked to the anion exchange protein (band 3) by ankyrin and to glycophorin by band 4.1, which also binds to actin and adducin (protein band numbers relate to migration in SDS-PAGE electrophoresis). (Adapted from Norman and Lodwick, 1999.)

Intestinal epithelium

Absorption is increased by microvillous projections, which increase intestinal surface area (Fig. 4.7).

Axonal transport

Kinesins and cytoplasmic dynein transport materials along axons, each moving in a different direction. Organelle movement away from the cell body is driven by kinesin, which moves toward the plus end of the microtubule. Conversely, movement toward the cell body is driven by cytoplasmic dynein, which moves toward the minus end of the microtubule. Transport is normally at a rate of 25 mm/day (Fig. 4.8). Vesicles containing newly synthesized neurotransmitters are transmitted to the cell terminal by this means.

Muscle contraction

In skeletal muscle, the arrangement of parallel actin and myosin into sarcomeres allows maximum efficiency of contraction. In smooth muscle, the contractile subunits resemble sarcomeres, but they are not as organized. (See *Crash Course, Musculoskeletal System* for further details.)

Motility of phagocytes

Phagocyte motility is achieved by the projection of foot-like pseudopodia, which are associated with actin gel–sol transition at the tip. Transition from a gel phase (where the actin in the cytoskeleton is polymerized) to a sol phase (where it is soluble) allows the pseudopodia to advance.

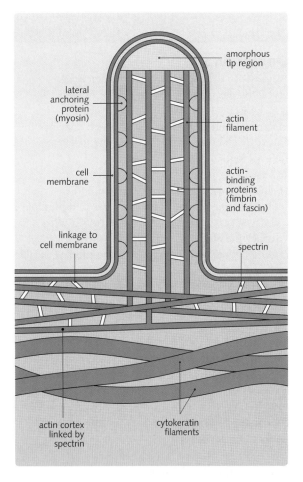

Fig. 4.7 Structure of a microvillus. A helical arrangement of myosin molecules binds the actin bundle to the inner surface of the cell membrane. (Adapted from Stevens and Lowe, 1997.)

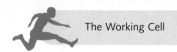

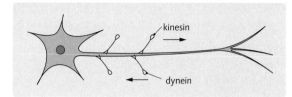

Fig. 4.8 Axoplasmic flow. Kinesin and dynein transport materials along axons.

Mitotic spindle

The spindle is a polar arrangement of microtubules across the equator of the cell. Chromosomes attach to the spindle via a kinetochore protein, at their centromeres. Separation of chromatids occurs as the microtubules contract, pulling them to separate poles (see Chapter 5).

Lysosomes

Definition

A lysosome is a membrane-bound organelle visible by electron microscopy that contains acid hydrolases capable of breaking down macromolecules. Confinement of such enzymes in this organelle protects the rest of the cell from their potentially damaging effects.

Lysosomes have:
- Diameters ranging from 50 nm to 1 μm.
- A single membrane consisting of a phospholipid bilayer that undergoes selective fusion with other membranous organelles.
- An ATP driven H^+ pump in the membrane, which acidifies the lysosomal matrix to pH 4.5–5.5.
- Hydrolases in the inner matrix that are active at acid pH and break down carbohydrates, lipids, and proteins.

New lysosomes are derived from the Golgi complex and are called primary lysosomes. Secondary lysosomes are formed from fusion with a vesicle containing substrate (Fig. 4.9). Most cells have hundreds of lysosomes, with phagocytic cells containing thousands. However, erythrocytes do not contain any lysosomes.

Functions of lysosomes

Lysosome functions are (see Fig. 4.9):
- Autophagy—digestion of material of intracellular origin (i.e., fuses with vacuoles from inside the cell).
- Heterophagy—digestion of material of extracellular origin (i.e., fuses with vacuoles from outside the cell—pinocytic, endocytic, or phagocytic).

Endocytosis is uptake of material into the cell, and it can be specific (receptor-mediated endocytosis) or nonspecific (pinocytosis). Pinocytosis is sometimes called "cell drinking" and results in uptake of extracellular molecules at their extracellular concentrations. Phagocytosis is the internalization of membrane-bound particulate molecules by engulfment. It only occurs in specialized cells. The endocytic vesicles that result from endocytosis fuse with primary lysosomes.

The lysosome has hydrolytic enzymes, which catalyze the breakdown of macromolecules into component residues. If allowed to leak out, as in lytic cell death, the hydrolases break down tissues. The products are of low molecular mass and they are transported across the lysosomal membrane by appropriate transport proteins. Over 60 different lysosomal enzymes have been identified, some of which are:
- Nucleases (e.g., acid RNase, acid DNase).
- Glycosidases (e.g., β-glucuronidase, hyaluronidase).
- Carbohydrate degradation enzymes (e.g., β-galactosidase, α-glucosidase).
- Proteases (e.g., cathepsins, collagenase).
- Phosphatases (e.g., acid phosphatase).
- Sulfatases (e.g., aryl sulfatase).
- Lipases.

Following synthesis in the rough endoplasmic reticulum (RER), lysosomal enzymes are modified by glycosylation in the RER lumen followed by covalent modification in the Golgi apparatus. Covalent modification includes phosphorylation of mannose groups to produce mannose-6-phosphate groups, which act as recognition markers and direct the enzymes specifically to primary lysosomes.

Receptor-mediated endocytosis

Receptor-mediated endocytosis occurs when ligands that bind specific surface receptors are internalized in clathrin-coated pits (Fig. 4.10). In general, the ligand is degraded in the lysosome and its receptor is recycled to the cell surface. A variety of receptors and their ligands undergo receptor-mediated endocytosis (Fig. 4.11).

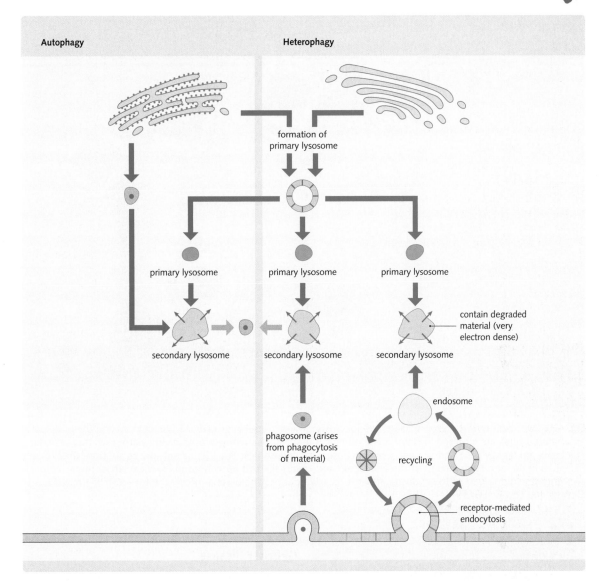

Fig. 4.9 Multiple pathways of exocytosis, endocytosis, and membrane recycling. The lysosome is common to all these pathways.

Lysosomal storage diseases

Lysosomal storage diseases are disorders of lysosomal function and result in macromolecules becoming trapped inside the lysosome. The lysosome enlarges, causing the tissue to enlarge, resulting in pathological features. The causes of storage disorders are:

- Enzymatic—resulting from deficient or defective acid hydrolases, or absence of a crucial activator.
- Nonenzymatic—caused by transporter defects.

Each disorder is rare, but together they affect 1 in 4800 live births. They are commonly fatal, but they can be diagnosed prenatally. All show recessive inheritance, most being autosomal, except for two that are X-linked. Features leading to suspicion of a lysosomal storage disorder are:

- Progressive neurologic degeneration.
- Hepato(spleno)megaly.
- Skeletal dysplasia with or without short stature.
- Coarse facies.
- Eye changes (e.g., cherry red spot, corneal clouding).

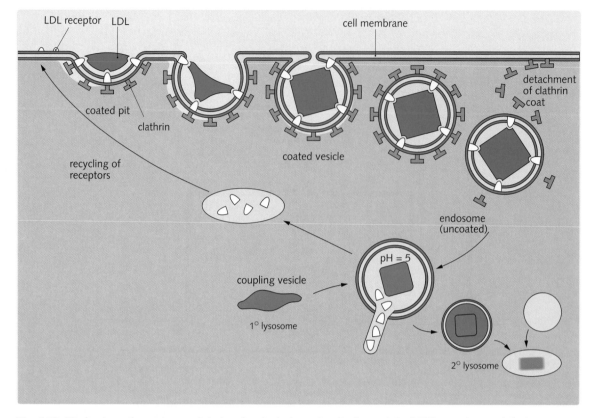

Fig. 4.10 Mechanism of receptor-mediated endocytosis. Low-density lipoprotein (LDL) receptors and their associated ligands are localized in clathrin-coated pits and are subsequently internalized in clathrin-coated vesicles. The coats are rapidly shed and uncoated vesicles fuse with endosomes. The LDL ligands dissociate from their receptors in the acid environment of the endosome and eventually end up in lysosomes. Meanwhile, the receptors are sequestered in a part of the endosome that is recycled back to the plasma membrane for reuse. (Adapted from Stevens and Lowe, 1997.)

Functions of receptor-mediated endocytosis	
Molecules taken up	**Function**
Low-density lipoprotein (LDL)	Transports TAGs and cholesterol
Transferrin	Transports iron
Insulin	Affects cell metabolism
Fibrin	Removes injurious agents

Fig. 4.11 Functions of receptor-mediated endocytosis.

Gaucher disease

Gaucher disease is the most common lysosomal storage disorder (incidence 1 in 25,000 live births). Inheritance is autosomal recessive, with a high incidence seen in Ashkenazi Jews, who have a carrier frequency of 1 in 60. There is a deficiency of β-glucosidase, resulting in accumulation of its substrate glucocerebroside. The enzyme is encoded on chromosome 1. There are three types of Gaucher disease.

- Type I—adult type, nonneuronopathic.
- Type II—severe infantile, rare, neurological signs seen at 3 months, die by 2 years of age.
- Type III—subacute, neuronopathic, variable presentation from childhood to 70 years of age.

Treatment approaches for Gaucher disease that have been tried include enzyme replacement therapy and bone marrow transplantation. Modification of the β-glucoside enzyme by adding mannose-b-phosphate (which targets the enzyme to macrophage lysosomes) has led to a dramatic reduction in symptoms of people affected with type I Gaucher disease. The treatment, however, is expensive, with an annual cost of $150,000 to $300,000.

Tay–Sachs disease

This is due to lack of the hexosaminidase A α-chain, resulting in accumulation of ganglioside GM2. The hexosaminidase A α-chain is encoded on chromosome 15 position q22–25, and inheritance is autosomal recessive. There is an increased incidence in Ashkenazi Jews (carrier frequency is 1 in 25 compared with the US general population carrier frequency of 1 in 200). Affected children are normal at birth, with symptoms beginning at 4–8 months of age, and death occurring by 3–4 years. Carrier screening is available, using an enzyme assay of the hexosaminidase system. Treatment is not yet available.

Cell surface and cell adhesion

Importance of cellular interaction and adhesion

If groups of cells are to combine together to form part of an organ, it is imperative that each cell is held in its proper place and is able to communicate with its neighbors. Interactions between cells, and with the extracellular matrix (ECM), largely carry out such a structural role, but may also facilitate cell–cell communication in several biological processes including migration, growth, immunological functioning, permeability, cell recognition, tissue repair, differentiation, and embryogenesis.

Cells such as those in connective tissue bind via specific adhesion molecules to the ECM, which provides elasticity and resistance to mechanical forces. However, epithelium has little ECM (only the basement membrane), so cell–cell interactions are adapted to bear tensile and compressive stresses and show several types of cell–cell junctions.

Types of cell junction	
Group	**Members**
Occluding junctions	Tight junctions

Anchoring junctions	Actin filament attachment sites: (adherens junctions)
	    cell–cell (e.g., adhesion belts)
	    cell–matrix (e.g., focal contacts)
	
	Intermediate filament attachment sites:
	    cell–cell (e.g., desmosomes)
	    cell–matrix (e.g., hemidesmosomes)

Communicating junctions	Gap junctions Chemical synapses

Fig. 4.12 Types of cell junction.

Types of junction

Junctions are found between cells, and between cells and the ECM. There are three groups of cell junction (Fig. 4.12), which comprise six types (Fig. 4.13). A junctional complex consists of a tight junction, an adhering junction, and a desmosome.

Tight junctions

All epithelia act as selectively permeable barriers, with tight junctions blocking diffusion of membrane proteins between apical (top) and basolateral (sides at the bottom) domains of the plasma membrane and sealing neighboring cells together so that water-soluble molecules cannot leak between cells (Fig. 4.14). Cell–cell contact at these junctions is mediated by the protein occludin. The ability to restrict ion passage increases logarithmically with the number of strands (e.g., small intestine tight junctions are 10,000 times more leaky than bladder tight junctions are). The degree of permeability offered by tight junctions is under physiologic control, and it is influenced by intracellular signals.

Anchoring junctions

Anchoring junctions are responsible for maintaining tissue integrity, and they are, therefore, most abundant in cells under stress (e.g., cardiac muscle). They are made up of:

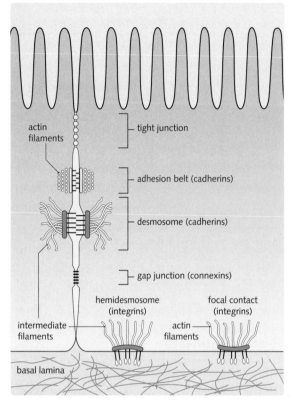

Fig. 4.13 Cell–cell and cell–matrix junctions. There are six distinct types of junctions in epithelial tissue. (Adapted from Norman and Lodwick, 1999.)

- Intracellular attachment proteins.
- Transmembrane linker glycoproteins.
- ECM or transmembrane linker glycoproteins on another cell (Fig. 4.15).

Thus, they link the cytoskeletons of adjoining cells to each other or the ECM. Anchoring junctions containing actin filament connections are called adherens junctions. These junctions appear as focal adhesions, and they are formed from clusters of integrins that bridge between the ECM and actin accessory proteins, which in turn bind to actin.

Adherens cell–cell junctions occur as streak-like attachments in nonepithelial cells and as continuous belts just below tight junctions in epithelial cells. These junctions attach the cytoskeletons (actin cell cortex) of adjacent cells together. The membranes are held together by a Ca^{2+}-dependent mechanism mediated by cadherins.

Desmosomes act as anchoring sites for intermediate filaments and thus provide tensile strength (Fig. 4.16). Cell–cell contact is mediated by desmogleins, which are a type of cadherin. Autoimmune disease against desmogleins causes pemphigus, a blistering skin disorder. Hemidesmosomes have a similar structure to desmosomes, but they link cellular intermediate

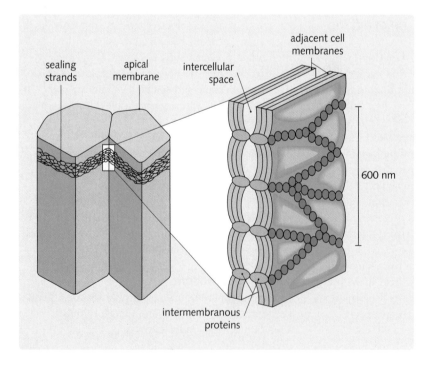

Fig. 4.14 Structure of a tight junction. The tight junction forms a continuous band around the cell and it is, therefore, also called zonula occludens. The integral membrane protein occludin mediates cell–cell interaction. Each junction is made up of multiple pairs of this protein, one of each pair coming from each cell. (Adapted from Stevens and Lowe, 1997.)

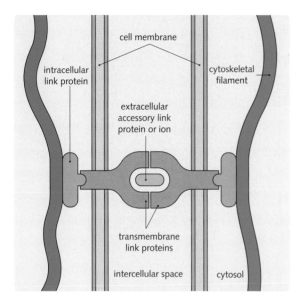

Fig. 4.15 General structure of an anchoring junction. Different (or multiple) link proteins and transmembrane proteins operate for the different classes of junction. (Adapted from Stevens and Lowe, 1997.)

filaments to the ECM (basement membrane) via integrin protein attachment (see Fig. 4.12).

Gap junctions

These are communicating junctions that allow cells in a tissue to respond as an integrated unit. Inorganic ions carrying current and water-soluble molecules are able to pass directly from one cell to another through these structures, permitting electrical and metabolic cell coupling.

Four α-helices form a connexin. Six connexins form a connexon, the pore of which is formed from one α-helix of each protein. Connexons of neighboring cells align to form a continuous aqueous channel (Fig. 4.17). Molecules of up to 1300 D can pass through the 1.5 nm pore. Several thousand connexons form a gap junction. Some pores are gated, with opening related to a three-dimensional change, which is often mediated via extracellular signals. Electrical coupling via gap junctions is important in:

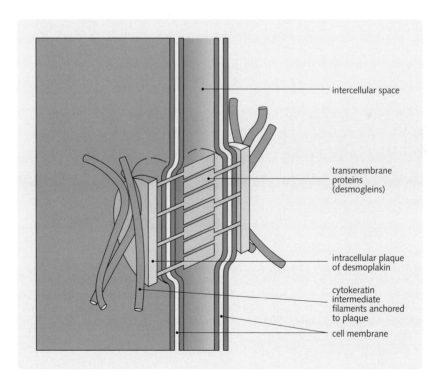

Fig. 4.16 Structure of a desmosome. On the cytoplasmic surface of each interacting cell is a dense plaque composed of desmoplakin that is associated with attached intermediate filaments on one side and desmoglein (a type of cadherin) on the other. Cell–cell interaction is mediated by homophilic binding between adjacent desmoglein proteins. (Adapted from Stevens and Lowe, 1997.)

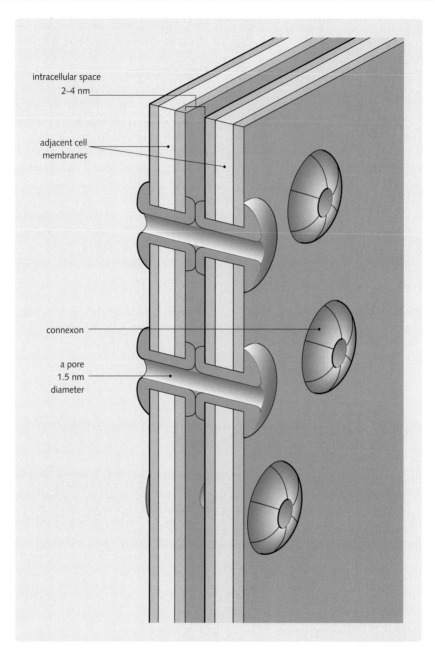

intracellular space
2–4 nm

adjacent cell
membranes

connexon

a pore
1.5 nm
diameter

Fig. 4.17 Structure of part of a gap junction. The junction consists of several hundred pores, which are aligned on adjacent cells. Each pore is comprised of two connexons, one from each cell, which join across the intercellular gap to form a continuous aqueous channel. This channel facilitates electrical and chemical cellular coupling, since electrical currents and second messengers can pass freely through it. The cell can regulate permeability of gap junctions. (Adapted from Stevens and Lowe, 1997.)

- Peristalsis.
- Synchrony of heart contractions.
- Coordination of ciliated epithelium.

Gap junctions play a role in embryogenesis by allowing gradients of morphogens to form across blocks of cells.

Glycoproteins and cell labeling

Surface glycoproteins are important in cell recognition processes, with specific oligosaccharide chains allowing cells to recognize each other. Examples are:

- ABO blood groups.
- Major histocompatibility complex (MHC) antigens.

The ABO blood groups are determined by the carbohydrates (agglutinogens) found on the erythrocyte membrane. Antibodies to the agglutinogens not present on the host erythrocytes are contained in plasma. If a transfusion contains erythrocytes with agglutinogens that are not found on the recipient's erythrocytes, the donor red blood cells will be agglutinated and then hemolyzed (Fig. 4.18). Group O is the "universal donor" and AB the "universal recipient."

The MHC codes for glycoproteins that are found on all of an individual's cells (except erythrocytes), and this mechanism helps host immunity distinguish between "self" and "foreign" cells (see *Crash Course, Immune, Blood, and Lymphatic Systems*).

Adhesion molecules

There are four major cell adhesion molecule families (Fig. 4.19):

- Cadherins.
- Immunoglobulin superfamily.

A	Agglutination in blood transfusion			
Donor	**Recipient**			
	O ab	A b	B a	AB –
O ab	–	–	–	–
A b	+	–	+	–
B a	+	+	–	–
AB –	+	+	+	–

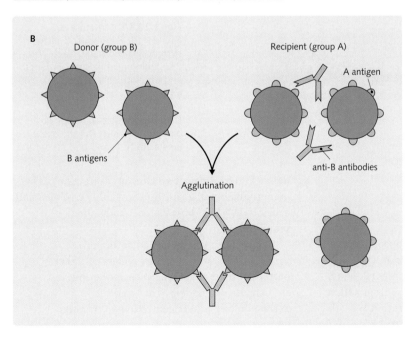

Fig. 4.18 Agglutination in blood transfusion illustrated (A) in table form, and (B) diagrammatically. Agglutinogens are denoted by capital letters, and plasma antibodies by small letters.

Families of adhesion molecules				
Family	Members	Ca²⁺/Mg²⁺ dependent	Cytoskeletal association	Associated cell function
Cadherins	E-CAD, N-CAD, P-CAD, desmosomal CAD	Yes	Actin filaments	Adhesion belt, desmosomes
Immunoglobulin (Ig) family	N-CAM, V-CAM, Lt	No	Intermediate filaments (some members)	—
Selectins (blood and endothelial cells only)	P-selectin, E-selectin	Yes	—	Cell homing
Integrins	LFA-1 (β_2), MAC-1 (β_2)	Yes	Actin filaments, intermediate filaments	Focal contacts, hemidesmosome

Fig. 4.19 Families of adhesion molecules. The characteristics of the four main families of adhesion molecules.

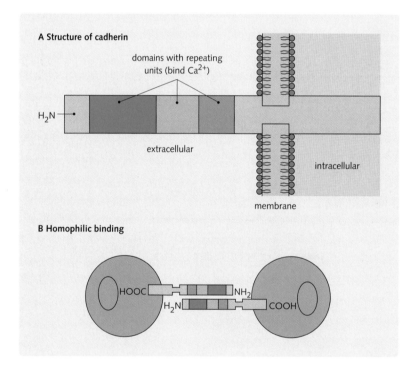

Fig. 4.20 (A) Structure of cadherin. It is composed of five extracellular domains, each 700–750 amino acid residues in length, and one intracellular domain. The intracellular portion is not present in T-CAD (T, truncated). (B) Cadherin exhibits homophilic binding, in which the molecule acts as both ligand and receptor.

- Selectins.
- Integrins.

Cadherins

The cadherins are single-pass glycoproteins that mediate communication and adhesion (Fig. 4.20). Cadherins form homophilic attachments, which is where two cells with the same protein adhere to each other through the same protein (i.e., the protein is both the ligand and the receptor, and it must therefore have two sites of interaction). The homophilic binding site is near the N-terminus, and it has HAV (histidine, alanine, and valine) sequences.

Cadherins are attached to actin and cytoplasm inside the cell by a class of linker proteins called catenins. Since cadherins are calcium dependent, changing the extracellular Ca²⁺ concentration alters their interactions.

There are four main classes of cadherins:

- E-CAD, which is found in the epithelium and early nervous tissue.
- P-CAD, which is found in epithelium and chicken placenta.
- N-CAD, which is found in nervous tissue and skeletal muscle.
- L-CAD, which is found in liver.

Other cadherins have been identified (e.g., R-CAD in the retina), and proteins related to cadherins have been found in *Drosophila* and desmosomes.

Immunoglobulin (Ig) family

These adhesion molecules are characterized by:

- Antibody fold in each domain.
- β-barrel structure.
- Two β-pleated sheets joined by cysteine–cysteine disulfide bonds, which are 60–80 residues apart.
- Loop regions without β-structure (variable expressed regions).

There is Ca^{2+}-independent adhesion, and the Ig proteins have homo- and heterophilic binding sites. Heterophilic binding occurs where a protein on one cell acts as a receptor and a different protein on another cell acts as the ligand. Ig members are involved in:

- Adhesion.
- Signaling.
- Axonal growth and fasciculation (fasciculation means that axons grow along other axons by homophilic binding).

N-CAM is an Ig member found in nervous tissue, which can undergo alternative splicing, so expression of exons can vary. It exists in transmembrane, lipid anchored, or secreted forms. Other important Ig family members are listed in Fig. 4.21.

Selectins

Selectins are Ca^{2+} dependent and undergo heterophilic binding to carbohydrate ligands (Fig. 4.22). P-selectin and E-selectin are cell–cell adhesion molecules expressed by endothelial cells during inflammatory responses, expression being induced by local chemical mediators:

- E-selectin is activated by tumor necrosis factor (TNF), interleukin-1 (IL-1), and endotoxin.
- P-selectin is activated by histamine, thrombin, platelet activating factor, and phorbol esters.

The lectin domain recognizes specific oligosaccharides on the surface of neutrophils, the oligosaccharides Lewis X and sialyated Lewis X are recognized by P-selectin and E-selectin respectively. Neutrophils thus stick to the endothelial lining of blood vessels via these weak affinity interactions until integrins are activated. L-selectin is constitutive on the surface of polymorphonuclear neutrophils, monocytes, and lymphocytes. Selectins are important in the homing of these cells to lymph nodes and subendothelial capillaries.

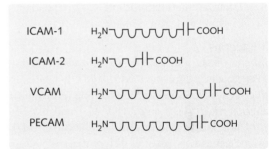

Fig. 4.21 Ig family members. (ICAM, intracellular adhesion molecule; VCAM, vascular adhesion molecule; PECAM, platelet endothelial cell adhesion molecule.)

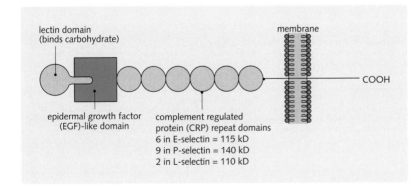

Fig. 4.22 Structure of a selectin molecule.

Integrins

Integrins are the major receptors for binding to the ECM, and also contribute to some cell–cell interactions. The structure is a heteroduplex of α- and β-glycoproteins (Fig. 4.23) with a similar structure to transmembrane proteoglycans.

There are 16 known α-chains and nine known β-glycoproteins, each β-chain forming an integrin subfamily. Each β has 2–4 α-subunits attached (e.g., α4β1 is a β1-chain with four α-chains attached). The integrins differ from other receptors in that they bind their ligand with low affinity, and they are present at high concentration. Interactions are heterophilic and Ca^{2+} dependent (Fig. 4.24). β2 and β1 are important integrins.

β2 integrins

These are leucocyte-specific. β2αL is also called LFA1 (leucocyte function-associated). It mediates direct cell–cell interactions by binding intracellular adhesion molecules 1 and 2 (ICAM-1 and ICAM-2). MAC1 is also a β2 integrin and binds ICAM-1. Surface antigen ("cluster of differentiation") nomenclature is also used (e.g., CD18 is β2).

β1 integrins

These are found on most cells. Several are called VLAs (very late acting) as they are expressed late in lymphocyte activation (e.g., VLA4, which binds VCAM—vascular adhesion molecule).

Integrins binding

Integrins usually bind actin-based cytoskeleton inside the cell. Outside the cell, integrins can bind:
- ECM (e.g., fibronectin).
- Cell surface molecules (e.g., ICAM-1).
- Soluble molecules (e.g., fibrinogen).

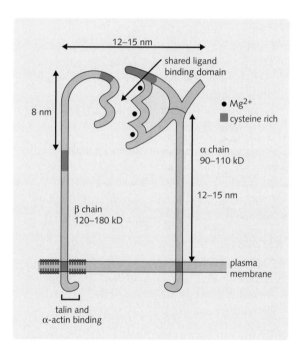

Fig. 4.23 Structure of integrin.

Integrins and transmembrane proteoglycans				
Family	Members	Ca^{2+}/Mg^{2+} dependent	Cytoskeletal association	Associated cell function
Integrins	Many	Yes	Actin filaments	Focal
Transmembrane proteoglycans	$α_6β_4$	Yes	Intermediate	Hemidesmosomes
	Syndecans	No	Actin	None

Fig. 4.24 Integrins and transmembrane proteoglycans.

Integrins have recognition sites for ligands, e.g., Ig-like domains bind ICAMs and the tripeptide RGD (arginine, glycine, aspartic acid), which is a sequence commonly expressed in fibronectin and other ECM proteins. Cells can vary their binding properties by varying integrin affinities and specificities.

Integrins take part in signal transduction in cells (e.g., clustering of $\beta1\alpha5$ by fibronectin causes cytoplasmic alkalization).

Basement membrane

Basement membrane is a sheet of ECM underlying epithelial and endothelial cells and surrounding adipocytes, Schwann cells, and muscle cells. It acts to isolate these cells from the mesenchyme or connective tissue. It is also called the basal lamina and it is composed of type IV collagen, heparan sulfate, proteoglycans, entactin, and laminin. Functions of basement membrane are:

- Cell adhesion.
- To act as a porous filter in the kidney's glomeruli.
- To inhibit the spread of neoplasia.
- To regulate cell migration.
- Growth and wound healing.
- Differentiation.

Extracellular matrix

ECM is a hydrated polysaccharide gel containing a meshwork of glycoproteins. It is composed of:

- Proteoglycans—which form a gel.
- Structural proteins—collagen, elastin.
- Fibrous adhesive proteins—laminin, fibronectin, tenascin.

ECM components are secreted by local fibroblasts in most tissues, but chondroblasts and osteoblasts are also involved in cartilage. ECM influences cell division, development, differentiation, migration, metabolism, and shape. Connective tissues rely on the properties of the local ECM, which is:

- Calcified in bone and teeth.
- Rope-like in tendon.
- Transparent in the cornea.

Proteoglycans

These form the hydrated polysaccharide gel that acts as a ground substance and allows diffusion of substances such as nutrients and hormones from the blood to the tissue and vice versa. Glycosaminoglycans (GAGs) are unbranched polysaccharide chains of repeating disaccharide

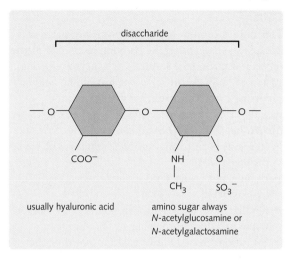

Fig. 4.25 Glycosaminoglycan disaccharide subunit.

units (Fig. 4.25). Proteoglycans are formed in the Golgi apparatus where:

- The core protein is linked via a serine to a tetrasaccharide.
- Glycosyl transferases add sugar residues.
- Ordered sulfation and epimerization reactions occur.

The main types of GAGs are:

- Hyaluronic acid—found as a lubricant in synovial fluid (up to 8×10^6 D).
- Chondroitin sulfate—in cartilage.
- Dermatan sulfate.
- Heparin sulfate—an anticoagulant.
- Heparin.
- Keratin sulfate—in skin.

Chondroitin sulfate, dermatan sulfate, and heparin sulfate are all between 500 and 50,000 D.

GAGs are very hydrophilic, and they have an extended coil structure, which takes up extensive space. GAGs have a negative charge and attract cations; consequently Na^+, which is osmotically active, is attracted, so water is sucked into the matrix giving turgor pressure able to withstand forces of many hundreds of times atmospheric pressure.

Proteoglycans function to:

- Provide hydrated space.
- Bind secreted signaling molecules.
- Act as sieves to regulate molecular trafficking.

Proteoglycans and glycoproteins are compared in Fig. 4.26.

Collagen

This fibrous protein has great tensile strength, and it is resistant to stretching. It comprises 25% of the protein in mammals, and it is rich in proline (ring structure) and glycine (the smallest amino acid and occurring every third residue so allowing the strands to fit together). Collagen synthesis is carried out in the ER. Synthesis occurs as follows:

- It begins with formation of an amino acid proline α-chain.
- Proline and lysine residues are then hydroxylated.
- Finally, interchain hydrogen bonds form a stable triple helix (i.e., procollagen, Fig. 4.27).
- Secretion from the ER causes removal of the propeptides forming collagen. This stage is omitted in type IV collagen.

There are 20 collagen α-chains, each encoded by separate genes, but only 10 types of collagen. Types I, II, and III are fibrillar collagen, and they are found in connective tissue (Fig. 4.28).

Fibrils are collagen aggregations of 10–300 nm in diameter and aggregate to form collagen fibers of a few millimeters in diameter. Organization is tissue specific; for example:

- "Wickerwork" pattern in skin resists multidirectional stress.
- Parallel layers in bone and cornea.

Type IV collagen forms a sheet-like meshwork, and it is only found in the basal lamina (Fig. 4.29).

Osteogenesis imperfecta (brittle bone disease) is a heterogeneous group of conditions characterized by spontaneous fractures, bone deformity, and defective dentition. The substitution of a larger amino acid for glycine disrupts triple helix formation and causes a severe, dominantly inherited form of the disease.

Comparison of proteoglycans and glycoproteins	
Proteoglycans	**Glycoproteins**
Up to 95% carbohydrate	1–60% carbohydrate by weight
Unbranched carbohydrate	Branched carbohydrate
80 sugar residues	13 sugar residues
Larger than 3×10^5 D	No larger than 3×10^5 D

Fig. 4.26 Comparison of proteoglycans and glycoproteins. (GAG, glycosaminoglycan.)

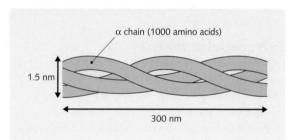

Fig. 4.27 Structure of collagen. Collagen is a right-hand triple helix (superhelix).

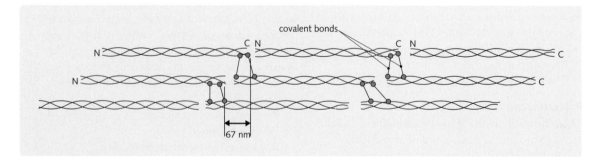

Fig. 4.28 Structure of fibrillar collagen. Collagen molecules are positioned side by side, staggered from adjacent molecules by one-quarter of their length. (Adapted from *Molecular Cell Biology*, 2nd edn, by Darnell, Lodish, and Baltimore, Scientific American Books, 1990.)

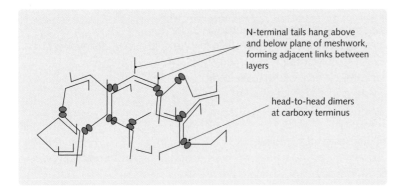

Fig. 4.29 Structure of type IV collagen, which assembles into multilayered sheets. (Adapted from *Molecular Biology of the Cell*, 3rd edn, by B. Alberts *et al.*, Garland Publishing, 1994, with permission of Routledge, Inc., part of The Taylor & Francis Group.)

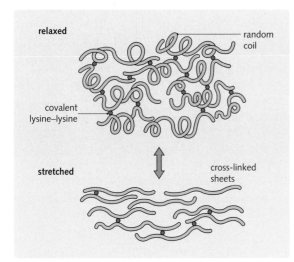

Fig. 4.30 Structure of relaxed and stretched elastin. (Adapted from Stevens and Lowe, 1997.)

Elastin

Elastin is found in places that need elasticity (e.g., skin, blood vessels, lungs). It is a highly glycosylated, hydrophobic protein (Fig. 4.30) that is rich in the nonhydroxylated forms of proline and glycine. The sheets are organized with the help of a microfibrillar glycoprotein, fibrillin, which is secreted before elastin. Fibrillin deficiency results in Marfan syndrome.

Laminin

Laminin is a complex of three polypeptide chains held together in a "cross shape" by disulfide bonds.

Fibronectin

This is an adhesive glycoprotein with binding sites for cells and matrix. It is a dimer of two subunits, which are folded into globular domains. Forms of fibronectin involved in wound healing and embryogenesis appear to promote cell proliferation and migration.

Tenascin

This protein, which can promote or inhibit cell adhesion and migration, is only produced by embryonic tissue and glial cells.

Role of the fibroblast

Fibroblasts are members of the connective tissue cell family. Members of the connective tissue family are all of common origin and interchangeable under appropriate conditions, other members being chondrocytes, osteocytes, adipocytes, and smooth muscle cells. Connective tissue differentiation is controlled by cytokines, especially hormones and growth factors. Interchangeability allows them to support and repair most tissue types. Fibroblasts:

- Secrete the fibrous proteins of the ECM in most tissues (except in cartilage and bone where they are produced by chondrocytes and osteocytes, respectively).
- Are involved in the organization of ECM, enabling the configuration of ECM into tendons and other structures.

71

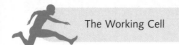

- List the three components of the cytoskeleton.
- Describe the basic structure of actin, microtubules, and intermediate filaments.
- Name three actin accessory proteins and their function.
- Draw a diagram of the erythrocyte cytoskeleton.
- Describe the structure and function of cilia.
- Draw the structure of a microvillus, and discuss its function.
- Describe axonal transport.
- Outline the salient features of a lysosome.
- Define primary lysosome, secondary lysosome, autophagy, and heterophagy.
- Describe endocytosis, pinocytosis, and phagocytosis.
- List five lysosomal enzymes.
- Describe receptor-mediated endocytosis, and give two examples.
- Describe the salient clinical and pathological features of a lysosomal storage disorder.
- Draw a diagram to show the six types of cell–cell and cell–matrix junction.
- Describe the structure of tight junctions, and list two of their functions.
- Discuss the role of actin and intermediate filaments in resisting mechanical stress.
- What is the difference between homophilic and heterophilic binding?
- Describe the structure of a cadherin and an integrin molecule, and list the junctions each is involved in.
- List the components of the extracellular matrix, and summarize their functions.
- Discuss how fibroblasts control ECM composition.

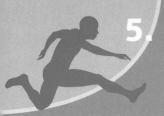

5. The Molecular Basis of Genetics

Organization of the cell nucleus

Electron microscopy has made visible detailed features of cellular ultrastructure that can not be observed using light microscopy (see Chapter 1).

The nucleus is the largest structure in eukaryotic cells. The nucleoplasm is in constant contact with the cell cytoplasm via pores in the nuclear membrane. The nucleus consists of DNA, proteins, and RNA, and it plays a vital role in:

- Protein synthesis.
- The passage of genetic information from one generation to the next.

Structures in the nucleus
Nuclear envelope
The nuclear envelope encloses the nucleus. It consists of two layers of membrane, the outer being continuous with the endoplasmic reticulum (Fig. 5.1). The space between the inner and outer membranes is called the periplasm and this forms a continuum with the lumen of the endoplasmic reticulum (ER). Ribosomes are attached to the outer layer of the nuclear envelope as well as to the ER.

Nuclear pores
Nuclear pores are found at points of contact between the inner and outer membranes (Fig. 5.2). They are electron-dense structures consisting of eight protein complexes arranged around a central granule. They control the passage of metabolites, macromolecules, and RNA subunits between the nucleus and the cytoplasm. Molecules up to 60 kD pass freely through these pores. However, transport of larger molecules is ATP-dependent, and it requires the receptor-mediated recognition of a nuclear targeting sequence by the pore complex.

Chromatin
Chromatin is the collective name for the long strands of DNA and their associated nucleoproteins. Two types of chromatin can be seen when a cell is viewed under an electron microscope (see Chapter 1):

- Heterochromatin, which is electron dense and is distributed around the periphery of the nucleus and in discrete masses within the nucleus. The DNA is tightly condensed, making these regions generally inaccessible to transcription factors necessary for RNA synthesis, and is transcriptionally inactive.
- Euchromatin, which is electron lucent and represents DNA that is less condensed and actually or potentially active in RNA synthesis.

Nucleoli
Nucleoli are extremely dense structures in the nucleus that represent the sites of ribosomal RNA synthesis and assembly. There may be one, several, or no visible nucleoli in a cell nucleus.

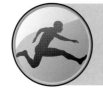

Cells that are not active in protein synthesis tend to have nuclei rich in heterochromatin and no nucleoli.

Nuclear matrix
The nuclear matrix consists of DNA, nucleoproteins, and structural proteins. Nucleoproteins are proteins closely associated with DNA. They are defined as histones and nonhistones. Histones are strongly basic globular proteins around which DNA winds in a regular fashion, like beads on a string, to form chromatin (see Fig. 5.16). Chromatin is thought to interact with the protein filaments associated with the inner nuclear envelope called lamins. The lamins—a type of intermediate filament—are arranged in a lattice, forming a thin shell that underlies the inner nuclear membrane. A less regularly organized network of intermediate filaments surrounds the outer membrane, and together these networks provide mechanical support for the nuclear envelope.

Cell cycle

Concept of the cell cycle

The cell cycle can be regarded as the life cycle of an individual cell. It can be divided into two phases:

• Mitosis (or cell division)—which results in the production of two daughter cells.
• Interphase—the interval between divisions during which the cell undergoes its functions and prepares for mitosis.

Interphase can be further subdivided into G_1, S, and G_2 phases as shown in Fig. 5.3. Nondividing cells, such as neurons, do not go through this cycle, and they remain in a resting state called G_0.

Regulation of the cell cycle

There are three points of control in the cell cycle where progression through the cycle may be regulated:

• The restriction point is the point at the end of G_1 at which the cell becomes committed to completing a cycle of division. The cell will not proceed beyond this point if there are inadequate nutrients or growth factors.
• Mitosis entry occurs at the beginning of the M phase. Cells will not progress beyond this point if there is DNA damage.
• Mitosis exit occurs at the end of mitosis. Cells will become arrested at this stage if the mitotic spindle fails to assemble adequately.

Progression through these checkpoints is controlled by the activity of cyclins, which are proteins that govern the transition from one phase to another. The intracellular concentrations of cyclins vary throughout the cell cycle.

Cyclins

Cyclins control the cell cycle by regulating cyclin-dependent kinases (CDKs). CDKs become active when they bind and form a complex with cyclin proteins. Activated CDKs stimulate cell cycle progression by phosphorylating (and therefore activating) specific proteins in the cell required for transition to the next stage. For example:

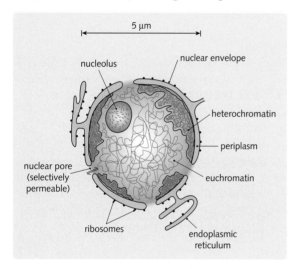

Fig. 5.1 Structure of the nucleus.

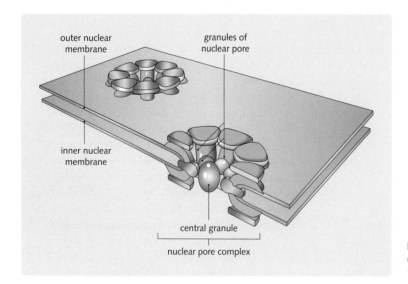

Fig. 5.2 Structure of a nuclear pore. (Adapted from Stevens and Lowe, 1997.)

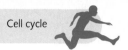

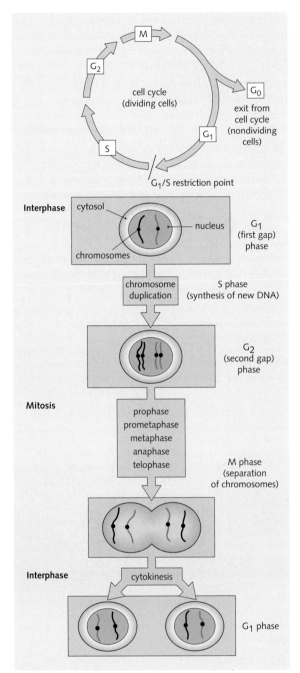

Fig. 5.3 The cell cycle. In G_1 there is cell growth and performance of functions specific to the tissue involved. The length of G_1 varies, depending upon the cell type. (Adapted from Stevens and Lowe, 1997.)

Cyclins and CDKs involved in cell cycle progression

Cyclin	Kinase	Function
D	CDK4, CDK6	Progression past restriction point at G_1/S boundary
E, A	CDK2	Initiation of DNA synthesis in early S phase
B	CDK1	Transition from G_2 to M

Fig. 5.4 Cyclins and cyclin-dependent kinases (CDKs) involved in the cell cycle. Cyclin C does not exist.

- At the beginning of prophase of mitosis, nuclear membrane breakdown is initiated by phosphorylation of lamins, which form part of the nuclear skeleton.
- Chromosome condensation at the beginning of mitosis is initiated by the phosphorylation of H1 histone, a nuclear-associated protein.
- G_1–S transition is initiated by CDK-dependent phosphorylation of Rb protein. Unphosphorylated Rb protein forms a complex with the transcription factor E2F. On phosphorylation of Rb, E2F is released and activates transcription of genes required for G_1–S transition.

Human cyclins are designated A, B, D, and E. Each one accumulates at a different time in the cell cycle (Fig. 5.4).

It is thought that specific CDK inhibitors are always present in the cell. When cyclin levels rise above a threshold the inhibitors can no longer exert their effect, hence the 'spikes' of CDK activity.

Maturation-promoting factor (MPF) is an example of a cyclin–CDK complex. It initiates transition from G_2 into mitosis, and it is controlled by cyclin B. A small increase in cyclin levels produces a big increase in MPF kinase activity, which promotes chromosome condensation. It is a very powerful factor, and it can even initiate mitosis in nonreplicating cells. It is, therefore, under tight control within the cell so that its effects are produced quickly and transiently. Entry into S phase is controlled by availability of the E2F transcription factor as described above.

The activity of CDKs, and thus progression through the cell cycle, is further influenced by several extracellular signaling pathways that facilitate coordinated cell division in the multicellular organism.

Cyclins are so called because of their cyclic accumulation and disappearance throughout the cell cycle.

Extracellular regulation of the cell cycle

A mitogen is an agent that induces mitosis. In addition to the activity of cyclins, the cell cycle is influenced by a multitude of factors including:
- Growth factors.
- Hormones.
- Cell–cell interactions.

The huge variety of factors involved allows cell growth and replication to be finely controlled, responding to changes in the environment. Growth factors are soluble substances that can act locally or over long distances to affect cell growth. In common with the effects of hormones and cell–cell interactions, growth factors exert their action by binding to specific target receptors on the cell surface. This in turn initiates the phosphorylation of target proteins within the cell in a cascade that ultimately results in changes in gene expression (see Chapter 3).

The cell cycle and cancer

Cancer is characterized by uncontrolled cellular growth. Normal cells are in equilibrium, and there is a balance between proliferation, quiescence, and death. Malignant cells may have the ability to grow autonomously, and they are not subject to the normal controls that regulate cell division.

Malignancy occurs as a result of DNA mutations that result in either increased or decreased expression of genes associated with cell cycle control. The most common causes of altered gene expression are:
- Chemical damage (e.g., by benzene, nitrosamines).
- Radiation (e.g., ultraviolet light).
- Integration of viral DNA into the host genome.
- Inherited defects.

The first three causes listed are "wear-and-tear" effects, which means that the mutations tend to accumulate with age.

Cancer represents clonal expansion of a cell in which there has been sufficient change to the genomic DNA to transform the cell's phenotype from a normal to a malignant cell. Usually in the progression to cancer there is an accumulation of mutations that together cause malignant transformation (see Fig. 7.33).

The genes that when mutated are associated with cancer can be grouped into two categories:
- Oncogenes (e.g., *Ras, Fos, Myc*) are mutated or up-regulated versions of normal cellular genes (proto-oncogenes) that induce uncontrolled growth. Proto-oncogenes are frequently components of cell signaling pathways (see Chapter 3).
- Tumor suppressor genes (e.g., *p53, Rb, GAP*) are genes expressed in normal cells, with loss of their activity resulting in uninhibited growth. Many of these genes code for proteins that are normally involved in the regulation of cell division and differentiation.

Mutations in genes that code for DNA repair proteins are also associated with cancer; for example, patients with xeroderma pigmentosum (see Chapter 8) have a tendency to develop skin tumors.

Mutations in *BRCA1* and *BRCA2* genes are associated with familial breast cancer. The proteins coded by these genes are thought to be important in the repair of double-strand DNA damage by a process called homologous recombination.

p53

p53 is an important tumor suppressor that has been dubbed the "guardian of the genome." Its basic function is to restrict the entry of cells with damaged DNA into S phase (i.e., it regulates progression of the cell cycle past the restriction point). Cells with mutant for p53 are not arrested in G_1 and progress through the cell cycle and division with damaged DNA. The gene for p53 lies on chromosome 17 and codes for a nuclear phosphoprotein of 53kD. Three major roles of p53 have been identified:

- Transcription activator—regulating certain genes involved in cell division.
- As a G_1 restriction point for DNA damage—if there has been excess DNA damage (e.g., ultraviolet damage) it inhibits cell division.
- Participation in the initiation of apoptosis (programmed cell death).

Mitosis and meiosis

Definitions
Karyotype
This is the chromosome complement of a cell. In a standard karyotype the chromosomes are conventionally arranged in an order depending upon size. Chromosomes are distinguished individually by their size, centromere position, and banding pattern.

Genome
This is the entire genetic complement of a cell.

Gamete
The reproductive cell formed by meiosis containing half the normal chromosome number.

Ploidy
This refers to the number of complete sets of chromosomes in a cell. A haploid cell contains a single set of chromosomes (e.g., gametes); a diploid cell contains two copies of each chromosome (e.g., somatic cells); a polyploid cell contains more than two sets of chromosomes (sometimes this occurs normally in plants and in some animal cells such as megakaryocytes).

Overview of cell division
Cell division is the process by which a cell, including the nucleus, undergoes replication and splits to produce two daughter cells. Many somatic cell types are continually replenished by cell division. In order to be viable, each daughter cell must contain a complete set of genetic material so that all its proteins can be expressed at the appropriate levels.

In addition to its role in directing protein synthesis, DNA enables the passage of genetic information from one generation to the next. Therefore, in the sexually reproducing multicellular organism, cells must have two mechanisms of cell division, resulting in both diploid and haploid daughter cells.

- Mitosis is the type of cell division that occurs in somatic cells and results in the production of two genetically identical daughter cells.
- Meiosis occurs in gamete formation (e.g., sperm and ova). Each daughter cell contains half the genetic information of the parent cell, and genetic recombination ("crossing-over") ensures a reassortment of genetic material between homologous ("paired") chromosomes.

Mitosis
Two identical diploid daughter cells are formed as a result of mitosis.

Mitosis: $2n \rightarrow 2n$

There are four distinct phases in mitosis (Fig. 5.5).

Prophase
There is condensation of chromosomes and the centrioles duplicate and migrate toward opposite poles of the cell. A spindle of microtubules is formed simultaneously.

Dissolution of the nuclear membrane marks the end of prophase.

Metaphase
The chromosomes become attached to the spindle. The area of attachment is called the kinetochore. The chromosomes become arranged along the spindle, forming the equatorial plate.

Anaphase
Chromatids separate at the centromeres, and are pulled to opposite poles by the spindle. The end of anaphase is marked by the clustering of two groups of identical chromatids at opposite poles of the cell.

Telophase
The chromosomes begin to uncoil. The nuclear membrane re-forms and nucleoli reappear. The cytoplasm is divided into two by the process of cytokinesis.

Each sister chromatid of a metaphase chromosome is a double helix, because both strands were replicated in the preceding S phase. Thus, after separation in mitotic anaphase each daughter cell receives a complete copy of the genome. (It is a common misconception that the strands of the double helix are separated at anaphase, in which case the genome would only be complete after S phase.)

Meiosis

In the first division of meiosis two genetically different haploid cells are formed (Fig. 5.6). In the second division, each haploid cell is duplicated by the separation of sister chromatids.

Meiosis: $2n \rightarrow n$

Prophase I

There are five stages during which homologous chromosomes come together and exchange segments in homologous recombination:

- Leptotene—chromosomes begin to condense.
- Zygotene—homologous chromosomes pair, shorten, and thicken, and form bivalents (pairs of homologous chromosomes).
- Pachytene—meiotic recombination ("crossing-over") occurs, in which homologous regions of DNA are exchanged between homologous chromosomes.
- Diplotene—the homologous chromosomes begin to separate but remain connected at points where crossing over has occurred. These are known as chiasmata and serve to physically link homologs until anaphase of meiosis I.
- Diakinesis—recombinant chromosomes are maximally condensed at this point.

Metaphase I

Chromosomes become attached to a spindle and align at the equatorial plane ("the metaphase plate").

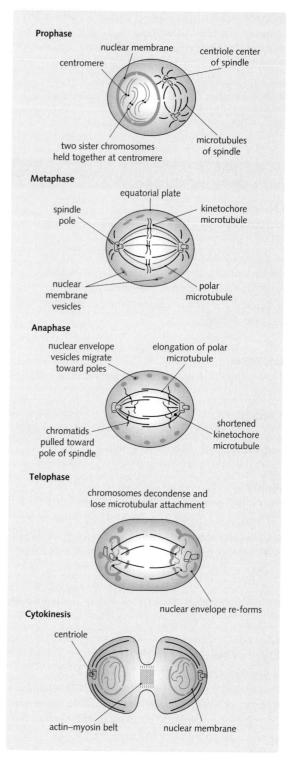

Fig. 5.5 Mitosis. (Adapted from Stevens and Lowe, 1997.)

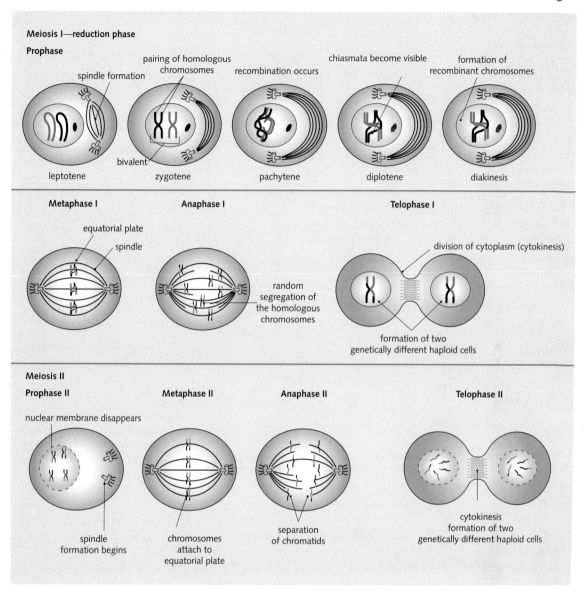

Fig. 5.6 Meiosis—see text for explanation of each phase.

Anaphase I

Each pair of homologous chromosomes migrates to opposite poles of spindle, hence "reduction division." Note that the sister chromatids do not separate at this point.

Telophase I

Two genetically different haploid cells are formed.

Second division

The second division is like mitosis, but a haploid number of chromosomes is involved. The chromatids separate in anaphase II.

Genetic diversity and gametogenesis

Two processes in meiosis are vital in the generation of genetic diversity:

- Meiotic recombination ("crossing-over"), which allows random exchange of genetic material between homologous chromosomes.
- Independent segregation of homologous chromosomes.

During anaphase I, homologous chromosomes segregate independently of each other. Since humans possess 23 pairs of homologous

Fig. 5.7 Oogenesis.

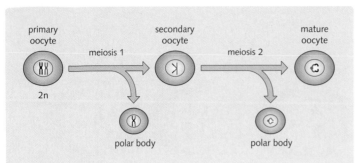

chromosomes, there are 2^{23} possible ways that the chromosomes can segregate to form a haploid set.

In humans, meiosis begins during gametogenesis. In females this occurs in the ovaries. The first ("reduction") meiotic division begins during month 5 of embryonic life, but it is arrested at diplotene of prophase I and completed just before ovulation. Meiosis II takes place after ovulation is completed at the time of fertilization. Therefore:

- There is a fixed number of oocytes.
- There is a period of arrest between the start of meiosis I and the completion of meiosis II of 12–45 years.

Oogenesis produces a single oocyte and two polar bodies (Fig. 5.7).

Male spermatogenesis occurs in the seminiferous tubules of the testes. After sexual maturity the spermatogonia continuously multiply by mitosis, subsequently undergoing meiosis to produce unlimited numbers of spermatocytes.

Endomitosis

Endomitosis is the process of repeated DNA replication in the absence of nuclear division and cytokinesis. It can generate huge nuclei with up to 16 copies of the DNA. Endomitosis occurs in the formation of megakaryocytes, which are cells in the bone marrow from which anucleate platelets bud off.

Nucleic acids

Structure of nucleic acids

Nucleic acids are linear polymers of nucleotides (Fig. 5.8). DNA (deoxyribonucleic acid) and RNA (ribonucleic acid) are nucleic acids that play an integral role in the growth and replication of all living cells.

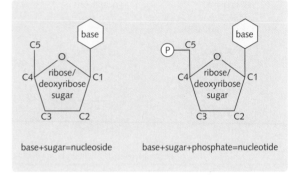

Fig. 5.8 Structure of nucleosides and nucleotides. Deoxyribose has an H group on C2 of the ribose moiety, whereas ribose has an OH group at this position. (Adapted from *Molecular Biology of the Cell*, 3rd edn, by B. Alberts *et al.*, Garland Publishing, 1994, with permission of Routledge, Inc., part of The Taylor & Francis Group.)

Nucleotides have three components:
- Base (purine or pyrimidine).
- Pentose sugar (deoxyribose in DNA, ribose in RNA; Fig. 5.9).
- Phosphate.

Purines and pyrimidines

The nucleotide bases in nucleic acids are heterocyclic molecules derived from either purine (A, G) or pyrimidine (C, U, T). They are planar aromatic rings that contain nitrogen (Fig. 5.10).

Purine and pyrimidine biosynthesis

Almost all eukaryotic cells are capable of synthesizing purines and pyrimidines *de novo*, which suggests an important role in cell survival.

Purines are synthesized in an 11-stage pathway with a starting chemical of α-D-ribose-phosphate. The process requires folate (tetrahydrofolate). The initial product is inosine monophosphate (IMP),

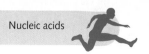

Comparison of DNA and RNA		
Feature	DNA	RNA
Sugar	Deoxyribose	Ribose
Base pairing	A–T/G–C	A–U/G–C
Structure	Double helix	Single-stranded structures

Fig. 5.9 Comparison of DNA and RNA. (A, adenine; C, cytosine; G, guanine; T, thymine; U, uracil.)

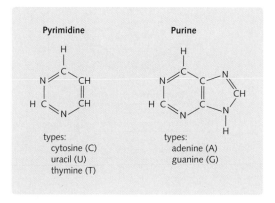

types:
cytosine (C)
uracil (U)
thymine (T)

types:
adenine (A)
guanine (G)

Fig. 5.10 Structure of pyrimidine and purine bases.

ribonucleoside or a deoxyribonucleotide (e.g., adenosine or deoxyadenosine, respectively).

A nucleotide is a compound of a sugar residue attached to a base and a phosphate group (see Fig. 5.8). Nucleotides are the subunits of nucleic acids. They are named according to whether the base is a ribonucleotide or a deoxyribonucleotide and the number of attached phosphate groups (e.g., adenosine monophosphate).

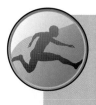

A nucleotide is a phosphorylated nucleoside. Do not be confused by notation, a nucleotide may alternatively be described as a nucleoside phosphate.

A nucleoTide has Three moieties.

which is rapidly converted to adenosine monophosphate (AMP) and guanosine monophosphate (GMP). A complex negative feedback control network operates to prevent excessive build-up of AMP and GMP.

Pyrimidine synthesis involves a six-step pathway, in which the ribose sugar is incorporated as one of the final steps. The final product is uridine triphosphate (UTP), which is converted to CTP (cytidine triphosphate) by amination of the uracil.

Pentose sugars
These are five-carbon rings (see Fig. 5.8). Deoxyribonucleotides are formed by the reduction of the ribose group of the corresponding ribonucleotide.

Nucleosides and nucleotides
A nucleoside is a compound of a sugar residue and a nucleotide base linked by a N-glycosidic bond between C1 of the sugar and an N atom of the base (see Fig. 5.8). The nucleosides of the various bases are named according to whether they are a

Production of nucleic acids
Nucleic acids are produced from the polymerization of nucleoside triphosphates. During synthesis a series of nucleic acid condensation reactions occur between phosphate and sugar groups to produce strong phosphodiester bonds. Long, unbranching chains form with linkages between C3 and C5 of each sugar, hence the notation $5' \rightarrow 3'$ or $3' \rightarrow 5'$ to describe the orientation of nucleotides in a nucleic acid chain. Each sugar is separated from the next by a phosphate group to form a strong and rigid sugar–phosphate backbone from which the bases project (Fig. 5.11).

DNA double helix
The structure of DNA was discovered by Watson and Crick in 1953. They showed that DNA consists of two intertwined polynucleotide strands held together by base pairing to form a double helix. Adenine and thymine pair via two hydrogen bonds between opposing strands, whereas guanine and cytosine have three. Base pairing results in two

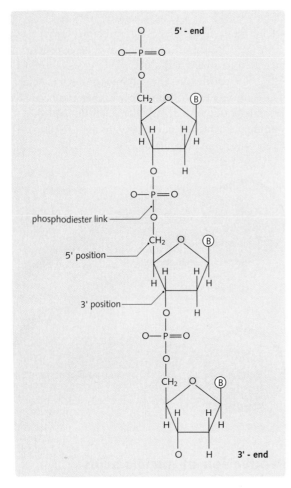

Fig. 5.11 Nucleic acids. The backbone of DNA is formed from deoxyribose sugars linked by phosphodiester bonds. B indicates the position of the base. (Adapted from Norman and Lodwick, 1999.)

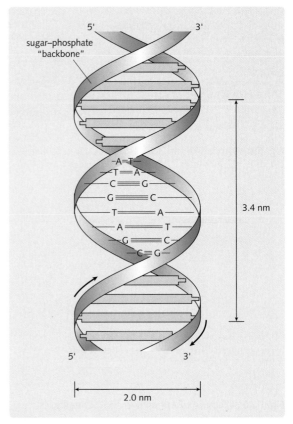

Fig. 5.12 The DNA double helix is a right-handed helix with a common axis for both strands. There are ten base pairs per turn. (A, adenine; C, cytosine; G, guanine; T, thymine.)

complementary polynucleotides, which run antiparallel to each other (i.e., one runs 5′ to 3′, the other runs 3′ to 5′; Fig. 5.12).

DNA as an information carrier

DNA is found predominantly in the nucleus but also in mitochondria. It acts as a template during transcription, and it is also the vehicle of inheritance (i.e., it is passed from one generation to the next).

RNA molecules

In eukaryotes, RNA is synthesized predominantly in the nucleus, but generally moves out into the cytoplasm to carry out its function. In eukaryotic cells, all RNA is produced from DNA by transcription.

Messenger RNA

Messenger RNA (mRNA) carries genetic information from the nucleus into the cytoplasm. In eukaryotes it is derived by splicing the initial RNA transcript, whereas it is produced directly by transcription in prokaryotes. It forms the template upon which polypeptides are manufactured during translation, and it is a single-stranded molecule without any intramolecular hydrogen bonds (Fig. 5.13).

Transfer RNA

Transfer RNA (tRNA):
- Carries specific amino acids to the site of protein synthesis.
- Has two active sites, which allow it to carry out its functions.
- Is a linear molecule with an average of 76 nucleotides.

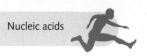

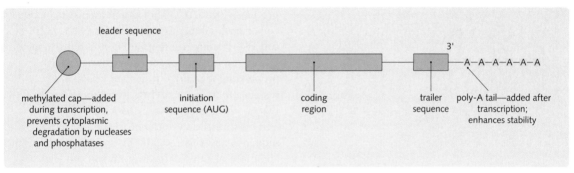

Fig. 5.13 Structure of eukaryotic mRNA. (A, adenine; C, cytosine; G, guanine; U, uracil).

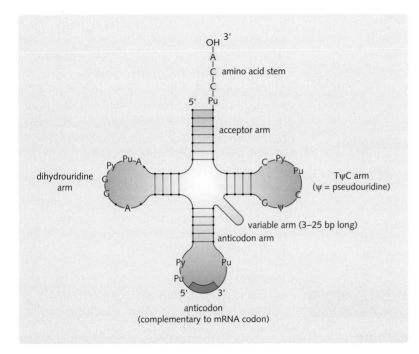

Fig. 5.14 Secondary structure of tRNA. It consists of five arms. The active sites are on the acceptor arm, where the 3′ terminal CCA group can accept a specific amino acid, and the anticodon is on the anticodon arm, which recognizes the corresponding mRNA codon. Specific base pairing within the five arms helps to maintain the secondary structure. (A, adenine; C, cytosine; G, guanine; Pu, purine; Py, pyrimidine.)

- Exhibits extensive intramolecular base pairing, which gives it a characteristic "clover-leaf-shaped" secondary structure.

Up to 20% of the bases undergo posttranslational modification. Their precise function is not known, but they may be involved in tRNA–protein interactions or stabilizing the tRNA molecule. Figure 5.14 shows the arrangement of the secondary structure of tRNA.

Ribosomal RNA
Ribosomal RNA (rRNA) is a component of ribosomes. In a eukaryotic cell each ribosome consists of two unequal subunits, made up of proteins and RNA, called the S (small) and L (large) subunits (Fig. 5.15). The RNA molecules undergo extensive intramolecular base pairing, which is important in determining the ribosomal structure. Ribosomes are capable of self-assembly under physiologic conditions with the correct complement of components.

Heteronuclear RNA
Heteronuclear RNA (hnRNA) is the primary transcript produced by eukaryotic cells. Unlike the final mRNA transcript it contains introns that are removed by RNA splicing.

83

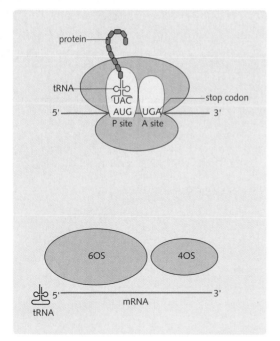

Fig. 5.15 Structure of a eukaryotic ribosome. Ribosomes consist of two unequal subunits, composed of RNA and protein, held together by magnesium ions. In rat cytoplasmic ribosome, the small (40S) unit is composed of 33 polypeptides and 18S rRNA, while the large (60S) unit is composed of 49 polypeptides and three rRNA molecules of 2.8S, 5.8S, and 5S. The ribosome has binding sites for mRNA, the peptidyl tRNA (P-site) and aminoacyl tRNA (A-site). (S, Svedberg unit of sedimentation.) (Adapted from Baynes and Dominiczak, 1999.)

DNA packaging and repair

DNA packaging in the nucleus

In the nucleus of a normal human cell, there are 46 chromosomes each containing 48–240 million bases of DNA. Watson and Crick's DNA double helix model predicts that each chromosome would have a contour length of 1.6–8.2 cm (i.e., the total length of the DNA would be about 3 m). However, the average nucleus has a diameter of approximately 5 µm! Therefore, an extremely high degree of organization is needed to fit this amount of DNA into the nucleus. DNA packaging in interphase cells can be described on three levels.

Nucleosomes

Nucleosome formation is the first level of packaging. A nucleosome is formed by 146 bp of DNA wound twice around an octamer of histone proteins (Fig. 5.16). The octamer consists of two copies each of the histone proteins H2A, H2B, H3, and H4. Histone proteins are conserved throughout eukaryotic evolution, and they contain a high proportion of positively charged amino acid residues that can, therefore, form ionic bonds with DNA, which is negatively charged.

This interaction does not depend on DNA sequence and theoretically histones can bind with any piece of DNA. However, in the cell the position of histone binding is influenced by:

- AT content (AT sequence bends more easily than GC).
- The presence of other tightly bound proteins.

DNase I is an endonuclease that breaks the internal phosphodiester bonds in DNA, irrespective of its base sequence. The regulatory regions of genes are frequently bound by regulatory proteins that prevent histones from binding. Since histone binding protects DNA from degradation with DNase I, the regulatory regions of genes are particularly sensitive to this enzyme, and they are sometimes called "nuclease-hypersensitive sites."

Nucleosome bound regions of DNA are separated by a region of linker DNA that varies from 0 to 80 bp in length. Consequently, on electron micrographs nucleosomes appear as 11 nm "beads" on a 2 nm DNA "string."

Chromatin

The second level of DNA packing is mediated by histone H1 that binds together adjacent nucleosomes to condense DNA into the 30 nm fiber, which is also called the solenoid (see Fig. 5.16).

Loop formation

The third level of organization is less clearly understood, but it is thought to involve the formation of DNA loops radiating from a central scaffold of nonhistone proteins. It is thought that the loops form transcriptional units.

Active chromatin

If nuclei isolated from different vertebrate cell types are treated with the enzyme DNase I, they show different patterns of degradation. This is attributed to actively transcribed genes (which differ between cell types) being more sensitive to the enzyme, which suggests that active chromatin

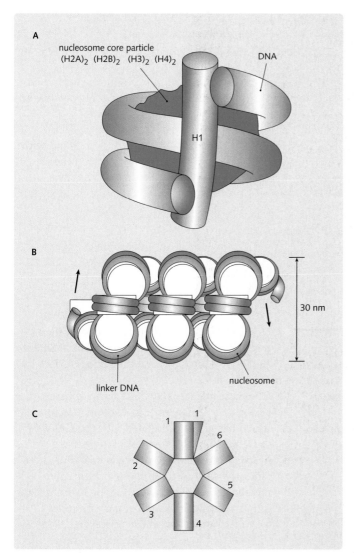

A

nucleosome core particle
(H2A)$_2$ (H2B)$_2$ (H3)$_2$ (H4)$_2$

DNA

H1

B

30 nm

linker DNA

nucleosome

C

Fig. 5.16 Chromatin fiber organization. (A) The nucleosome core particle is composed of pairs of histones—(H2A)$_2$ (H2B)$_2$ (H3)$_2$ (H4)$_2$. A fifth histone, H1, is also associated with the nucleosome. 166 base pairs of DNA wind around each nucleosome. Linker DNA runs between one nucleosome and the next. It consists of 8–114 base pairs. (B) Chromatin consists of nucleosomes bound together through their H1 proteins (not shown in this part of the figure). (C) Bound nucleosomes form a solenoid, with six nucleosomes per turn. (Adapted from *Molecular Biology of the Cell*, 3rd edn, by B. Alberts *et al.*, Garland Publishing, 1994, with permission of Routledge, Inc., part of The Taylor & Francis Group.)

and inactive chromatin are packaged differently. In contrast to inactive chromatin, active chromatin shows the following features:

- Histone H1 is less tightly bound.
- Nucleosomal histones are highly acetylated.
- Histone H2B is less phosphorylated.
- There is enrichment for a variant of H2A.

The differences between active and inactive chromatin suggest that chromatin structure is important in the regulation of gene expression. It is thought that large areas of the genome may be transcriptionally silenced during differentiation as a result of specialized packing. Although the precise details are not understood, it is thought that methylation status may influence chromatin structure.

Several neurodevelopmental disorders, namely Rett, fragile X and ICF (immunodeficiency, centromeric instability, and facial anomalies) syndromes, are thought to arise as a result of defective methylation.

Methylation

The CpG dinucleotide is generally underrepresented in the genome. However, it is found at the expected level in promoter regions. In the promoters of inactive genes the 5′ position of

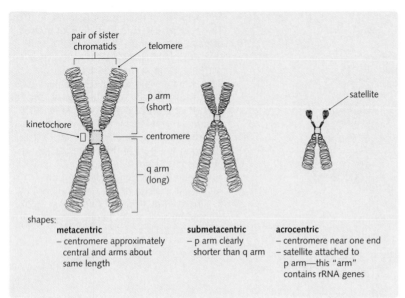

Fig. 5.17 Anatomy of a chromosome showing the three shapes: metacentric, submetacentric, and acrocentric.

cytosine is frequently methylated, whereas it is generally unmethylated in active genes. Methyl-CpG binding proteins bind to methylated regions and recruit histone deacetylase, which may trigger the formation of inactive chromatin. In this way, methylation may act to mark chromatin for inactivation, although the factors that prompt it to do so are unclear.

Chromosomes

At metaphase, chromatin is maximally condensed, and it forms 1400 nm fibers. After cell staining with biological dyes such as Giemsa, these are visible as chromosomes under light microscopy.

Each metaphase chromosome is composed of two identical sister chromatids. Chromatids are connected at a central region called the centromere, above and below which chromatin strands loop across between chromatids to hold them together (Fig. 5.17).

The kinetochore is an organelle located at the centromere region. It acts as a microtubule organizing center (MTOC) and facilitates spindle formation by polymerization of tubulin dimers to form microtubules during the early stages of mitosis (see Chapter 4).

DNA damage

Agents that cause DNA damage include:
- Ionizing radiation.
- Ultraviolet light, which promotes chemical cross-linking between two adjacent thymine residues on a DNA strand, resulting in the formation of a pyrimidine dimer. These distort the DNA double helix in the region of the dimer.
- Chemical mutagens, which can be of three types: base analogues (e.g., 5-bromouracil), which become incorporated into the DNA and cause misreading; chemical modifiers (e.g., hydroxylamine and compounds containing free radicals—such as those formed during the metabolism of polycyclic aromatic hydrocarbons in tobacco smoke), which react with bases to form derivatives that cause misreading; intercalators (e.g., some antibiotics), which slip between adjacent bases and inhibit RNA transcription.
- Parts of (or entire) viral genomes, which can become incorporated into eukaryotic chromatin. This can disrupt coding regions or promoting regions, or it can affect levels of expression of existing genes.

DNA can also change spontaneously under normal physiological conditions. For example, adenine and cytosine can undergo spontaneous deamination to produce hypoxanthine and uracil residues.

A mutation is a change in the base sequence of DNA (see also Chapter 7):
- If this is in a coding region and there is a change in the overall number of bases, this may result in a frameshift error in which the reading

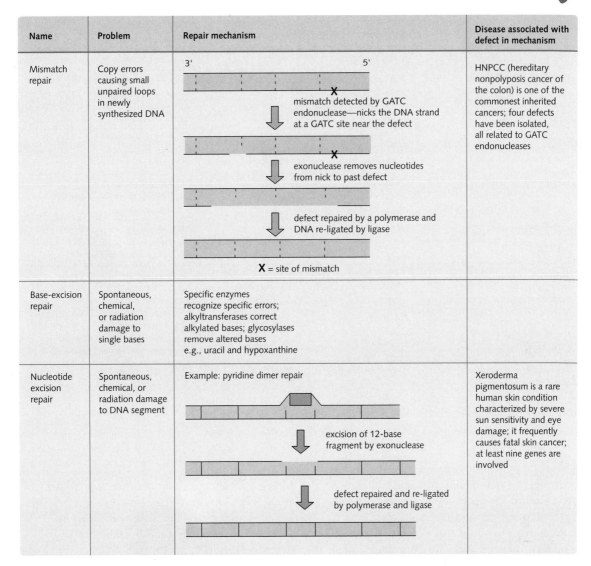

Name	Problem	Repair mechanism	Disease associated with defect in mechanism
Mismatch repair	Copy errors causing small unpaired loops in newly synthesized DNA	3' 5' **X** mismatch detected by GATC endonuclease—nicks the DNA strand at a GATC site near the defect **X** exonuclease removes nucleotides from nick to past defect defect repaired by a polymerase and DNA re-ligated by ligase **X** = site of mismatch	HNPCC (hereditary nonpolyposis cancer of the colon) is one of the commonest inherited cancers; four defects have been isolated, all related to GATC endonucleases
Base-excision repair	Spontaneous, chemical, or radiation damage to single bases	Specific enzymes recognize specific errors; alkyltransferases correct alkylated bases; glycosylases remove altered bases e.g., uracil and hypoxanthine	
Nucleotide excision repair	Spontaneous, chemical, or radiation damage to DNA segment	Example: pyridine dimer repair excision of 12-base fragment by exonuclease defect repaired and re-ligated by polymerase and ligase	Xeroderma pigmentosum is a rare human skin condition characterized by severe sun sensitivity and eye damage; it frequently causes fatal skin cancer; at least nine genes are involved

Fig. 5.18 Mammalian DNA defect repair mechanisms. GATC (guanine, adenine, thymine, and cytosine) exonuclease recognizes and binds to a GATC base sequence near to the DNA defect and nicks the DNA at this site.

frame (i.e., order of nucleotide codons) of amino acids is disrupted. This usually results in a truncated protein product.
- An altered base may result in a misreading error, which can result in an altered protein product. "Missense" mutations arise when the triplet code is altered to another amino acid, while "nonsense" mutations result if the triplet code is changed to a stop codon.
- The mutation may disrupt a regulatory region and affect the level of expression of a particular gene.

DNA repair

There are obvious evolutionary advantages to having cellular systems for the detection and repair of DNA damage. There are three mechanisms by which mammalian cells can replace abnormal regions of DNA (Fig. 5.18).

DNA replication

DNA replication is the process by which DNA molecules are divided longitudinally, such that each half is conserved to act as a template for the

DNA polymerases in *Escherichia coli* (Prokaryote)		
	DNA Pol I	**DNA Pol III**
Notes	First polymerase to be discovered by Kornberg in 1957	Discovered when a mutant strain of *E.coli* with very low Pol I activity was shown to have a normal rate of reproduction
Structure	Single polypeptide with 928 residues, 109 kD mass; forms one large ("Klenow") fragment and one small fragment	Three subunits with total 140 kD; subunits—a, e, q
Functions	Polymerase (Klenow fragment) 3′–5′ exonuclease (Klenow) 5′–3′ exonuclease (small fragment)	Polymerase (a subunit), 3′–5′ exonuclease (e subunit) 5′–3′ exonuclease
Associated proteins	Nil	At least seven other proteins associate to form a complex called the Pol III holoenzyme
Processivity (the number of consecutive reactions the enzyme is capable of performing)	At least 20 consecutive polymerization steps can occur before Pol I becomes dissociated from the DNA	In the holoenzyme the extra subunits interact with DNA and other proteins to clamp the polymerase onto the DNA, creating very high processivity (>5000 residues); Pol III alone has a processivity of 10–15 residues
Main biological function	Proofreading and error correction	DNA replication, proofreading

Fig. 5.19 Prokaryotic DNA polymerases. *E. coli* also has a Pol II. Its main physiologic function is unknown.

formation of a new strand. It is said to be semiconservative, since only one strand is newly synthesized in each daughter molecule.

Replication has been studied extensively in *Escherichia coli* because it has a single chromosome that divides every 20 minutes at 37°C. Moreover, it has been possible to isolate a range of replication deficient mutants, which can be used to identify and characterize the corresponding replication proteins.

Such studies suggest that, even in prokaryotes, replication is a complex process that requires about 30 proteins. Less is known about eukaryotic replication because of the increased complexity of the process and the difficulty in obtaining replication deficient mutants.

DNA polymerases

DNA polymerases are the enzymes responsible for DNA chain synthesis. They couple nucleoside triphosphates onto a growing DNA strand by adding a phosphate group onto the free 3′-OH group. New DNA molecules are thus synthesized in a 5′–3′ direction. Polymerization is driven thermodynamically by the elimination of a pyrophosphate (PP_i) and its subsequent hydrolysis:

$$(DNA)_n + dNTP \rightarrow (DNA)_{n+1} + PP_i$$

Three DNA polymerases have been characterized in *E. coli*, of which two are important in replication (Fig. 5.19). Four have been identified in eukaryotes (Fig. 5.20). RNA polymerase can begin a polynucleotide chain by linking two nucleoside triphosphates together directly. In contrast, DNA polymerase has an absolute requirement for a perfectly base-paired nucleotide, onto which it can then add nucleotides at the 3′-OH end. This has important consequences:

- DNA polymerase requires a primer on which to initiate extension.
- It will pause if an incorrect base is inserted.

Eukaryotic DNA polymerases				
	α	β	γ	δ
Notes	Multi-subunit protein; activity varies with rate of cell proliferation	Activity does not affect rate of cell growth	Chloroplasts contain similar enzymes	
Mass (kD)	120–220	30–50	150–300	140–160
Inhibitors				
Aphidicolin dideoxy	Yes	No	No	Yes
Didioxol NTPs	Weak	Strong	Strong	Weak
Arabinosyl NTPs	Strong	Weak	Weak	Strong
NEM	Strong	Weak	Strong	Strong
Functions	Polymerase, primase, NO exonuclease	Polymerase, exonuclease	Polymerase	Polymerase 3′–5′ exonuclease
Location	Nucleus	Nucleus	Mitochondrion	Nucleus
Processivity	Moderate (approximately 100 nucleotides)	?	Unlimited	?
Biological function	Initiates "lead strand" and "lag strand" replication	DNA repair	Replication of mitochondrial DNA	Complete elongation of lead and lag strand replication

Fig. 5.20 Eukaryotic DNA polymerases. (NEM, *N*-ethyl-maleimide; NTP, nucleoside triphosphate.)

The primers that are required for DNA polymerase activity are synthesized by RNA polymerase, since this enzyme does not itself require priming oligonucleotides. It synthesizes short stretches (10–20 nucleotides) of RNA primer sequence.

If Pol III, the main replication enzyme, inserts an incorrect base into the extending DNA chain, it cannot proceed until the erroneous nucleotide is excised. This is achieved by its own 3′–5′ exonuclease activity (see Fig. 5.19). In this manner, the enzyme corrects its own mistakes as it goes along. This function is called "proofreading," and it maintains the fidelity of DNA sequence after replication.

Mammalian polymerases are not capable of proofreading. Instead, mispaired bases are removed by endonucleases such as GATC endonuclease in mismatch repair (see Fig. 5.18).

Errors in replication occur at a rate of about 1 in 10^5 base pairs. This is reduced to about 1 in 10^8 by proofreading mechanisms.

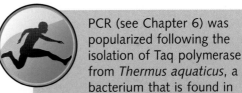

PCR (see Chapter 6) was popularized following the isolation of Taq polymerase from *Thermus aquaticus*, a bacterium that is found in hot springs. This enzyme is not denatured by the temperatures needed to separate DNA strands. Whereas Taq is added once at the beginning of PCR, polymerase isolated from nonthermophilic bacteria had to be added every single cycle (i.e., every 5 minutes over a 3 hour period).

DNA replication fork

Although there are some differences in prokaryotic and eukaryotic replication and their enzyme machinery (Fig. 5.21), the processes are broadly

Comparison of prokaryotic and eukaryotic DNA replication		
	E. coli (prokaryote)	**Mammalian (eukaryote)**
Site	Cytoplasm	Nucleus (and mitochondrion)
No. of proteins involved	30	100s
DNA polymerase	Pol I—fidelity and repair Pol III—DNA synthesis	Four enzymes identified
Initiation	Single origin of replication (OriC)	Multiple origins of replication (spatially and temporally separated during DNA replication)
Rate of replication	10^3 nucleotides/sec	10^2 nucleotides/sec
Postreplication	RNA primers removed from lag strand by Pol I 5'–3' exonuclease	RNA primers removed by 5'–3' exonuclease (NOT associated with α polymerase)
Timing of replication	Continuous DNA synthesis between cell divisions	DNA synthesis and cell division separated by G_1 and G_2 (gap) phases
Okazaki fragments	Large (1000–2000 bp)	Small (100–200 bp)
DNA polymerase	Same for leading and lagging strands	Alpha polymerase initiates replication; δ polymerase extends replication for both leading and lagging strands

Fig. 5.21 Prokaryotic and eukaryotic DNA replication.

similar. Replication is initiated at "origin of replication" that gives rise to two replication forks. Replication complexes assemble at both of these and proceed in opposite directions (Fig. 5.22).

Since DNA-dependent polymerases can only add nucleotides to the 3' end, DNA must be synthesized in a 5'–3' direction on both antiparallel strands. The leading strand can be synthesized in a continuous process from a single RNA primer. However, the lagging strand must be synthesized in pieces (called Okazaki fragments) from multiple RNA primers (see Fig. 5.22). These primers are later replaced with DNA and the pieces joined together by a DNA ligase.

Prokaryotic replication
Initiation

E. coli has a single origin of replication (*OriC*), which is a 245 bp DNA sequence. The addition of this sequence to any piece of circular DNA confers upon it the ability to replicate in *E. coli*.

Initially, sequence-specific protein binding around the origin causes the DNA to denature (strands dissociate) and unwind (Fig. 5.23). This produces a prepriming complex, which facilitates further unwinding and entry of the other components of the replication complex (Fig. 5.24):

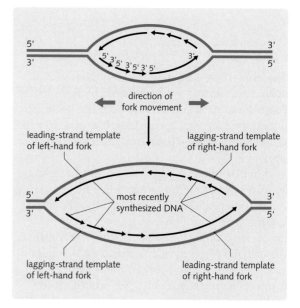

Fig. 5.22 The replication bubble. Two replication complexes form at each origin of replication and proceed in opposite directions. Note that the strand that is leading and the strand that is lagging depends upon the direction the replication complex is migrating.

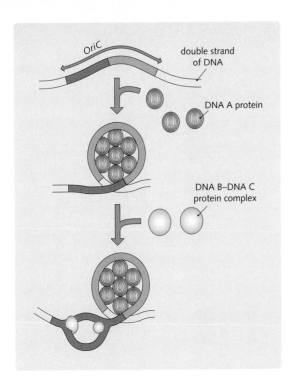

Fig. 5.23 Formation of prepriming complex for prokaryotic DNA replication. DNA A is a protein that recognizes and binds to 9 bp segments of *OriC*. The process is facilitated by Hu protein. The DNA A–DNA complex becomes negatively supercoiled. The DNA A–DNA complex guides the binding of DNA B–DNA C complex onto the adjacent region of *OriC*. DNA B has helicase activity and unwinds the DNA in the prepriming complex.

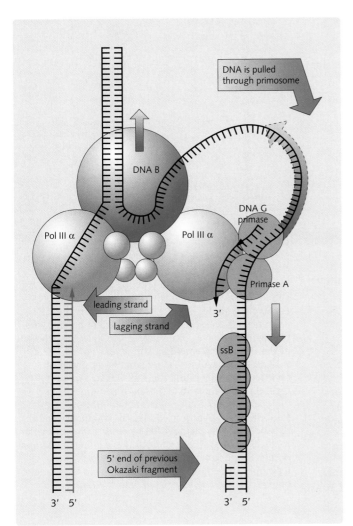

Fig. 5.24 Replication of DNA in *E. coli*. The replisome consists of two polymerase enzymes, one that binds to the leading strand and one that binds to the lagging strand. The holoenzyme moves continuously along the template for the leading strand while the lagging strand is "pulled through" by the primosome creating a loop in the DNA. Helicase (DNA B) creates the unwinding point as it translocates along the DNA. (© Oxford University Press and Cell Press 1994. Reprinted from *Genes V* by Benjamin Lewin (1994), by permission of Oxford University Press.)

- DNA helicase clamps to the lagging strand and unwinds the DNA helix.
- Primase binds to the helicase to form the primosome, which synthesizes the RNA primer.
- Single-strand binding (ssB) proteins stabilize ssDNA on the lagging strand.
- DNA polymerase III clamps to the leading strand and synthesizes DNA.
- A regulated sliding clamp protein holds DNA polymerase on the DNA.
- DNA topoisomerase relieves helical winding and tangling problems.

Two replication complexes (replisomes) are formed at each origin of replication. Note that each replisome contains two polymerases (see Fig. 5.24).

Elongation

The DNA chain is elongated by the action of DNA polymerase III (see above). Other enzymes are required to deal with the lagging strand:

- DNA Pol I removes RNA primer sequence and completes the DNA strand in the resulting gap.
- DNA ligase joins the fragments together.

Termination

Replication is complete when the replisomes, which set off around the circular chromosome in opposite directions, meet in the middle. Prokaryotic replication is summarized in Fig. 5.25.

Eukaryotic replication

The eukaryotic genome is much larger than the prokaryotic, and DNA replication involves multiple origins (Fig. 5.26). Other than for *Saccharomyces cerevisiae*, eukaryotic origins of replication have not been identified. Replication proceeds in two directions from each origin of replication and continues until neighboring forks fuse. Initiation at the various origins is separated spatially and temporally throughout S phase, with clusters of up to 100 origins undergoing initiation at the same time. The coordinating trigger is unknown, but there is thought to be an intrinsic factor in the DNA. Heterochromatin replicates later in S phase than euchromatin. The genome is replicated once only, and it is thought that the chromatin is marked after

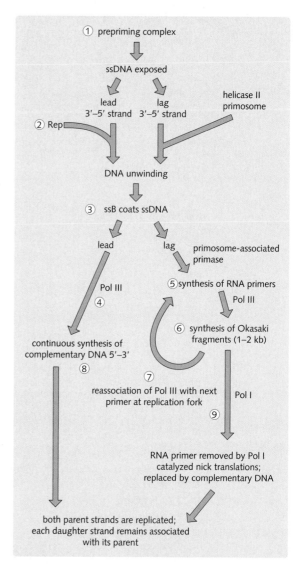

Fig. 5.25 Prokaryotic polymerization process in *E. coli*. (1) DNA is supercoiled around DNA A. DNA B and DNA C facilitate ssDNA exposure. (2) REP protein binds to the lead strand. Helicase II and primase bind to the lag strand. These produce further unwinding of the DNA. (3) Single-strand binding protein (ssB) coats the ssDNA and prevents reassociation. (4) The Pol III holoenzyme replicates DNA in *E. coli*. There is continuous synthesis of the DNA complementary to the lead strand (5'–3'). (5) Lag strand synthesis is initiated by synthesis of an RNA primer by a primase. (6) The lag strand is replicated in fragments (Okasaki fragments), each of which has a 5' RNA primer. (7) Pol III dissociates from the newly synthesized Okasaki fragment and reassociates with the next RNA primer at the replication fork. (8) DNA synthesis of both the lead and lag strands occurs on the same multiprotein that is called a replisome. Therefore, the lag strand has to loop around on itself to become associated with the replisome.

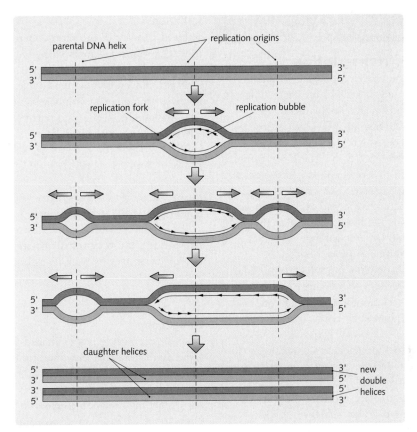

Fig. 5.26 Eukaryotic DNA replication. There are multiple origins of replication, but replication is initiated at specific points at specific times to ensure that the entire genome is replicated once, and once only. (Adapted from Jorde *et al.*, 1997.)

replication to prevent it being replicated a second time, possibly by DNA methylation.

The components of the eukaryotic replication fork are less well characterized than prokaryotic components. However, it is known that two distinct DNA polymerases are involved:
- Polymerase α is required for the initiation of replication and priming of Okazaki fragments during elongation.
- Polymerase δ is the primary enzyme responsible for elongation of replication for both leading and lagging strands.

After the replication fork passes, chromatin structure is reformed by the addition of new histones. The presence of histone proteins in eukaryotic chromosomes is thought to account for the slower rate of eukaryotic replication and shorter Okasaki fragments (see Fig. 5.21).

Telomerase

DNA polymerases require an RNA primer. This poses a potential problem at the ends of eukaryotic linear chromosomes because there is nowhere for the lagging strand primer to bind to facilitate replication of the terminal sequence. Thus, potentially the chromosome could become progressively shorter after successive rounds of replication, resulting in a loss of genetic information. Telomerase circumvents this problem by adding protective telomeres to the ends of each chromosome.

Although active in germ-line cells, telomerase is not normally active in somatic cells. It has been proposed that the progressive shortening of telomeres in somatic tissue is an important component of aging. Immortal cancer cells frequently show regained telomerase activity.

Transcription and RNA synthesis

Definition of transcription

Transcription is the process by which RNA is synthesized according to a DNA template. The process is catalyzed by DNA-dependent RNA polymerases, which unwind dsDNA to expose unpaired bases upon which DNA–RNA hybrids form. RNA is synthesized 5′–3′. The DNA template displays polarity in that only one strand can act as a template (template strand). The nontranscribed strand is called the coding strand as it has the same base composition as the RNA except that thymines (Ts) are substituted for uracils (Us).

The template strand is transcribed. It is identified by RNA polymerase, which binds to the specific DNA sequences that comprise the "promoter." Transcription of a gene may be influenced and regulated by both *cis* and *trans* acting factors:

- *Cis* acting factors are specific sequences of DNA that lie on the same molecule of DNA as the gene they regulate.
- *Trans* acting factors are proteins that bind to *cis* acting elements. They are transcribed from genes distinct from the ones they regulate.

Prokaryotic transcription

Transcription occurs in three phases:

- Initiation.
- Elongation.
- Termination.

E. coli RNA polymerase

E. coli RNA polymerase (RNAP) is a large holoenzyme that contains two Zn^{2+} ions, which the enzyme needs for its catalytic activity. It has a core subunit composition of $\alpha2\beta\beta'$, which associates with another subunit, sigma (σ), to form the initiation complex, $\alpha2\beta\beta'\sigma$. The σ-subunit is concerned specifically with promoter recognition and binds to the promoter TATAAT (Pribnow) box (sequences of bases: TATAAT). *E. coli* has a number of σ-factors that recognize the promoter regions of specific, coordinated sets of genes. The β-subunits form the catalytic center, while the α-subunits are important in the assembly of the complex.

Initiation

Subunit σ binds to the promoter region, which induces a conformational change in RNAP that allows nucleotides to associate with the β-subunit. This is followed by chemical initiation, which involves coupling of two nucleotide triphosphates. The first is almost always a purine, usually adenine:

$$pppA + pppN \rightarrow pppApN + PP_i$$

(pppA, adenosine triphosphate; pppN, nucleoside triphosphate; PP_i, pyrophosphate.)

After the enzyme has synthesized about eight nucleotides, the σ factor dissociates and a number of elongation factors become associated with the enzyme instead.

Elongation

The RNA molecule is synthesized 5′–3′. The DNA template is gradually unwound by RNAP pushing the DNA's coils ahead of it, creating positive superhelicity ahead of the complex and corresponding unwinding behind it (Fig. 5.27). Only about 17 bases are exposed at a time. The RNA quickly leaves the DNA template and the DNA reforms its double helix.

The overall equation for the polymerization process is:

$$(RNA)_n + XTP \rightarrow (RNA)_{n+1} + PP_i \rightarrow 2P_i$$

(XTP, nucleoside triphosphate; PP_i, pyrophosphate; P_i, inorganic phosphate.)

Termination

Elongation reactions continue until RNA polymerase encounters a transcription termination signal, such as:

- The formation of a hairpin loop in the transcript.
- The binding of a rho (ρ) subunit to the polymerase complex.

Prokaryotic posttranscriptional modification

In prokaryotes there is very little or no posttranscriptional modification of mRNA, and translation begins while the RNA transcript is still

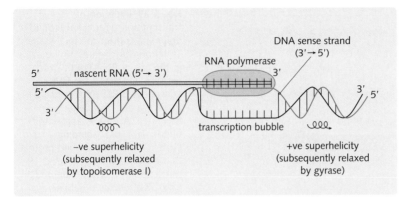

Fig. 5.27 RNA chain elongation. The RNA molecule develops in a straight line while DNA rotates. (Adapted from *Biochemistry*, by D. Voet and J.C. Voet, John Wiley & Sons, 1990.)

Eukaryotic RNA polymerases			
RNA polymerase	Localization	Cellular transcripts	Effect of α-amanitin
I	Nucleolus	18S, 5.8S, and 28S rRNA	Insensitive
II	Nucleoplasm	mRNA precursors and hnRNA	Strongly inhibited
III	Nucleoplasm	tRNA and 5S rRNA	Inhibited by high concentrations

Fig. 5.28 Eukaryotic RNA polymerases. These differ with respect to their template specificity, localization, and sensitivity to α-amanitin (the active ingredient in *Amanita phalloides*, a poisonous mushroom). (Adapted from *Biochemistry*, 3rd edn, by L. Stryer, W.H. Freeman and Company, 1988.)

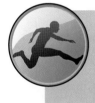

When answering questions on replication, transcription, or translation, consider the processes in three stages: initiation, elongation, and termination.

being produced. However, rRNA (ribosomal RNA) and tRNA (transfer RNA) transcripts do show a degree of posttranscriptional modification. They are synthesized as a continuous strand that undergoes posttranscriptional cleavage with a nuclease, which may be followed by base modification:
- CCA is added to the 3′ end of each tRNA.
- Bases in rRNA may be methylated.
- Bases in tRNA may be modified to produce inosine, pseudouridine, and dihydrouridine.

Eukaryotic transcription

Eukaryotes have three chromosomally encoded RNA polymerases, which recognize different promoters and, therefore, transcribe different types of RNA molecule. The TATA box (Hogness–Goldberg box) is found in the promoters of genes transcribed by RNA polymerase II. These polymerases can be identified because they differ in their sensitivity to a mushroom toxin, α-amanitin (Fig. 5.28).

Sequence of events
Initiation
Transcription in eukaryotes is more complicated than in prokaryotes, and it requires the presence of several transcription factors (these are defined as proteins that are required to initiate or regulate eukaryotic transcription). The polymerase II transcriptional complex that transcribes mRNA contains transcription factors (TF II) B, D, E, F, and H. It is assembled, and transcription initiated, as follows (Fig. 5.29):

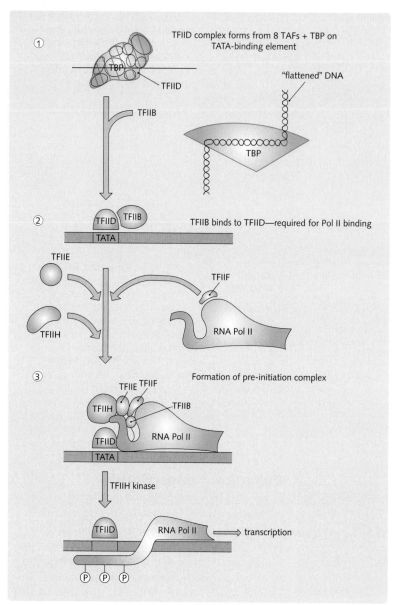

Fig. 5.29 Initiation of transcription with eukaryotic RNA polymerase II. In the final stage, TFIIH phosphorylates amino acids in the tail of RNA Pol II, which reduces its affinity for TAFs and releases RNA Pol II for transcription. (A, adenine; T, thymine; TAF, TATA-associated factor; TBP, TATA-binding protein—a saddle-shaped protein that unwinds the DNA helix; TF, transcription factor.) (Adapted from *The Journal of Molecular Biology* **150**: 92–120, by J. Engel, E. Odermatt, A. Engel, J.A. Madr and H. Furthmayr *et al.*, 1981.) (Courtesy of H. Furthmayr.)

- TFIID binds to the TATA box *via* its TBP (TATA-binding protein) subunit.
- TFIIB binds to TFIID.
- TFIIH, TFIIE, TFIIF, and Pol II bind.
- TFIIH phosphorylates Pol II.
- Pol II is released from the complex and begins transcription.

If the transcription complex contains only the five "basal" transcription factors highlighted above, the level of transcription is low. Physiological levels of transcription require the presence of enhancers. These are *cis* acting elements that may be located many kilobases away from the start of transcription in a 5′ or 3′ direction. Enhancers are bound by *trans* acting proteins, which are then able to associate with the polymerase complex to increase the level of transcription (Fig. 5.30).

Since the expression of transactivators is tissue specific, enhancers facilitate tissue-specific control of gene expression in multicellular organisms.

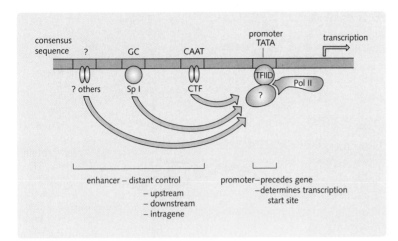

Fig. 5.30 Hierarchical control over gene expression in eukaryotes. Physiological levels of expression depend on the interaction between polymerase and transactivating and repressor proteins. There is sequence homology between TATAAT and eukaryotic TATA. Both form the site of the transcription initiation complex. (A, adenine; T, thymine; C, cytosine; G, guanine.)

Similarly, transcription from a gene may be reduced in a tissue-specific manner by the presence of silencers (the *cis* acting element) and repressor proteins (the *trans* acting element).

Elongation

The overall equation is the same as for prokaryotic elongation. However, the transcript is modified while it is still being transcribed by the addition of a 5′ cap (see below), which does not occur in prokaryotes.

The length of the primary RNA transcript (hnRNA) at an average of 7000 nucleotides is very much larger than the average prokaryotic transcript and, moreover, it is larger than the predicted 1200 nucleotides needed to code for average protein of 400 amino acid residues. This discrepancy reflects the presence of introns, which are not found in prokaryotic transcripts.

Termination

This is a far less precise process in eukaryotes than in prokaryotes because the 3′ end of the molecule undergoes posttranscriptional modification, where the transcript is cleaved at a highly conserved AAUAAA sequence. Transcription can sometimes carry on for hundreds of bases past this site. The precise signal for termination of transcription has not yet been found.

Eukaryotic post-transcriptional modification
Addition of a 5′ cap

This is a very early modification that occurs soon after transcription initiation. A cap structure containing 7-methylguanosine is enzymatically

added to the 5′ end of the growing transcript, using an unusual 6′ to 5′ phosphodiester bond. It is thought to have three functions:
- It protects the mRNA from enzymatic attack.
- It aids in splicing (i.e., the removal of introns from hnRNA).
- It enhances translation of the mRNA.

3′ cleavage at the AAUAAA sequence and addition of a poly(A) tail

Although RNA polymerase continues to transcribe the DNA, the transcript is cleaved by enzymes 10–20 nucleotides downstream from the polyadenylation signal (AAUAAA). The cleavage gives the 3′ end of the transcript a well-defined end. The 100–250 nucleotide poly(A) tail is generated from adenosine triphosphate (ATP) by the enzyme poly(A) polymerase. The poly(A) tail is believed to assist in transport of the MRNA to the cytoplasm for translation.

Splicing

Heterogeneous nuclear RNAs (hnRNAs) are the primary transcripts from genomic DNA. The production of mature eukaryotic mRNAs from hnRNA involves a process called gene splicing. This is the removal of noncoding introns and the joining together of the intervening exons. This process occurs in the nucleus by means of an RNA–protein complex called the spliceosome, which assembles immediately after the intron sequence has been transcribed. Spliceosomes consist of:
- A core structure made up of three subunits called small nuclear ribonuclear proteins (snRNPs; pronounced "snurps"). Each snRNP

contains at least one snRNA and several proteins. The protein subunits are named after the associated snRNAs: U1, U2, and [U4/U6, U5].
- Non-snRNP splicing factors and an hnRNA.

The role snRNPs play in splicing was revealed by the finding that antibodies specific for these ribonucleoproteins inhibit splicing. These were isolated from patients with the autoimmune disease systemic lupus erythematosus, which is characterized by the formation of antibodies against many nuclear components.

The splicing process depends on the existence of consensus sequences within the hnRNA intron, which are recognized by components of the spliceosome:
- The first two nucleotides of the intron are always GU, which binds U1 and forms the splice donor site.
- An "A" nucleotide approximately 30 nucleotides from the 3' end of the intron binds U2 and forms the branch site.
- The last two nucleotides of the intron are always AG, which binds U5 and forms the splice acceptor site.

The binding of the snRNPs to the intron causes it to form a loop. The splicing reaction then proceeds in two stages, with the first stage releasing the first exon and the second stage the second exon (Fig. 5.31):
- The nucleotide at the branch site attacks the donor site and cleaves it, such that the 5' end of the intron becomes covalently attached to the adenine nucleotide at the branch site, forming a "lariat-shaped" structure.
- The 3'–OH end of the first exon (generated in the previous reaction) adds to the beginning of the second exon sequence, cleaving the RNA at the splice acceptor site.

After the reaction is complete, the two exons are joined together and the intron sequence is released as a lariat.

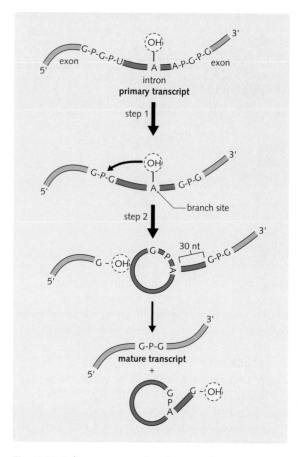

Fig. 5.31 Spliceosome mediated RNA splicing. The first stage in the reaction results in the breaking of the phosphate bond at the 5' exon/intron boundary and its joining to the adenine at the branch site. In the second step the phosphate bond at the 3' exon/intron boundary is cleaved, which is followed by the reformation of a phosphate bond between the terminal nucleotide of the first exon and the first nucleotide of the second exon. Note that, as shown here, in over 60% of cases, the exon ends with a "G" and the next exon begins with a "G." (Adapted from Baynes and Dominiczak, 1999.)

Comparison of prokaryotic and eukaryotic transcription

A comparison of prokaryotic and eukaryotic transcription is shown in Fig. 5.32.

Antibiotics and transcription

There are significant differences between eukaryotic and prokaryotic replication, therefore, prokaryotic replication machinery is a suitable target for antimicrobial action. Actinomycin inhibits both RNA and DNA polymerases by intercalating

Comparison of prokaryotic and eukaryotic transcription		
	Prokaryotic	**Eukaryotic**

Site of transcription	Cytoplasm	Nucleus:
		5.8S/18S/28S rRNA
		    in nucleolus
		5S rRNA, tRNA, mRNA
		    in nucleoplasm

RNA polymerase	Single species; RNAP (*E. coli*); large holoenzyme; core enzyme consists of four subunits; $\alpha_2\ \beta\beta'$	Three RNA polymerases in nucleus: Pol I transcribes rRNA; Pol II, mRNA; Pol III, rRNA and tRNA; consist of two large subunits with homology to the prokaryotic β subunits and a complex array of approximately 12 small subunits (e.g., Pol II assembly initiated by TFIID binding to promoter)
Initiation	S subunit associates with the core enzyme and facilitates binding to the promoter	Complex assembly of proteins
Termination	RNA forms stable hairpin loop between A–T-rich and G–C-rich region, then weak base pairing between poly(U) RNA and DNA encourages dissociation; the ρ factor is an enzyme that facilitates transcription termination with or without the hairpin loop	Termination is imprecise and signal is unknown
Posttranscriptional modification	mRNA requires little or no modification	hnRNA = mRNA precursor; 5' methyl cap added during transcription; 3' end cleaved at AAUAAA site and poly(A) tail added; introns removed by splicing
mRNA	Polycistronic; each transcript can code for more than one polypeptide	Monocistronic can code for only one polypeptide

Fig. 5.32 Comparison of prokaryotic and eukaryotic transcription. (A, adenine; C, cytosine; G, guanine; T, thymine; U, uracil.)

between G–C pairs in duplex DNA to inhibit nucleic acid synthesis. Rifampicin specifically inhibits prokaryotic RNA polymerases. It blocks chain elongation by remaining bound to the promoter to prevent new initiation complexes forming. It does not block eukaryotic RNA polymerases, so it is a useful bactericidal agent against Gram-positive bacteria and tuberculosis.

Translation and protein synthesis

Definition of translation

Translation is the mRNA-directed biosynthesis of polypeptides. It is a complex process that involves several hundred macromolecules.

The genetic code

In the translation process from mRNA to protein, amino acids are coded for by groups of three bases called codons. Since nucleic acids contain four bases, codons could specify 4^3 (64) amino acids. The same genetic code (Fig. 5.33) is seen in most living organisms, so it is said to be universal. It is nonoverlapping and comma free.

Since there are 64 codons but only 20 amino acids are commonly used in polypeptide synthesis, a large proportion of the codons could be considered redundant. However, the code is degenerate and more than one codon exists for each amino acid. Codons in the mRNA transcript are recognized by the three-nucleotide "anticodon" tRNA molecules charged with the appropriate amino acid.

99

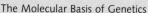

Standard genetic code								
First base (5′)	**Second base**							**Third base (3′)**
	U		C		A		G	
U	UUU phe	UCU ser		UAU tyr		UGU cys		U
	UUC phe	UCC ser		UAC tyr		UGC cys		C
	UUA leu	UCA ser		UAA stop		UGA stop		A
	UUG leu	UCG ser		UAG stop		UGG trp		G
C	CUU leu	CCU pro		CAU his		CGU arg		U
	CUC leu	CCC pro		CAC his		CGC arg		C
	CUA leu	CCA pro		CAA gln		CGA arg		A
	CUG leu	CCG pro		CAG gln		CGG arg		G
A	AUU ile	ACU thr		AAU asn		AGU ser		U
	AUC ile	ACC thr		AAC asn		AGC ser		C
	AUA ile	ACA thr		AAA lys		AGA arg		A
	AUG met	ACG thr		AAG lys		AGG arg		G
G	GUU val	GCU ala		GAU asp		GGU gly		U
	GUC val	GCC ala		GAC asp		GGC gly		C
	GUA val	GCA ala		GAA glu		GGA gly		A
	GUG val	GCG ala		GAG glu		GGG gly		G

Fig. 5.33 Standard genetic code. (A, adenine; C, cytosine; G, guanine; T, thymine; U, uracil.) To find out which amino acid a particular codon codes for, first select the 5′ end base (left column). Then read across to select the column corresponding to the second position base. Read down to find the 3′ end base (right column) and locate the row on which the corresponding amino acid lies. (Adapted from Nussbaum, McInnes, and Willard, 2001.)

Allowed wobble pairings in the third codon–anticodon position	
5′-anticodon base	**3′-codon base**
C	G
A	U
U	A or G
G	U or C
I	U, C or A

Fig. 5.34 Wobble hypothesis. Base pairing possibilities between the 3′ nucleotide of the codon and the 5′ nucleotide of the anticodon. For example, a tRNA that has U in the 5′ position will be able to recognize two different codons, XXA and XXG. (A, adenine; C, cytosine; G, guanine; I, inosine; T, thymine; U, uracil; X, the base recognized by a hypothetical tRNA.)

Codons that differ in the third base may be recognized by the same tRNA, while those that differ in the first or second bases are not. The "wobble hypothesis" seeks to explain this by suggesting that the third base in tRNA anticodons allows for a certain amount of play (or "wobble"), and so it may bind a variety of bases (Fig. 5.34).

Three codons (UAA, UAG, and UGA) are not recognized by tRNAs, and these are termed stop codons. They mark the end of a polypeptide and signal to the ribosome to stop synthesis.

Mitochondrial DNA

Mitochondria contain their own DNA, which differs from that in the rest of the cell. Human mitochondrial DNA consists of 16 kb of circular dsDNA. It codes for:
- 22 mitochondrial (mt) tRNAs.
- 2 mt rRNAs.
- 13 proteins synthesized by the mitochondrion's own protein-synthesizing machinery. All are subunits of the oxidative phosphorylation pathway.

The differences between mitochondrial DNA code and nuclear DNA code are shown in Fig. 5.35. Codon/anticodon pairings show more "wobble" pairings than in the process originating in the nucleus. This is made possible by unusual mt tRNA sequences such as mt tRNA^ser, which lacks a D arm.

Protein synthesis in prokaryotes

The components needed for translation are mRNA, tRNA, ribosome, GTP, initiation factors, and elongation factors.

Variations between mitochondrial and standard genetic code		
	Standard	Mammalian mitochondrion
UGA	Stop	Trp
AUA	Ile	Met (initiation signal)
CUN	Leu	—
AGA/AGG	Arg	Stop
CGG	Arg	—

Fig. 5.35 Summary of variations between mitochondrial and standard genetic code. (N, one of four nucleotides.)

Amino acids combine with their corresponding tRNA in a reaction catalyzed by a specific aminoacyl transferase:

Aminoacyl transferase

Amino acid + tRNA → Aminoacyl-tRNA

This incorporates a high-energy ester bond between the aminoacyl group and the 3′ CCA group of the tRNA. This is known as "charging" the tRNA. The energy released when this bond is broken drives the peptide bond formation step of chain elongation. Like transcription, translation consists of three stages: initiation, elongation, and termination.

Initiation

The initiation complex is composed of a ribosome, mRNA, and initiator tRNA. The process of initiation requires:
- Three initiation factors, IF-1, IF-2, and IF-3.
- A molecule of GTP.

In prokaryotic cells both transcription and translation take place in the cytoplasm. In eukaryotic cells, transcription takes place in the nucleus and translation occurs in the cytoplasm. The two processes are separate and DNA never comes into contact with ribosomes.

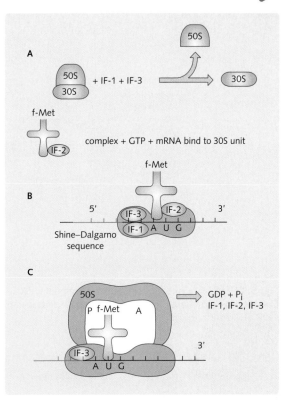

Fig. 5.36 Initiation factors of prokaryotic translation. (A) IF-1 and IF-3 bind to 30S subunit of ribosome to promote dissociation of 50S subunit. (B) f-Met–IF-2 complex and GTP and mRNA bind to 30S unit. IF-2 is required for f-Met-tRNA binding to mRNA. f-Met-tRNA–mRNA binding is not, therefore, dependent upon codon–anticodon association. IF-3 assists ribosomal binding to the Shine–Dalgarno sequence on mRNA. (C) IF-3 is released and GTP hydrolyzed. The 50S subunit associates and IF-1 and IF-2 are released. f-Met-tRNA lies in the P site so the A site is ready to accept incoming tRNA. (Note that f-Met-tRNA is the only tRNA that does not enter the ribosome via the A site.)

Initiator tRNA is f-met-tRNA. It carries a formylated methionine residue, and it recognizes an AUG codon on the mRNA. Each mRNA contains many AUG codons in its various reading frames. The one corresponding to the start of translation is preceded by a purine-rich tract of nucleotides called the Shine–Dalgarno sequence. This binds to a corresponding pyrimidine-rich sequence in the ribosomal S unit (Fig. 5.36).

Elongation

Chain elongation involves the addition of aminoacyl residues to the growing polypeptide. It is a three-stage process.

101

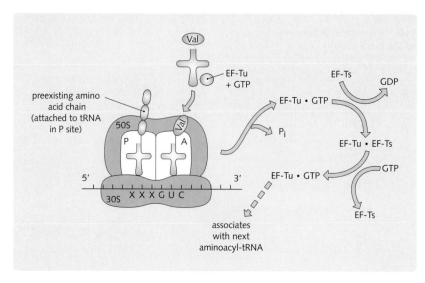

Fig. 5.37 Step one of chain elongation: aminoacyl-tRNA binding to ribosomal A site. Elongation factors EF-Tu and EF-Ts interact to liberate EF-Tu, which can then associate with another free aminoacyl-tRNA. GTP is hydrolyzed to GDP + P_i during this recycling process.

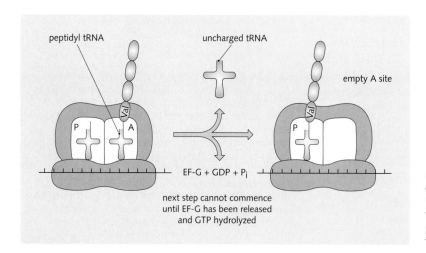

Fig. 5.38 Step three of chain elongation: translocation. Unchanged tRNA is expelled from the A site and the peptidyl-tRNA is transferred from the A site to the P site.

Step one

Aminoacyl-tRNA binds to the ribosomal A site (Fig. 5.37) as follows:

- Complex of aminoacyl-tRNA, GTP, and elongation factor Tu (EF-Tu) is formed.
- Codon–anticodon binding with concomitant hydrolysis of GTP.
- Release of GDP and inorganic phosphate (P_i) and EF-Tu.

Step two

Peptide bond formation is catalyzed by a peptidyl transferase in the 50S subunit. Peptidyl group in the P site is added onto the aminoacyl group in the

A site. The reaction is driven by a high-energy ester bond between the aminoacyl group and tRNA.

Step three

The translocation (Fig. 5.38) process occurs as follows:

- Uncharged tRNA is expelled.
- Peptidyl-tRNA is transferred from the A site to the P site. This requires EF-G and GTP.
- The tRNA is still bound to the mRNA codon, so, as the peptidyl-tRNA moves across from the A site to the P site, the mRNA moves with it. A new codon now lies in the A site. This

Comparison between prokaryotic and eukaryotic translation		
	Prokaryotes	**Eukaryotes**
Ribosome	Large subunit 50S, small subunit 30S, whole ribosome 70S	Large subunit 60S, small subunit 40S, whole ribosome 80S
Initiation	Three initiation factors called IF-1, 2, 3; initiator tRNA carries f-Met (formylated methionine); start codon AUG; Shine-Dalgarno sequence precedes the start site on the mRNA; binds to a complementary sequence on the ribosome's S subunit	Over 10 initiation factors with multiple subunits called eIFs ("e" for eukaryote); initiator IRNA carries Met (not N-formylated); start codon AUG; no Shine-Dalgarno sequence, mRNA 5'-methylated cap may have a binding site on ribosome S subunit to guide translation complex to start site
Type of mRNA code	Polycistronic (mRNA often codes for more than one protein)	Monocistronic (mRNA always codes for a single protein)
Elongation	Elongation factors called EF-Tu, EF-Ts, and EF-G	EF-Tu and EF-Ts are replaced by a single factor, eEF-1; EF-G replaced by eEF-2
Termination	Three release factors, RF-1, 2, 3; RF-3 is bound to GTP and the RF-3–GTP complex stimulates ribosomal binding of RF-1 and 2; GTP hydrolysis triggers complex to disassemble	Single release factor, eRF, which binds to the ribosome with GTP; GTP hydrolysis triggers eRF release from ribosome

Fig. 5.39 Comparison between prokaryotic and eukaryotic translation.

mechanism allows the reading frame to be maintained.

Termination
The termination codons, UAA, UAG, and UGA, are recognized by release factors (RFs) rather than tRNAs:
- RF-1 recognizes UAA and UAG.
- RF-2 recognizes UAA and UGA.
- RF-3, which binds GTP, stimulates ribosomal binding of RF-1 and RF-2.

The binding of an RF causes the peptidyl transferase to transfer the peptidyl group to water rather than to an aminoacyl group. This results in the release of a free polypeptide. The uncharged tRNA is released from the ribosome and the RFs are expelled.

Protein synthesis in eukaryotes
Protein synthesis is very similar in eukaryotes, but more associated factors are involved. Figure 5.39 compares prokaryotic and eukaryotic translation.

Endoplasmic reticulum
Endoplasmic reticulum (ER) is a diffuse system of membrane-bound cisternae in the cytoplasm of eukaryotic cells (see Chapter 1). There are two types—rough endoplasmic reticulum (RER) and smooth endoplasmic reticulum (SER). The membranes of RER have ribosomes attached to them, and they are specialized for the synthesis and secretion of proteins. The SER is devoid of ribosomes. It is responsible for the synthesis of cholesterol and phospholipids, and it is prominent in cells that are active in lipid biosynthesis such as liver cells.

Proteins bound for organelles, plasma membrane, or export enter the ER lumen as they are translated, following interactions between specific proteins on the ribosome, ER membrane, and in the cytoplasm.

Factors affecting protein synthesis
Elongation factors and bacterial toxins
EFs are vital to the process of translation. For example the *E. coli* factor EF-Tu controls the rate-limiting step of translation. In the cytoplasm of normal *E. coli* cells, every aminoacyl-tRNA is sequestered by an EF-Tu protein. In the absence of this factor the rate of protein synthesis is too slow to support cell growth.

Bacterial toxins can block translation. The toxin produced by *Corynebacterium diphtheriae* (the

103

Antibiotics that inhibit translation		
Antibiotic	Site of action	Process inhibited
Streptomycin	Prokaryote ribosomal 30S subunit	Initiation/elongation (causes mRNA misreading)
Erythromycin	Prokaryote 50S subunit	Translocation
Chloramphenicol	Prokaryote 50S subunit	Peptidyl transferase
Cycloheximide	Eukaryote 60S subunit	Peptidyl transferase
Tetracycline	Prokaryote 30S subunit	Aminoacyl tRNA binding to ribosome A site
Puromycin	Ribosome	Peptide transfer causes premature termination as it mimics an aminoacyl tRNA

Fig. 5.40 Antibiotics that inhibit translation.

organism causing diphtheria), for example, inhibits translation by inactivating EF-2.

Antibiotics and protein synthesis

Many antibiotics block protein synthesis, either by blocking translation or by other means. Some are particularly useful therapeutically because they specifically target prokaryote translation (Fig. 5.40).

Antibiotics and mitochondria

The translation process in eukaryotic mitochondria is very similar to that in prokaryotes. Antibiotics that inhibit prokaryotic protein synthesis can also affect mitochondrial protein synthesis. Antibiotics, however, do not harm their mammalian host because:

- Some antibiotics are unable to cross the inner mitochondrial membrane.
- Mitochondria are replaced at cell division. This occurs relatively slowly in most cells so mitochondria are depleted only with long-term antibiotic use.
- In rapidly dividing cells, the local environment can sometimes prevent uptake of antibiotic (e.g., in bone, high calcium levels cause the formation of calcium–tetracycline so the drug cannot be taken up by cells in the bone marrow).

Control of gene expression and protein synthesis

Control of protein synthesis is synonymous with control of gene expression. In the prokaryote, control can be at the level of transcription or translation. The situation is more complex in eukaryotes and a total of six control points have been identified (Fig. 5.41).

Constitutive, inducible, and repressible enzymes

Constitutive enzymes are present at fixed concentrations in the cell, irrespective of changes in the cell environment. They are examples of products of housekeeping genes in multicellular organisms.

The level of expression of inducible/repressible enzymes is altered by the cellular environment. A certain chemical may induce the expression of a gene, while another chemical may repress its expression.

Enzyme induction can be a side effect of drug treatments that cause important drug interactions, for example, treatment with phenytoin and warfarin. Phenytoin is a liver enzyme inducer and it causes increased levels of the enzyme system that metabolizes warfarin, so if the drugs are taken together the warfarin is rapidly metabolized and high doses are required to keep it in the therapeutic range. Subsequent withdrawal of the phenytoin will cause the enzyme induction to cease, and this can cause a rebound hemorrhage due to the massively increased systemic levels of warfarin.

Transcriptional regulation

Control at the level of transcription is important in the regulation of gene expression in both prokaryotes and eukaryotes.

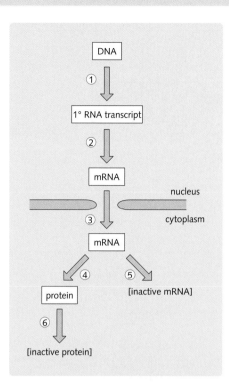

Fig. 5.41 Eukaryotic control of gene expression. (1) Transcription control. (2) Processing of transcript. (3) Transport control. (4) Translational control by selection of ribosomes by mRNA. (5) mRNA degradation control. (6) Protein activity control and posttranslational modification.

Prokaryotes

Prokaryotes live in environments where competition for the available nutrients is fierce. It is clearly advantageous for bacteria to have the ability to metabolize a wide variety of nutrients. However, synthesizing proteins consumes energy and so bacteria regulate the proteins they are expressing at any one time.

Some enzymes, such as those required for lactose catabolism, are only synthesized when the appropriate substrate is present (in this case lactose). The control of expression of these genes is said to be by induction.

Other enzymes, such as those required for the synthesis of tryptophan, are controlled by repression. Tryptophan is essential for cell survival, so the enzymes that synthesize this amino acid are expressed constitutively. However, if tryptophan happens to be present in the growth media, expression of these genes is turned off.

Regulation of genes in response to changes in nutrient supply is very efficient in bacteria because all the functionally related genes in a metabolic pathway are regulated by one promoter. A series of genes whose regulation is coordinated is called an operon (Fig. 5.42).

Eukaryotes

Transcriptional regulation in eukaryotes is much more complex than in prokaryotes. In multicellular organisms, although the DNA complement in all cell types is the same, the genes expressed from it vary immensely. Whole sections of the genome are permanently repressed during the process of differentiation (see Chapter 1). The details of this are poorly understood, but it is thought that chromatin packing and epigenetic mechanisms are important.

Difference in chromatin structure between cell types determines whether specific transcriptional activators and repressors are expressed. These bind to enhancers and silencers respectively and influence the levels of transcription of individual genes in a tissue-specific manner.

Even within active euchromatin the expression of genes is subject to regulation according to the needs of the whole organism. Thus, signaling cascades initiated by hormones in response to changes in the external environment will ultimately alter gene expression (see Chapter 3). Similarly, changes in the cellular internal environment may result in changes in gene expression (for example, an accumulation of DNA damage will trigger the expression of apoptosis genes).

Micro RNA and small interfering RNA

Gene expression can also be regulated through the action of RNA interference (RNAi). Micro RNA (miRNA) and small interfering RNA (siRNA) molecules are both small, double-stranded RNA fragments with a high degree of homology to specific genes. Under certain conditions, these molecules are capable of silencing or modulating gene expression by inhibiting translation of the RNA transcript. Hypothesized as a cellular defense mechanism against viruses, RNA interference is conserved across a wide range of organisms, including mammals.

Double-stranded RNA introduced into the cytoplasm can be cleaved into short RNA

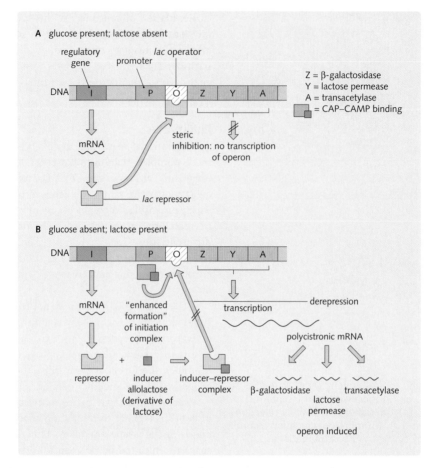

Fig. 5.42 The *lac* operon. (A) The "*lac* repressor" binds to the "*lac* operator" with great affinity. The *lac* operator is formed by a stretch of DNA that overlaps with the operon's initiation site. *lac* repressor binding prevents the formation of a transcription initiation complex so transcription cannot occur. (B) Lactose binds to the *lac* repressor and changes its shape so it has a much lower affinity for the *lac* operator, and derepression occurs. An initiation complex forms and transcription begins. At the same time, low levels of glucose cause an increase in intracellular cAMP, which binds to catabolite activator protein (CAP). The CAP–cAMP complex binds to the *lac* operon promoter region and encourages the formation of an RNA initiation complex. (A, Y, Z, are genes for transacetylase, lactose permease, and β-galactosidase, respectively.)

fragments (19–25 nucleotides long) by a specific endonuclease called dicer. The subsequent short RNAs, now known as siRNA, are incorporated into a multiprotein RNA-induced silencing complex (RISC). The single-stranded siRNA molecule, now bound to RISC, searches through the cytoplasmic pool of RNA transcripts for complementary full-length mRNAs. The identified mRNAs are then cleaved by slicer, an endonuclease contained within RISC. The cleavage effectively silences gene expression. Micro RNAs (miRNAs) are also short, single-stranded RNAs that are generated by dicer cleavage of longer pre-miRNA fragments. Unlike

siRNA, however, miRNA fragments are not transcribed from the genes they ultimately silence, but from other regions of the genome—areas where no genes are currently believed to exist. Additionally, although the miRNAs do bind RISC, the entire complex does not cleave and degrade the target mRNA but rather binds the mRNA and inhibits its translation. It is estimated that between 200 and 300 miRNAs exist in the human genome.

In model systems, RNAi techniques have been used to effectively target and "knock down" the expression of specific genes. Consequently, the therapeutic potential of RNAi (delivered as RNA in liposomes or in a viral expression vector) for infectious and cancerous disease is now being actively investigated.

Epigenetic mechanisms

When a specific cell type replicates, the daughter cells retain the structural characteristics of the parent cell. This suggests that the changes in chromatin structure initiated in differentiation can be transmitted. Epigenetic mechanisms are those that exert a heritable influence on gene activity that is not accompanied by a change in DNA sequence. Examples include histone modification and methylation.

Posttranslational modification of proteins

Concepts

Posttranslational modification is the alteration of proteins after translation. These modifications give the mature protein functional activity and include peptide cleavage and covalent modifications, such as glycosylation, phosphorylation, carboxylation, and hydroxylation of specific residues.

A newly synthesized protein may be destined for extracellular secretion, the cytoplasm, or organelles such as the plasma membrane, nucleus, or lysosomes. Proteins are directed to the appropriate location by:

- Conserved amino acid sequence motifs (e.g., the signal peptide and the nuclear targeting signal).
- Moieties added by posttranslational modification (e.g., mannose-6-phosphate for lysosomal delivery).

Signal peptide

The signal peptide (or leader sequence) is not strictly related to posttranslational modification, but it is involved in a process vital to it. It is a characteristic hydrophobic amino acid sequence of 18–30 amino acid residues near the amino terminus of the polypeptide that directs noncytoplasmic polypeptides into the ER lumen as they are translated (Fig. 5.43).

Inside the ER lumen the polypeptide can undergo posttranslational modifications specific to each protein. Proteins destined for extracellular secretion are transported to the Golgi apparatus in vesicles that bud off the ER. Further modification may take place here and the secreted protein is packaged into vesicles that fuse with the cell plasma membrane, releasing their contents to the exterior.

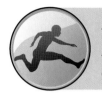

All proteins are translocated into the ER lumen except those destined for the cytoplasm.

Glycosylation of proteins

Glycosylation occurs in the ER lumen or the Golgi apparatus, and it involves the addition of an oligosaccharide to specific amino acid residues. There are two types of glycosylation, designated N-linked and O-linked, that employ specific glycosyltransferases:

- N-linked—the oligosaccharide is added to the polypeptide by a β-N-glycosidic bond to an aspartate residue.
- O-linked—the oligosaccharide is an α-O-glycosidic bond to a serine or threonine residue.

Glycosylation is important for the functioning of some proteins and the correct compartmentalization of others:

- O-linked glycosylation is involved in the production of blood group antigens.
- N-linked glycosylation is involved in the transfer of acid hydrolase to lysosomes and the production of mature antibodies.

Other modification of proteins

Proteins may be modified by (Fig. 5.44):

- Phosphorylation, which targets Ser or Tyr residues and tends to regulate enzyme activity (Ser) or protein activity (Tyr). Kinases transfer phosphate groups from ATP onto the target residue.
- Sulfation, which targets Tyr. It is important in compartmentalization (e.g., marking proteins for export) and biological activity.
- Hydroxylation, which targets Lys and Pro residues. It is very important in the production of collagen (and extracellular matrix protein). The hydroxylation of Lys and Pro residues occurs during translation, and it is essential for the formation of the collagen triple helix.

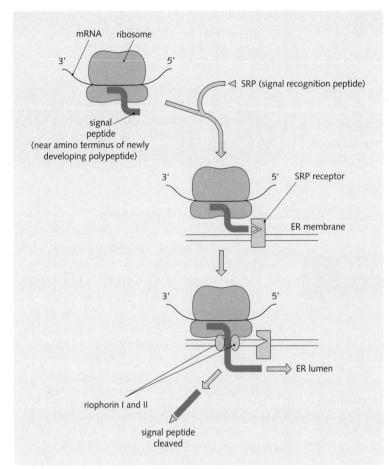

Fig. 5.43 Role of the signal peptide in translocation into the endoplasmic reticulum (ER) lumen. The signal peptide is near the amino terminus of the newly developing polypeptide. It associates with a cytoplasmic signal recognition peptide (SRP) and then with an SRP receptor ("docking protein") on the ER membrane. The ribosome then interlocks between two membrane-associated proteins, riophorin I and II, which drive the developing polypeptide into the ER lumen.

Summary of some posttranslational modifications				
Destination	**Protein function**	**Modification**	**Residue**	**Example**
Secreted	Structural	Hydroxylation	Lys/Pro	Collagen
	Enzyme	Hydrolytic cleavage	(peptide bond)	Pepsinogen → pepsin
	Hormone	Hydrolytic cleavage	(peptide bond)	Proinsulin → insulin
	Clotting factor	Carboxylation	Glu	Prothrombin → thrombin
	Antibody	Glycosylation (*N*-linked)	Asp	IgG
Membrane	Receptor	Lipidation	Gly/Cys	Antibody receptors
	Cell recognition	Glycosylation (*O*-linked)	Ser	Blood group antigens
	Receptor activation	Phosphorylation	Tyr	Growth factor receptor activation
Cytoplasm	Enzyme	Phosphorylation	Tyr	Activation
Lysosome	Hydrolytic enzymes	Glycosylation (*N*-linked)	Asp	Acid hydrolases

Fig. 5.44 Summary of some posttranslational modifications.

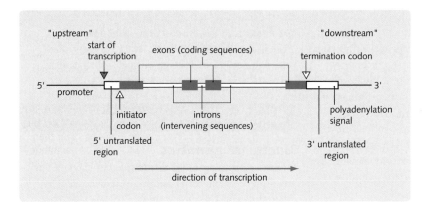

Fig. 5.45 Structure of a typical eukaryotic gene. The first and final exons include sequence that is transcribed and present in the mature mRNA, but not translated. These are called the 5′ and 3′ UTR (untranslated regions) respectively. Note that this diagram is not to scale and in reality the average intron is much longer than the average exon. (Adapted from Nussbaum, McInnes, and Willard, 2001.)

- Lipidation of Cys and Gly residues, which is necessary for anchoring proteins such as antibody receptors into the membrane.
- Acetylation of Lys, which can change the charge of the residue. In histone H4, this alters its binding properties to DNA.
- Cleavage, which activates some enzymes and hormones.

Disorders of posttranslational modification

I-cell disease is a lysosomal storage disease characterized by psychomotor retardation, skeletal deformation, and early death. It results from a deficiency of mannose-6-phosphate glycosyltransferase, which is responsible for glycosylation of enzymes destined for lysosomes. All the cells' lysosomal enzymes lack their recognition markers, so they are secreted into the extracellular matrix rather than being taken up by lysosomes. Consequently, undigested substrates accumulate within the lysosomes with severe pathological consequences (see also Chapter 4).

Structure of genes

Eukaryotic genes

A protein-coding gene is a nucleotide coding sequence that results in the production of a functional mRNA and polypeptide. The "one gene, one polypeptide" hypothesis states that the base sequence of DNA determines the amino acid sequence in a single corresponding polypeptide.

The typical eukaryotic gene contains both exons and introns (Fig. 5.45). Exons are expressed sequences (i.e., ones that code for amino acids) and introns are the noncoding intervening sequences. The length of a typical exon is a few hundred base pairs whereas introns tend to be several kilobases long. Introns are:

- Rare in prokaryotic genes.
- Uncommon in lower eukaryotes such as yeast.
- Abundant in higher eukaryotes (vertebrate structural genes rarely lack introns).

The 3′ untranslated region (3′ UTR) contains a consensus polyadenylation signal. The promoter region lies in the 5′ DNA immediately preceding a gene and is sometimes called the "upstream flanking region." Sequence analysis studies have revealed "consensus" sequences in prokaryotes and eukaryotes, which are vital for promoter function. The most conserved sequence in the *E. coli* promoter is the TATAAT box, which forms the initial binding site for the transcription enzyme RNAP. The situation is more complex in eukaryotes. More consensus sequences have been detected and include the GC box (GGGCGG), the TATA box, and the CAAT box. Each region has been shown to bind specific transcription factors. Eukaryotic genes may also require enhancer sequences for physiological expression that may be situated many kilobases from the start of transcription.

Gene structure and evolution
Introns

Eukaryotic genes contain introns, whereas prokaryotic genes do not. Given that eukaryotes are thought to have evolved from prokaryotes, it seems intuitive that introns arose at some point in this process. However, many believe that ancient

109

prokaryotes did have introns, but have since lost them.

Exons often encode functional protein domains. If these are separated by long introns, then any chromosome break is likely to be in a noncoding region. Such breakage may lead to recombinational exchange between genes, "shuffling" new combinations of exons together, to produce new, potentially advantageous proteins. If this process were to occur in the absence of introns, it is likely that the new protein would be out of frame, and the functional domains would be lost.

Prokaryotes typically exist in environments where competition for resources is fierce and replication of large amounts of DNA places a huge energetic burden. It is proposed that introns were consequently lost after prokaryotes had evolved most of their current repertoire of proteins.

Gene duplication
Gene duplication is a rare consequence of normal recombinational events. Duplicated genes are free to mutate and evolve new functions and patterns of expression, since they are not required for the survival of the organism. The mechanism of gene duplication events means that some functionally related proteins, such as the family of β-globin genes and the human leucocyte antigen (HLA) complex, are each clustered close together on the same chromosome.

HLA complex
The HLA complex on the short arm of chromosome 6 is an example of a gene cluster. The term haplotype describes a cluster of alleles (alleles are alternative versions of a gene) that occur together on a DNA segment and are inherited together. The HLA haplotype genes:
- Are mostly members of the immunoglobulin superfamily—a family of hundreds of genes, which occur throughout the human genome and are involved in cell surface recognition.
- Share sets of related exons that they have evolved from an ancestral gene by duplication.
- Are characterized by the presence of immunoglobulin "domains" (or folds) consisting of 110 amino acid residues stabilized by a disulfide bridge.

There are three classes of HLA genes. Classes I and II are also known as the histocompatibility

or transplant rejection genes as they are responsible for organ transplant rejection, although their principal function seems to be in "presentation" and recognition of foreign antigens (Fig. 5.46).

Genetics of bacteria and viruses

Bacterial genetics
There are fundamental differences in the cellular machinery of bacterial and mammalian cells, so mammals can tolerate some chemicals that are toxic to bacteria. Humans can take antimicrobial agents in appropriate amounts to treat bacterial infections without harming the host. (NB an antibiotic is an antimicrobial agent manufactured by living organisms rather than by chemical synthesis.) A summary of the differences between bacterial and human cells is given in Fig. 5.47.

Antimicrobial agents
Inhibitors of nucleic acid synthesis
These agents:
- Target the folic acid synthesis pathway. (This pathway produces tetrahydrofolate, which is essential for base synthesis.)
- Do not affect mammalian cells because mammals obtain folic acid from their diet.
- Are bacteriostatic—they halt bacterial growth but do not kill them.

Sulfonamides (e.g., sulfadiazine) are analogs of γ-aminobenzoic acid. Trimethoprim inhibits bacterial but not eukaryotic dihydrofolate reductase. It is used in the treatment of urinary tract infections.

Inhibitors of DNA gyrase
Quinolones (e.g., ciprofloxacin) inhibit DNA gyrase, the enzyme that causes DNA unwinding. They are bactericidal, i.e., they kill bacteria.

Inhibitors of cell-wall synthesis
The bacterial cell wall is rigid, and it contains linear peptidoglycans, which are cross-linked by peptides. An important group of antimicrobials disrupt cell-wall synthesis by inhibiting formation of cross-links. They all contain a β-lactam ring that gives them their antimicrobial activity. They are bactericidal, and they are not effective against Gram-negative bacteria because they cannot penetrate the phospholipid-rich outer membrane.

Fig. 5.46 (A) Diagram to illustrate the classification of human leucocyte antigen (HLA) haplotype genes. (B) Features of different classes of HLA genes.

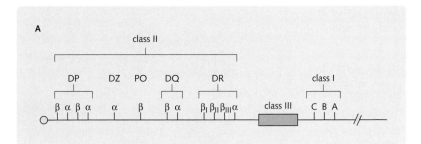

B	Classification of the HLA haplotype genes		
	Class I	**Class II**	**Class III**
Main products	A, B, C code for α_1, α_2, α_3 proteins, which complex with β_2 microglobulin coded for on chromosome 15	DR, DP, DQ	Complement components C4a, C4b, TNF, etc.
Expressed	On surface of all cells except erythrocytes	By antigen-presenting cells (e.g., macrophages and B lymphocytes)	
Structure		Each has an α and a β domain	Sequence homologies with class I and class II

	Differences between bacterial and human cells	
	Bacterial	**Human**
Form of genetic material	Prokaryotic, no nucleus or nucleolus, single DNA thread tightly coiled by topoisomerases, extrachromosomal elements called plasmids, double stranded	Eukaryotic, linear DNA, associated with proteins to form chromosomes, double stranded
Cell size	Average diameter 0.5–5μm	Up to 40μm
Protein synthesis	Ribosomal subunits 50S and 30S	Subunits 60S and 40S
Nucleic acid synthesis	Folate must be synthesized *de novo* for base synthesis	Folate can be obtained from the diet
Organelles	Few, associated with respiration and photosynthesis	Many and diverse

Fig. 5.47 Summary of the differences between bacterial and human cells.

Penicillins were the first group of antibiotics to be discovered, and they are still important clinically. Benzylpenicillin:
- Is used in the treatment of pneumococcal, streptococcal, and meningococcal infections.
- Is not effective orally so it is given by injection.

Cephalosporins have a similar spectrum to penicillin, although individual agents are active against certain bacteria. Cefuroxime is used prophylactically in surgery. It is active against *Staphylococcus aureus* (Gram positive) and is resistant to bacterial β-lactamase. Ceftazidime is active against *Pseudomonas aeruginosa*, which can cause infections in immunosuppressed patients.

Inhibitors of protein synthesis

Protein synthesis is an important site for antibiotic action. Clinically used protein synthesis inhibitors such as tetracycline, kanamycin, and erythromycin target prokaryotic ribosomes (50S L subunit and 30S S subunit), and they do not affect mammalian ribosomes (60S L subunit and 40S S subunit).

Transfer of genetic material

Although bacteria are not strictly capable of sexual reproduction, they may exchange genetic material by three mechanisms:

- Transformation—certain bacteria release DNA into the environment that can be taken up by other bacteria via specific receptors. If the DNA is compatible, it is incorporated into the bacterial genome; otherwise, it is degraded by exonucleases.
- Transduction—a fragment of bacterial DNA may become incorporated into a bacteriophage (a virus that infects bacteria) during its assembly. One in 10^6 bacteriophages contain such bacterial DNA. This may be introduced into the host cell along with viral genes during the infection process. Again, if the bacterial DNA is compatible it can be integrated into the host's genome.
- Conjugation—this is sometimes loosely called bacterial sexual reproduction. Bacteria may be designated F positive (F^+) or F negative (F^-). F^+ cells possess a plasmid (extra-chromosomal piece of genetic material) called the F factor, which includes genes for a cytoplasmic projection called a pilus. The pilus gives F^+ cells the ability to attach to other bacterial cells. In this way it forms cytoplasmic bridges through which genetic material may then be transferred after it has been replicated by "rolling circle replication." This process is called conjugation (Fig. 5.48).

Usually F plasmids exist as extrachromosomal circles of DNA. However, occasionally one may become integrated into the bacterial genome, resulting in Hfr (high frequency of recombination) cells. When this happens, the whole bacterial chromosome may be replicated by rolling circle replication, starting at an origin in the F factor. The replicated DNA, that now includes bacterial chromosomal material,

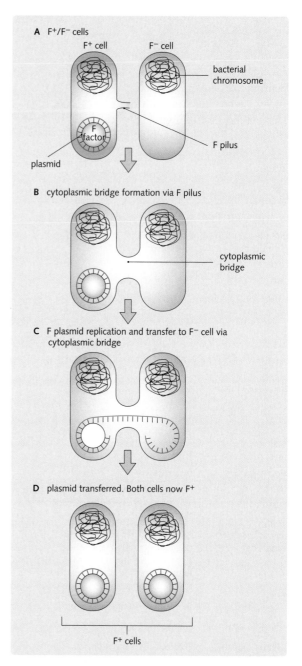

Fig. 5.48 Bacterial conjugation. (A) The ability to conjugate is conferred by a plasmid called the F factor. Bacteria with the plasmid are F^+. (B) F^+ cells contain thread-like projections called F pili, which can attach to F^- cells to form a cytoplasmic bridge. (C) F plasmid is replicated and a single-stranded replica is transferred along the bridge. (D) Within the recipient, the transferred material is replicated to form a new plasmid.

is passed along the cytoplasmic bridge into the recipient cell. Variable amounts of DNA are transferred because the bridge invariably breaks down before the whole chromosome has been transmitted. The transmitted material may then undergo recombination with the host chromosome. This process has been exploited to "map" the order of genes on bacterial chromosomes.

Occasionally, an F plasmid that has integrated into the genome may "pop-out" again, taking part of the bacterial chromosome with it. These are called F′ plasmids and may act as a vehicle to transmit bacterial genes to new hosts.

The conjugation process is another way for prokaryotes to "mix up" their gene pool and adapt to their environment. This process is important because it can contribute to the spread of antibiotic resistance genes such as those in methicillin-resistant *S. aureus* (MRSA), which is resistant to most clinically used antibiotics.

Viral genetics

Viruses are infectious particles consisting of a nucleic acid enclosed in a protein coat called the capsid, which may or may not be surrounded by a phospholipid envelope. They adsorb onto the surface of susceptible cells and inject their nucleic acid. They are ultimate parasites as they have no metabolism of their own and rely entirely on their host for replication and production of new virus particles. They contain either DNA or RNA, never both. The life cycle of a virus has ten stages (Fig. 5.49).

One of the most significant challenges in gene therapy is getting the therapeutic piece of DNA through the plasma membrane to the nucleus, while avoiding lysosomal degradation. Viruses have evolved very efficient mechanisms for doing this and, therefore, many gene therapy protocols exploit viral vectors (see Chapter 6).

DNA viruses

The viral DNA is transcribed into mRNA using host RNA polymerase (in the nucleus). The mRNA diffuses into the cytoplasm, associates with ribosomes, and is translated into viral proteins. These are either:

- Structural—used to assemble new virions (individual virus particles).
- Nonstructural—mainly enzymes involved in replication of the viral genome.

Details of some important DNA viruses are given in Fig. 5.50.

RNA viruses

There are two types of ssRNA viruses, designated positive- and negative-sense viruses.

In positive-sense viruses, the RNA can act as mRNA, and it is immediately translated into viral proteins.

Negative-sense RNA cannot act as mRNA. Positive-sense RNA is synthesized from the negative strand with an RNA-dependent polymerase, which assembles from the nucleoprotein subunits in the viral particle when the virus first infects its host.

Examples of some important RNA viruses are given in Fig. 5.51.

Retroviruses (including HIV)

Retroviruses are positive-sense ssRNA viruses that produce a DNA intermediate with a unique enzyme called reverse transcriptase (Figs 5.52 and 5.53).

Human immunodeficiency viruses HIV-1 and HIV-2 are important retroviruses. They are responsible for the worldwide pandemic of acquired immune deficiency syndrome (AIDS). HIV-1 has spread worldwide; HIV-2 is localized to West Africa. In 1995, an estimated 18 million people were HIV positive. By December 2005 this figure had risen to nearly 41 million. HIV is transmitted:

- In blood (needlestick injury, sharing needles).
- By sexual contact (heterosexual and homosexual).
- From mother to baby.

HIV attacks the immune system and progressively destroys it. It specifically targets CD4-positive (CD4+) cells (T helper cells and macrophages) by binding onto the CD4 receptor. The viral DNA

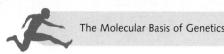

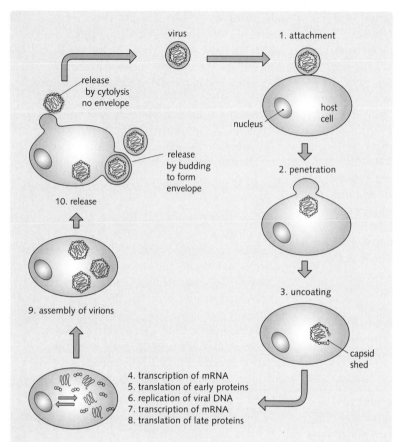

Fig. 5.49 Life cycle of a virus. In order to replicate, each virus must infect a host cell and "hijack" its cellular machinery. For the cycle to continue, the newly assembled virions must escape from the original host cell so that they can go on to infect new host cells. The ten stages that the virus must successfully pass through to complete this cycle are shown.

Some important DNA viruses			
Class	**Family**	**Species**	**Disease**
Double-stranded DNA	Papovaviridae	Papillomavirus	Human warts
	Adenoviridae	Adenovirus	Pharyngitis, acute respiratory disease, acute gastroenteritis
	Herpesviridae	Herpes simplex (HSV)	Cold sores (type I), genital herpes (type II)
		Varicella zoster virus (VZV)	Chickenpox (varicella), shingles (zoster)
		Epstein–Barr (EBV)	Glandular fever (infectious mononucleosis)
		Cytomegalovirus (CMV)	CMV retinitis (immunocompromised)
	Poxviridae	Variola virus Vaccinia virus	Smallpox Vaccinia
Single-stranded DNA	Parvoviridae	Human parvovirus B19	Aplastic crisis in sickle cell disease patient

Fig. 5.50 Some important DNA viruses.

Some important RNA viruses			
Class	Family	Species	Disease
Double-stranded RNA	Reoviridae	Human rotavirus	Acute gastroenteritis
	Enteroviruses	Poliovirus	Polio
	Togaviridae	Coxsackie B virus Echovirus	Myocarditis, aseptic meningitis Aseptic meningitis, exanthematous disease
	Orthomyxoviridae	Rhinovirus	Common cold
	Paramyxoviridae	Hepatitis A Yellow fever virus Rubella virus Influenza A Influenza B Measles virus Mumps virus	Acute hepatitis Yellow fever Rubelia (German measles) Influenza epidemics Influenza epidemics Measles Mumps
Positive-sense single-stranded RNA	Arenaviridae	Respiratory syncytial virus (RSV)	Acute infantile bronchiolitis
		Parainfluenza virus	Croup
Negative-sense single-stranded RNA	Rhabdoviridae	Lassa virus	Lassa fever
		Rabies virus	Rabies

Fig. 5.51 Some important RNA viruses.

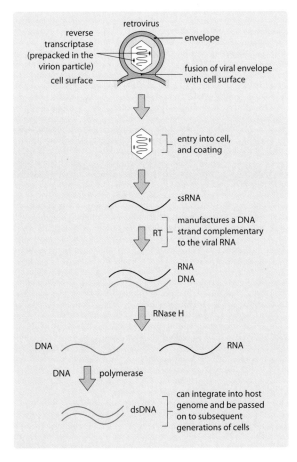

Fig. 5.52 Replication of retroviruses.

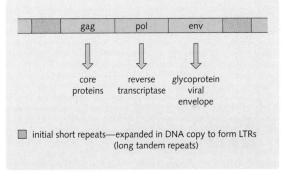

Fig. 5.53 Retrovirus genome—codes for three genes. These are preceded by a noncoding region containing enhancer and promoter regions that facilitate expression of the viral genome by host "machinery."

integrates into the host genome and new virus particles are manufactured.

AIDS is characterized by features of severe immunodeficiency—severe and overwhelming infections and opportunistic cancers.

Drug treatment of HIV/AIDS

Current drug treatments aim to disable the HIV by inhibiting its enzymes. Combinations of drugs can greatly reduce virus load, but it has yet to be proved that they can eradicate the virus from a person who has HIV.

Zidovudine (also called azidothymidine, AZT) is a reverse transcriptase inhibitor. It is an analog of thymidine that is phosphorylated in the host cell and competes with cellular nucleotide triphosphates in the reverse transcription process. Host mitochondrial DNA polymerases are also susceptible to AZT and this probably brings about the side effects. These include anaemia and neutropenia, gastrointestinal disturbance, headache, fever, and skin rash.

Didanosine (ddI) is a synthetic purine dideoxynucleoside that works in the same way as AZT to inhibit reverse transcriptase.

Protease inhibitors such as ritonavir target the enzyme that cuts up newly translated viral multiproteins into individual proteins to allow assembly of new viral particles.

Retroviruses have no mechanism for proofreading, so they have a very high rate of uncorrected mutation: a new mutation occurs approximately every time the 9000 bp genome is replicated. This leads to changes in the proteins of the viral coat and enzymes. Mutations tend to lead to resistance to drug treatments: for example, resistance to AZT developed over 12–18 months.

Combinations of three drugs are, therefore, given to avoid the emergence of a resistant strain of the virus. Trials have shown that a combination of AZT, ddI, and a protease inhibitor can slow disease progress. This treatment regimen is known as HAART (highly active antiretroviral therapy).

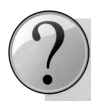

- Describe the structure and function of a nuclear pore.
- Define nucleoli, and explain the significance of a cell having no discernible nucleoli.
- Draw a diagram to show the stages of the cell cycle.
- Explain the role of cyclins in the regulation of the cell cycle.
- Explain the difference between a proto-oncogene and an oncogene. List two examples of oncogenes.
- List the three functions of p53 and with reference to them suggest why p53 is called "the guardian of the genome."
- Define mitosis and meiosis, and highlight the differences between them.
- Define karyotype, genome, haploid, diploid, and gamete.
- List the stages of meiosis (including the five stages of prophase I).
- Describe how nucleosides differ from nucleotides.
- Draw a diagram of the DNA double helix that includes strand polarity. State how many base pairs there are per turn. Describe which bases pair with one another and how many hydrogen bonds are involved.
- Draw a diagram of a tRNA.
- Describe the three levels of DNA packing.
- List four features of active chromatin compared with inactive chromatin.
- Discuss the three mammalian DNA repair mechanisms.
- Draw an annotated diagram of a replication fork.
- List the components of the prokaryotic replisome and their functions.
- List four differences between prokaryotic and eukaryotic replication.
- What is the function of the eukaryotic telomere?
- Describe the structure and function of RNA polymerase in *E. coli*.
- Discuss the function of the spliceosome, and describe the two stages of the reaction it mediates.
- Explain the wobble hypothesis.
- Draw a diagram of a typical eukaryotic gene.
- Discuss why some genes with related functions are clustered together on the same chromosome.
- Summarize the salient features of initiation, elongation, and termination of protein synthesis.
- Compare eukaryotic protein synthesis with the prokaryotic process.
- List five control points for the regulation of gene/protein expression in eukaryotes.
- What is the role of chromatin in the regulation of eukaryotic transcription?
- Explain the role of the signal peptide.
- Describe *N*- and *O*-linked glycosylation with examples.
- Explain the mechanisms of action of four types of antimicrobial agents with examples.
- List three means by which genetic material may be introduced into bacteria.
- Draw a diagram highlighting the various stages in the life cycle of a virus.

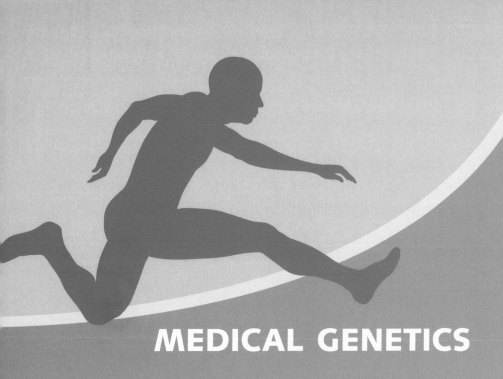

MEDICAL GENETICS

6.   Molecular Genetics as
     Applied to Medicine   121

7.   Genetic Disease   139

8.   Principles of Medical Genetics   177

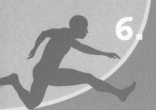

6. Molecular Genetics as Applied to Medicine

Basic techniques of molecular genetics

The increase in our understanding of the molecular basis of disease since the 1950s follows the discovery of the structure of DNA and the development of new technologies that permit the detailed analysis of normal and abnormal genes. In addition to providing the basis for theoretical advances, the techniques of molecular genetics permit the detection and laboratory diagnosis of genetic disease.

Molecular genetics is the study of the structure and function of genes at the molecular level. The basic techniques of molecular genetics concern:

- The separation of nucleic acids from the other components of the cell.
- The characterization of DNA sequence.
- The study of gene expression.
- The manipulation and modification ("engineering") of DNA.
- Gene cloning.

Molecular geneticists face two principal problems:
- Obtaining sufficient quantities of nucleic acid with which to work.
- Identifying specific sequences within a complex mixture of sequence.

Most of the techniques of molecular genetics address one or both of these issues.

Isolation of nucleic acids

The major constituents of any cell type are protein, lipid, carbohydrate, DNA, and RNA. There are many different methods of separating these components from one another, depending on the type of cells used, how much material is required, and the experiments in which they are to be used.

Most strategies for extracting nucleic acids from cells exploit their differential solubilities compared with the other cellular constituents or rely on synthetic resins that reversibly bind them.

DNA digestion with restriction enzymes
Restriction enzymes
Restriction enzymes are produced by microorganisms and named according to a symbol that corresponds to the bacterial species from which they were isolated, followed by a number (Fig. 6.1). Restriction enzymes:
- Cut double-stranded DNA.
- Recognize specific sequences of bases (frequently palindromes, i.e., sequences read the same forward as backward).
- Produce "sticky" or "blunt" ends (Fig. 6.2).

Most type II restriction enzymes (those used for genetic analysis) have recognition sites consisting of four, six, or eight base pairs, and they cleave the molecule at this site. Assuming a random distribution of bases in a piece of double-stranded DNA, a sequence of eight specific base pairs will occur much less frequently than a sequence of six base pairs (Fig. 6.3). Therefore, whereas a "six base pair cutter" such as *Eco*RI is only likely to cut once or twice in a 10kb plasmid, it will cut many times within the haploid human genome.

Gel electrophoresis
The fragments produced by digestion with restriction enzymes are separated by gel electrophoresis. The products of digestion are loaded into the well of an agarose gel, across which an electric field is applied:
- DNA is negatively charged, so it migrates toward the positive electrode.
- Small pieces of DNA migrate more quickly than large pieces, so fragments become sorted according to their size.
- Small DNA fragments end up furthest away from the wells at the end of electrophoresis.

DNA is visualized on agarose gels under ultraviolet light after staining with ethidium bromide, a

Examples of restriction endonucleases and their restriction sites	
Restriction endonucleases	**Restriction sites**
*Eco*RI	G↓AA*TTC CTTAA↑G
*Hpa*II	C↓CGG, CGC↑C
*Alu*I	AG↓CT, TC↑GA
*Taq*I	T↓CGA*, AGC↑T

Fig. 6.1 Some examples of restriction endonucleases and their restriction sites. (A*, N^6-methyladenine.)

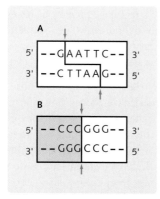

Fig. 6.2 Sticky and blunt ends after restriction enzyme digestion. (A) *Eco*RI cuts to produce staggered termini ("sticky ends"). (B) *Sma*I cuts to produce blunt ends. (Adapted from Mueller and Young, 2001.)

chemical which is easily inserted into the DNA strand and fluoresces upon exposure to ultraviolet light. The size of the fragments produced by restriction enzyme digestion can be determined by reference to a "marker" lane that contains fragments of known size.

Electrophoresis of digested human DNA

The digestion of human DNA with a six base pair cutter produces multiple fragments with an average size of 4 kb (Fig. 6.3). However, since the sequence of bases in much of the genome is random, the size of fragment varies about this mean, and many different sizes of fragment are produced. These appear as a "smear" on an appropriately treated agarose gel (Fig. 6.4).

Electrophoresis of digested plasmid DNA

In contrast, digestion of a 10 kb plasmid with a six base pair cutter cuts the plasmid twice on average, to produce two bands. An enzyme that cleaves once within the circular plasmid will linearize it, producing a single band. Thus, the products of digestion of plasmid DNA give distinct bands that can be visualized directly on appropriately treated agarose gels (Fig. 6.5A).

Restriction maps

A restriction map is a diagram depicting the linear arrangement of restriction enzyme cleavage sites on a piece of DNA. Such maps provide a means of characterizing DNA, so that naturally occurring or experimentally induced changes can be detected. Furthermore, identified restriction sites act as useful landmarks that serve a variety of purposes, such as orientating cloned segments of DNA. A restriction map is a type of physical map.

Fragment size produced and cutting frequency of restriction enzymes				
Restriction enzyme recognition sequence	**Average size of restriction fragment**	**Average number of cuts in 10 kb plasmid**	**Average number of cuts in *S. cerevisiae* (1.4×10^4 kb)**	**Average number of cuts in haploid human genome (3×10^6 kb)**
4 bp	4^4 bp (0.2 kb)	50	7.0×10^4	1.1×10^7
6 bp	4^6 bp (4.1 kb)	2	3.4×10^3	7.3×10^5
8 bp	4^8 bp (65.5 kb)	0	2.1×10^2	4.5×10^4

Fig. 6.3 Fragment size produced and cutting frequency for the digestion of human, *Saccharomyces cerevisiae*, and plasmid DNA with restriction enzymes that recognize four, six, and eight base pair sequences.

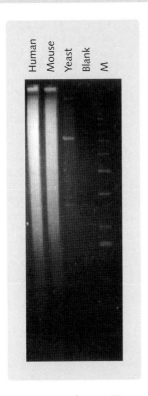

Fig. 6.4 Human, mouse, and yeast (*S. cerevisiae*) genomic DNA cut with a restriction enzyme that recognizes a six base pair sequence (*Hind*III). The marker lane contains DNA fragments of known size. (Courtesy of Dr. Steve Howe.)

Restriction maps are produced by digesting the piece of DNA with a variety of restriction enzymes and sizing the products that result. They can be produced directly from agarose gels for simple sequences such as plasmids (Fig. 6.5B). However, identifying and sizing individual fragments within the smears that result from digestion of human DNA is impossible, and so hybridization with a labeled probe is necessary.

Southern analysis
Hybridization

Hybridization enables the identification of individual sequences of DNA within a mixture that contains many sequences, using specific probes. A probe is a radioactively (or fluorescently) labeled piece of single-stranded DNA of defined sequence. Probes may be derived from:

- Cloned fragments of DNA.
- The products of polymerase chain reaction (PCR).
- Synthetically manufactured DNA.

Hybridization requires both the target and probe sequences to be first denatured (i.e., made single

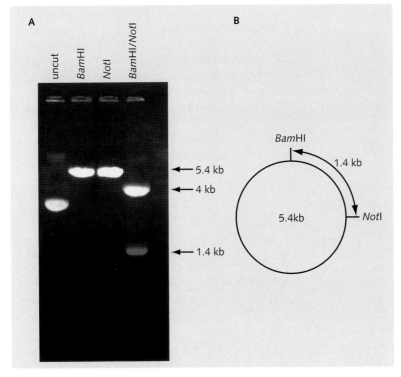

Fig. 6.5 (A) Plasmid DNA cut with restriction enzymes. The wells are labeled with the enzyme used to digest the plasmid. *Bam*HI and *Not*I each cut the plasmid once and linearize it. Digestion with both enzymes produces two bands. The lane labeled "uncut" contains plasmid DNA that has not been digested. Note this contains two bands that correspond to supercoiled and open circular forms of the plasmid, and that these forms migrate differently to the linearized plasmid. The restriction fragments are sized by comparison to a lane containing fragments of known size (not shown). (B) Restriction map of the plasmid based on the restriction enzyme digestion. (Courtesy of Dr. Ajay Mistry.)

123

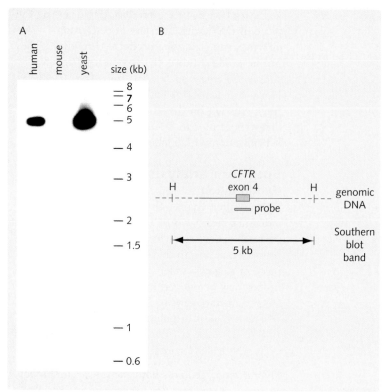

Fig. 6.6 (A) Autoradiograph obtained after the DNA digest pictured in Fig. 6.4 is hybridized with a single copy probe that hybridizes to exon 4 of the human *CFTR* (cystic fibrosis) gene. The probe is specific for human sequence, so hybridization to a 5 kb fragment occurs with human DNA, but there is no hybridization with mouse DNA. The probe anneals to a fragment in the yeast lane because this clone contains a yeast artificial chromosome (YAC) that includes the human *CFTR* gene. (B) Map depicting probe annealing on human genomic DNA. A 5 kb fragment results because exon 4 is flanked by two *Hind*III fragments (H) that are 5 kb apart. (Courtesy of Dr. Steve Howe.)

stranded). They are then mixed together under stringent conditions that only permit pairing of complementary strands of DNA. Thus, the labeled probe sequence binds specifically with complementary target sequence to form a hybrid, but it does not bind to noncomplementary sequence. The presence of such hybrids can be detected because the label will "expose" x-ray film (Fig. 6.6) or use some other detection method.

Southern blotting
Although DNA within agarose gels can be subjected to hybridization directly, it is only possible to do so once, because gels are fragile. Southern blotting is a technique by which DNA is transferred from the agarose gel to a nylon membrane (Fig. 6.7). Having the products of a restriction enzyme digestion on a nylon membrane is highly desirable, since it can be used in many consecutive hybridization experiments without the need to repeat the tedious digestion and electrophoresis steps. The steps required for sizing a band of restriction enzyme digested human DNA by Southern blotting and hybridization are summarized in Fig. 6.8. Although its use has

become more limited in recent years, Southern blotting is still used when working with DNA regions that are difficult to study with more conventional methods.

Northern blotting
Northern blotting is a technique used to study the expression of genes. It is analogous to Southern blotting, except that molecules of RNA, as opposed to DNA, are separated by electrophoresis and transferred to a nylon membrane, which can then be used in hybridization experiments.

Southern blotting was named after its developer, Ed Southern. Northern blotting and Western blotting (a technique for characterizing proteins) were named as a pun on the points of a compass.

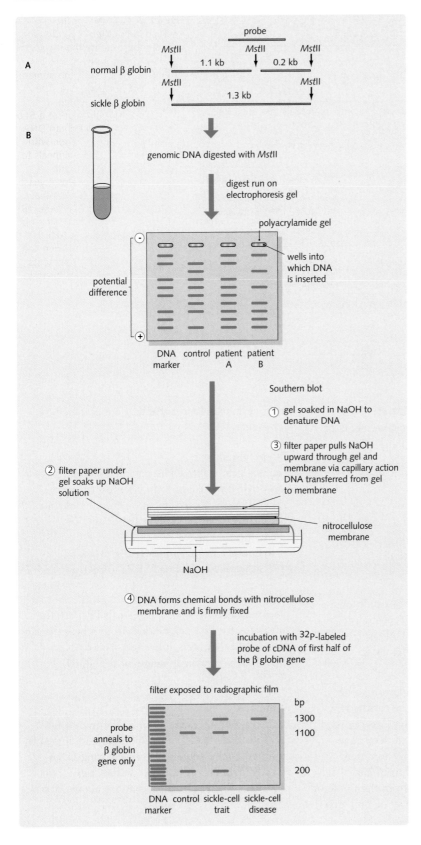

Fig. 6.7 Restriction map (A) and Southern blotting (B) showing a clinical example of diagnosis of sickle-cell disease: a point mutation in the gene for β-hemoglobin that destroys a restriction site for *Mst*II. Genomic DNA is digested with *Mst*II and run on an electrophoresis gel. The gel separates the DNA fragments, making the small ones travel further. The DNA is stained with ethidium bromide and viewed under ultraviolet light. The DNA can be transferred onto nitrocellulose film by Southern blotting. (1) Gel soaked in NaOH to denature DNA. (2) The filter paper under gel soaks up NaOH solution. (3) The filter paper draws NaOH upward through gel and membrane and so transfers DNA from gel to membrane. (4) DNA forms a chemical bond with nitrocellulose membrane and is firmly fixed. Radiolabeled probes on the Southern blot can be used to detect the β-globin gene. The mutation is detected by a single large *Mst*II fragment. (Normal genes have two smaller *Mst*II fragments because the probe spans this restriction site.)

125

Southern hybridization		
Day	Step	Description
1	1	Digestions set up and allowed to proceed for approximately 2 hours
	2	Products of digestion loaded onto agarose gel and subjected to electrophoresis for approximately 2 hours
	3	Gel stained, visualized under ultraviolet light, and photographed
	4	Gel soaked in sodium hydroxide and Southern transfer set up (see Fig. 6.7) and allowed to proceed overnight
2	5	Southern blotting apparatus dismantled and DNA fixed to membrane
	6	Radioactively labeled probe prepared
	7	Probe and membrane allowed to hybridize overnight
3	8	Membrane washed to remove nonhybridized probe
	9	Membrane exposed to x-ray film
4 or 5	10	Film developed

Fig. 6.8 A summary of the steps involved in Southern hybridization with an approximate time scale.

Polymerase chain reaction

PCR is a means of amplifying short segments of DNA (<2 kb using standard methods). Since its discovery in 1985, this technique has revolutionized molecular genetics. Its many uses include:

- Library screening.
- Probe preparation.
- Cloning.
- Genotyping polymorphic markers.
- Diagnostic detection of mutations.

PCR reagents

PCR hinges on the manipulation of conditions so that a DNA polymerase enzyme repeatedly replicates a specific sequence of DNA (Fig. 6.9). There are five reagents essential for PCR:

Target DNA

The target DNA is the sequence that is to be amplified, which acts as a template for the first round of replication. Very little DNA is required. If the purpose of the reaction is to determine whether a patient carries a specific mutation, sufficient DNA can be extracted from buccal cells, which can be painlessly scraped from the inside of the cheek. Alternatively, DNA may be prepared from peripheral leucocytes that are obtained by venepuncture.

Taq polymerase

Taq is a heat stable DNA polymerase enzyme that was originally isolated from *Thermus aquaticus*, a thermophilic bacterium that naturally inhabits hot springs. Like all DNA polymerases, *Taq* polymerase:

- Requires a primer to initiate synthesis.
- Synthesizes DNA in a 5′ to 3′ direction.

dNTPs

Deoxynucleotide triphosphates (dNTPs) are the substrates for *Taq* polymerase, from which the new strands of DNA are synthesized. The reaction should include equal amounts of dATP, dTTP, dCTP, and dGTP.

Primers

Each reaction includes 5′ and 3′ primers that together flank the target sequences and anneal to complementary sequences on opposing DNA strands. Primers are usually synthetically produced oligonucleotides that are about 20 bases in length.

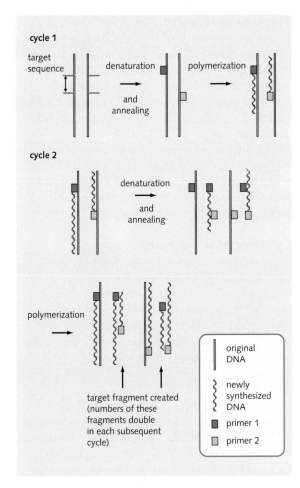

cycle 1

target sequence

denaturation and annealing

polymerization

cycle 2

denaturation and annealing

polymerization

target fragment created (numbers of these fragments double in each subsequent cycle)

original DNA

newly synthesized DNA

primer 1

primer 2

Fig. 6.9 Mechanism of action of the polymerase chain reaction (PCR). Each primer is complementary to sequence on opposing strands, flanking the target sequence. *Taq* polymerase catalyzes the addition of dNTPs onto the 3′ ends of both primers so that each round of PCR doubles the amount of target DNA.

Buffer

The buffer maintains the optimum pH and chemical environment for the polymerase enzyme.

Thermocycling

Tubes or, more recently, plates with 96, 384, or 1536 wall-like depressions containing the various reagents are placed in a thermocycling machine. This heats and cools the tubes in a cyclical manner, each cycle consisting of heating and cooling to three distinct temperatures.

Denaturing temperature

The reagents are heated to about 96°C for approximately 15 seconds. At this temperature, double-stranded DNA is denatured.

Annealing temperature

The reagents are cooled to about 60°C for around 1 minute. Primers anneal specifically to complementary sequence in the target DNA at this temperature.

Extension temperature

The reagents are heated to 72°C for about 1 minute. This is the optimum working temperature for *Taq* polymerase.

Each cycle theoretically doubles the amount of DNA, although the reaction becomes less efficient when residual amounts of reagents such as dNTPs eventually become limiting. Typically 30 cycles are performed, after which about 10^5 copies of the target sequence are present. This is sufficient DNA to be visualized on an agarose gel and used in genotyping or sequencing procedures.

Visualizing the products of PCR

The products of the PCR reaction can be visualized directly on an agarose gel under ultraviolet light after staining with ethidium bromide (Fig. 6.10). They appear as distinct bands, the size corresponding to the number of base pairs between the 5′ and 3′ ends of the two primers. The original template DNA is not visible because such a small amount is used in the PCR reaction.

Controls

Compared with Southern blotting, PCR is a quick method of genotyping polymorphic markers or identifying disease-causing mutations that is well suited to automation (Fig. 6.11). However, it is extremely sensitive to contamination, and small amounts of template DNA in any of the reagents will generate spurious results. Furthermore, for reasons that are often difficult to determine, artifacts (e.g., unexpected bands) are common or the amplification may fail completely. For this reason every experiment should include a minimum of two controls, as described below.

Negative control

The negative control (or "blank") contains all the reagents except for the target DNA. A band in the

127

lane that corresponds to this reaction suggests contamination.

Positive control

The positive control is DNA known to contain the target sequence, and has ideally produced the expected band in the same PCR reaction on a previous occasion. If the lane that corresponds to this reaction contains no band or unexpected bands, the experiment should be repeated.

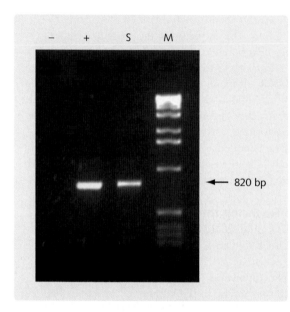

Fig. 6.10 The products of a PCR reaction. A 820bp band results because the primers are separated by this amount of sequence. The lane marked "−" is the negative control that contains all the components necessary for PCR except DNA. The lane marked "+" is the positive control, which is known to contain the sequence to which the primers anneal. The 820bp band is seen in the sample lane (S), suggesting that this clone also includes the sequence to which the primers anneal. "M" represents the marker lane that contains DNA fragments of known size. (Courtesy of Dr. Steve Howe.)

Reverse transcriptase PCR

This is a modification of PCR that is used to study gene expression. RNA cannot be used directly in PCR because *Taq* polymerase is unable to recognize it as a template. However, the viral enzyme reverse transcriptase (RT) can use RNA as a template for the production of a strand of DNA. In the first step of RT-PCR, RNA is incubated with this enzyme in the presence of dNTPs and an appropriate primer to allow the synthesis of a strand of cDNA. The products of this reaction are then used directly in a PCR reaction as described above.

Cytogenetic techniques

Cytogenetics is concerned with the study of chromosomes. Chromosomes derived from specially treated metaphase cells can be viewed directly by microscopy. Techniques such as G-banding and fluorescence *in situ* hybridization (FISH) enable individual chromosomes, or specific sequences within them, to be identified.

G-banding

G-banding is the most commonly used chromosome staining technique. Chromosomes are subjected to a controlled digestion with trypsin and stained with Giemsa. This results in a pattern of dark and light bands that is specific for each chromosome, and which, therefore, allows each chromosome to be identified. It is used in the diagnosis of:

- Monosomies and trisomies.
- Translocations.
- Large deletions and insertions.

For many of its applications, G-banding is being superseded by FISH.

PCR compared with Southern hybridization		
Consideration	**PCR**	**Southern hybridization**
Amount of DNA required	Small amount (100 ng)	Larger amount (5 μg)
Typical time taken	1–2 days	4–5 days
Suitability for automation	Yes	No
Spurious results	Frequent	Infrequent
Contamination problems	Common	Rare

Fig. 6.11 The relative advantages and disadvantages of PCR and Southern hybridization.

Fluorescence *in situ* hybridization

FISH is a method of visualizing specific regions of metaphase or interphase chromosomes. The DNA that constitutes chromosomes is fixed to a microscope slide and denatured. It is then hybridized with fluorescently labeled probe DNA that binds specifically to complementary sequence. The region of the chromosome where hybridization has occurred can be visualized under a fluorescent microscope. FISH probes may bind to a single genomic sequence (Fig. 6.12), or else they may stain an entire chromosome (such probes are called "chromosome paints"). In addition to being used in research laboratories to assist in gene mapping, FISH is used diagnostically to identify a variety of chromosome abnormalities, including:

- Monosomies and trisomies.
- Translocations.
- Microdeletions and insertions.

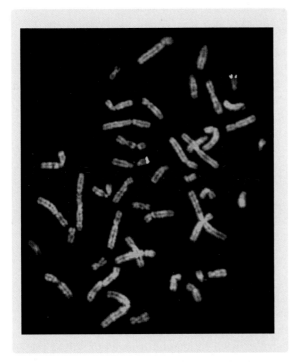

Fig. 6.12 Fluorescence *in situ* hybridization (FISH) using a single copy probe. Although the probe is said to be single copy, this refers to the haploid genome. On the metaphase spread illustrated, two pairs of dots are visible that correspond to hybridization of the biotin-labeled probe to both chromatids on a pair of homologous chromosomes. (Courtesy of Dr. Paul Scriven, GSTT.)

FISH is more sensitive than G-banding and may be used to identify microdeletions that cannot be detected by this technique.

DNA sequence analysis

Sequencing is the determination of the order of bases in a piece of DNA. DNA sequencing is used to identify the normal sequence of genes and to detect variation or mutation within a gene. This is often referred to as the gold standard of mutation screening, as it allows DNA sequencing by nucleotide examination of a DNA region. Prior to the Human Genome Project, sequencing was performed manually and was an expensive and time-consuming process. A major contribution of the Human Genome Project was the creation of a technology to automate and analyze more rapidly the sequencing protocol. Today's systems use fluorescent labels that are detected by a computerized laser system (Fig. 6.13), increasing the sequencing capacity to more than 1 million bases a day.

The sequencing process is based on dideoxy chain termination and begins with a single-stranded DNA template, usually created by PCR. An appropriate 15–20 nucleotide primer is used, along with a DNA polymerase and the four normal deoxynucleotides. The key to dideoxy sequencing, however, is the addition of a small quantity of each of the four nucleotides, altered to lack a hydroxyl group at the 3′ carbon position (the "dideoxynucleotides"). These altered molecules, each labeled with a different fluorescent dye, can be incorporated into the newly synthesized complementary strand of DNA but are unable to bond with any additional nucleotides, effectively ending strand elongation. The small proportion of dideoxynucleotides results in a mixture of synthesized DNA fragments, each terminating at random positions across the sequence. These fragments can be separated by gel electrophoresis on the basis of size and "read," according to the specific fluorescent label found at the end of each terminated dideoxynucleotide. The correct DNA sequence is generated by computer software and the identification of a variant nucleotide can be highlighted.

Microarray resequencing chips

Microarray, a major advance in genomic analysis, can examine DNA, RNA, or protein at a high-throughput level, depending on the design. DNA

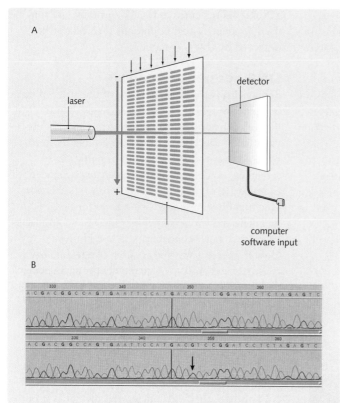

Fig. 6.13 Automated DNA sequencing using fluorescent primers. (A) A laser beam detects the four different fluorochromes that are used for each ddNTP as individual DNA fragments migrate past. (B) An example of a fluorescent DNA sequencing output (only G sequence is shown). The two traces are two different DNA sequences for the same portion of a gene. The arrow marks an allele that differs between the two sequences. In the top trace a T is found in this position, so the top sequence does not include the peak marked in the lower trace, which has a G at this allele. (Adapted from Mueller and Young, 2001.)

microarrays are able to examine the sequence of several thousand nucleotides simultaneously for a given sample. Thousands of synthetic DNA probes (oligonucleotides), representing both normal sequence and all possible single nucleotide substitutions, are placed on a microchip in a structured arrangement. This "resequencing" chip is then hybridized with the DNA of the patient, which has first been amplified by PCR and fluorescently labeled. A computer records and interprets the pattern of hybridization and produces a corresponding sequence for the sample DNA, including DNA variations or known mutations that may have clinical consequences.

The Human Genome Project

Introduction

The Human Genome Project (HGP) was a 13-year international cooperative research effort to investigate the human genome in its entirety. The specific aims of the HGP, completed in 2003, included:

- Mapping human genes and markers.
- Sequencing the human genome.
- Comparing the human genome with the genomes of model organisms (*E. coli*, *S. cerevisiae*, *C. elegans*, etc.).
- Developing new technologies (e.g., automated sequencing).
- Developing bioinformatics (systems for collecting, storing, and disseminating the information generated by the project).
- Addressing the ethical, legal, and social issues that arise from the HGP.

Although the initial work has been completed, analysis of the data and an understanding of how the sequence relates to health, disease, and behavior will continue for many years. Along the way, the HGP has overseen the development of several types of map of the human genome and of the genomes of model organisms.

Genetic maps

The genetic map of the human genome is based on the probability of recombination between paternally derived and maternally derived chromosomes at meiosis:

- Loci are assigned to linkage groups.
- Distances are quoted in recombination units (centimorgans).

One centimorgan (1 cM) is equivalent to a 1% chance of recombination (a Morgan is defined as a length of chromosome segment that undergoes one exchange with its homolog per meiosis).

Recombination is more frequent in female meiosis, so the male and female maps are different, with markers appearing further apart on the female version. Some areas of the genome are more prone to recombination than others, so there is not a perfect correlation between genetic and physical maps.

Genetic maps were fundamental to developing the scaffold of the human genome. The most recent high-resolution genetic maps have polymorphic markers spaced at intervals of less than 1 cM.

Genetic and physical maps are not perfectly correlated, but on average 1 cM is equivalent to 1 Mb.

Physical maps

Physical maps locate genes at cytogenetically defined locations, and they give distances in bp, kb, or Mb. Methods of physical mapping include:

- Restriction mapping.
- Sequencing.
- FISH.

The physical map of the human genome is based on the analysis of a set of ordered, overlapping DNA fragments that together span almost the whole human genome. These arrays of clones are anchored to specific named chromosomes.

Sequencing the genome

The base sequence of the genome is the most detailed type of physical map. This was the ultimate aim of the HGP: the production of single, continuous sequence of bases for each of the human chromosomes and the delineation of the position of all the human genes. The first drafts of the human

genome sequence were released in 2001, and the genome was declared "finished" in 2003. The sequence of the HGP is stored at the National Center for Biotechnology Information (NCBI) and can be viewed online at www.ncbi.nlm.nih.gov/.

The human proteome

The proteome is the complete set of proteins encoded by the genome. Compared with invertebrates, vertebrate proteins have a larger repertoire of motifs and domains available, and they include more complex domain architectures and multidomain proteins with multiple functions.

A surprise revealed by the HGP is that humans appear to require only 20,000–25,000 protein-coding genes, which is only double the number that flies and worms have. However, human genes are more complex, and it is believed that processes such as alternative splicing greatly increase the number of proteins produced (Fig. 6.14). This, in

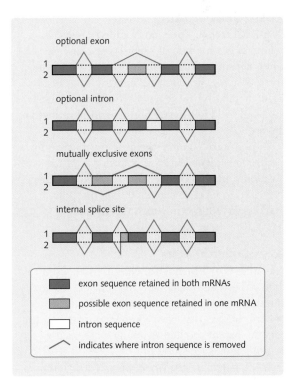

Fig. 6.14 Alternative splicing. Nonconsecutive exons are spliced together in some, but not all, of the transcripts produced from the gene. With each of the four mechanisms, a single type of RNA transcript is spliced in two alternative ways to produce two distinct mRNAs (1 and 2).

association with the greater complexity of protein domains, may be sufficient to account for the increased phenotypic complexity of vertebrates.

Cloning and characterizing human disease genes

The successful identification of the genes that are mutated in monogenic disorders has a number of possible consequences:
• Definitive diagnosis.
• More accurate assessments of risk or prognosis.
• Presymptomatic diagnosis.
• Prenatal diagnosis.

Furthermore, an increased understanding of the molecular basis of the disease may lead to the identification of new drug targets, enable rational drug design, and facilitate the production of animal models of the disease on which such therapies can be tested.

Positional cloning

Positional cloning (previously called reverse genetics) is a method of identifying a disease gene when nothing is known about the nature of the corresponding protein. This approach has been used to identify the genes responsible for many diseases, including cystic fibrosis and Huntington disease.

In positional cloning, the gene responsible for a condition is identified from knowledge of its position in the human genome. This knowledge comes from linkage analysis of polymorphic markers in families in which the disease is segregating (see "genetic linkage analysis," below).

Polymorphic markers

A marker is any Mendelian characteristic used to follow the transmission of a segment of chromosome through a pedigree. DNA polymorphisms that have a known position on the genetic map of the human genome are used as markers in linkage studies:
• DNA polymorphisms are inherited differences in DNA between normal, healthy people.
• They frequently arise in noncoding regions of the genome.
• Examples include restriction fragment length polymorphisms (RFLPs), microsatellites, and single nucleotide polymorphisms (SNPs).

Restriction fragment length polymorphisms

RFLPs are detected by Southern restriction analysis. Classically, they arise as a result of sequence variation within the recognition site of a restriction enzyme.

RFLPs may also arise if the restriction site spans a variable number tandem repeat (VNTR). These are tandemly repeated sequences that vary in length by multiples of the basic repeating unit, which is 10–100 bp in length. Many different lengths of sequence are possible, depending on how many copies of the basic repeat are included, so such markers are highly polymorphic, and they have multiple alleles.

Since the development of methods for analyzing microsatellite markers, RFLPs are not routinely used in genetic linkage experiments because Southern analysis requires more DNA per sample, and it is not as well suited to a high throughput of samples as PCR.

Microsatellite markers

Microsatellites are stretches of DNA consisting of repeating units of two, three, or four nucleotides. They are an extremely useful type of marker that is well suited to genetic linkage analysis for several reasons:
• They can be detected by PCR.
• They are extremely polymorphic.
• Tens of thousands of microsatellite polymorphic loci have been identified scattered throughout the genome.

An example of the results obtained after PCR with a pair of primers that spans a microsatellite is shown in Fig. 6.15.

Detection of the alleles present at these sequences via PCR forms the basis of "genetic fingerprinting" used in paternity testing and forensic studies.

Genetic linkage analysis
Linkage

Linkage analysis uses pedigree data to determine whether loci are linked and to estimate the recombination fraction (see below). At meiosis, homologous chromosomes exchange segments before separating into two daughter cells.

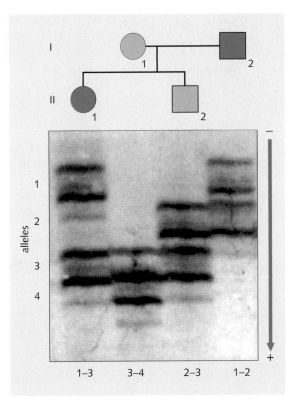

Fig. 6.15 An autoradiograph showing the results of a PCR using primers that span a microsatellite repeat. The microsatellite is closely linked to a gene that causes a dominant disorder and allele 1 is segregating with the condition. Note that each allele gives rise to multiple bands, which is due to an artifact of PCR. (Adapted from Mueller and Young, 2001.)

> Make sure that you can interpret microsatellite, RFLP, and PCR data from autoradiographs, gels, and computer scans of fragment peaks. Examiners will often present you with them and ask you to use the data to answer questions on genetic counseling, recombination, or even Hardy–Weinberg equilibrium.

Linked markers segregate together in meiosis more frequently than expected by chance because they lie close together on the same chromosome (Fig. 6.16). Crossovers are statistically unlikely to form between markers that are close together. However, if markers are sufficiently far apart on a chromosome it is likely that a crossover will form between them and recombination will occur. A Morgan is defined as the length of chromosome segment that undergoes, on average, one crossover per meiosis.

Recombination

Recombination occurs as a result of the formation of chiasmata (crossovers) during meiosis. Recombinants are seen in children who inherit a different combination of alleles at two loci compared with the combination found in the gametes that made the parent.

The recombination fraction (RF) is the proportion of recombinants. For unlinked loci it is 0.5, for linked loci it lies between 0 and 0.5. Tightly linked loci only rarely exhibit recombination between them, leading to low recombination fraction.

The LOD score

The random assortment of chromosomes at meiosis means that unlinked alleles on different chromosomes will segregate together on average 50% of the time. Thus, even in large families with many meioses, markers may appear to be linked because they have repeatedly segregated together by chance. The LOD score is a statistical test that expresses the likelihood of linkage compared with nonlinkage for different recombination fractions. A LOD score of 3 or greater is taken as statistical evidence for linkage. LOD scores from several families can be added together to provide strong evidence for or against linkage between a specific DNA marker and the disease of interest.

Family selection and pedigree analysis

The first step in identifying a disease gene is identifying sufficient families with the gene to identify linkage. The role of the clinician is vitally important at this stage, as it is imperative that all affected members of the family are identified and that all the families included in the study have the same disease. The mode of inheritance of the disease (recessive, dominant, etc.) should also be considered, as this information is required for linkage analysis.

Establishing linkage to a chromosome

To establish linkage to a specific chromosome, all members of the family are genotyped with respect to at least 400 polymorphic markers:

133

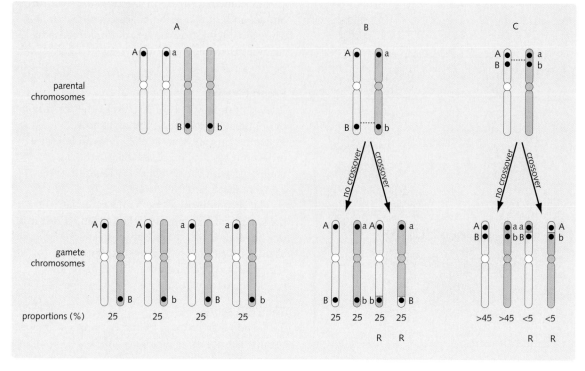

Fig. 6.16 Segregation at meiosis of alleles at two loci. Recombinants are marked (R). (A) The loci are on different chromosomes. (B) The loci are on the same chromosome but widely separated (>1 M apart). (C) The loci are closely adjacent and so segregate together most of the time (i.e., they are linked). (Adapted from Mueller and Young, 2001.)

- These polymorphic markers are nearly always microsatellites; however, SNP-based marker sets are on the horizon and may supplant the microsatellite-based marker sets.
- The sequence of these markers is freely available through the HGP.
- They are scattered throughout the whole genome.
- They have known positions on genetic and physical maps.

The data generated are reviewed to determine whether any one of these markers is segregating with the disease (Fig. 6.17).

Fine genetic mapping
Once linkage to a particular chromosome or chromosomal region has been identified, all the members of the family are genotyped with respect to a further set of more densely packed markers that map to the appropriate chromosomal region. This aims to:

- Confirm linkage is genuine.
- Narrow the region of the genetic map in which the disease gene can be shown to lie.

Even before the disease-causing mutations have been identified, closely linked genetic markers (5 cM or less) can be used to track the inheritance of a disease gene in individual families for diagnostic purposes.

From linked genetic marker to cloned gene
At this point, using the information provided by the HGP, the region of interest is examined for previously characterized genes that may serve as potential candidates for the disease under study. Such a candidate would be expressed in the tissues affected by the disorder. Ideally, there should be further biologic evidence available (for example, knowledge of the appropriate biochemical pathway) that would make it plausible that mutations in the candidate gene

might result in the specific disease. This method of locating disease genes is called the positional candidate gene approach. Otherwise, the region known to contain the gene must be progressively narrowed down by genetic and physical mapping techniques until a suitable candidate gene can be identified.

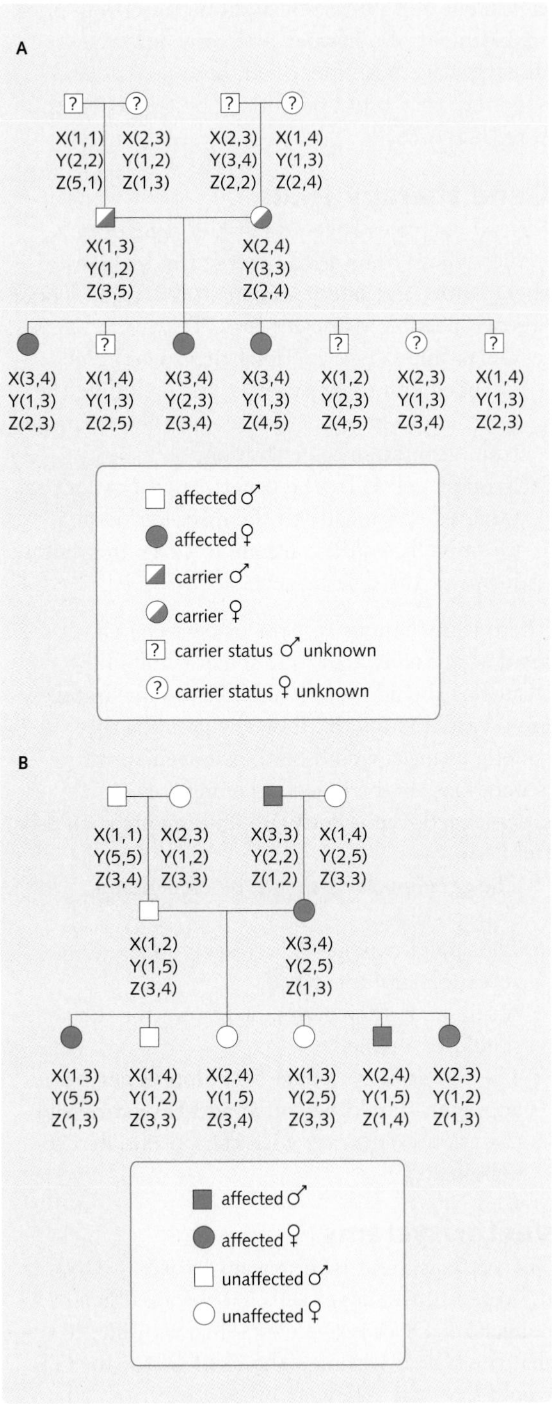

The data generated by the Human Genome Project have greatly simplified positional cloning. When the approach was first suggested in the 1980s, individual research groups had to identify polymorphic markers themselves with which to establish linkage. Once linkage was found, they then had to construct their own arrays of overlapping clones in order to construct physical maps before they could even begin to look for the disease-causing gene. Now, all this information is freely available thanks to the efforts of the Human Genome Project.

Other methods of identifying human disease genes

In addition to positional cloning, two other strategies have been employed to identify the genes that are mutated in genetic diseases.

Functional cloning

Functional cloning (also called forward genetics) is the identification of a gene responsible for a disease based on knowledge of the underlying molecular defect. For example, if the nature of the deficient protein is known, it is often possible

A

```
  [?]──(?)      [?]──(?)
X(1,1) X(2,3)  X(2,3) X(1,4)
Y(2,2) Y(1,2)  Y(3,4) Y(1,3)
Z(5,1) Z(1,3)  Z(2,2) Z(2,4)

    X(1,3)         X(2,4)
    Y(1,2)         Y(3,3)
    Z(3,5)         Z(2,4)
```

```
 ●      [?]     ●      ●     [?]    (?)    [?]
X(3,4) X(1,4) X(3,4) X(3,4) X(1,2) X(2,3) X(1,4)
Y(1,3) Y(1,3) Y(2,3) Y(1,3) Y(2,3) Y(1,3) Y(1,3)
Z(2,3) Z(2,5) Z(3,4) Z(4,5) Z(4,5) Z(3,4) Z(2,3)
```

□ affected ♂
● affected ♀
◪ carrier ♂
◑ carrier ♀
[?] carrier status ♂ unknown
(?) carrier status ♀ unknown

B

```
  □──○          ■──○
X(1,1) X(2,3)  X(3,3) X(1,4)
Y(5,5) Y(1,2)  Y(2,2) Y(2,5)
Z(3,4) Z(3,3)  Z(1,2) Z(3,3)

    □──────────────●
  X(1,2)         X(3,4)
  Y(1,5)         Y(2,5)
  Z(3,4)         Z(1,3)
```

```
 ●      □      ○      ○      ■      ●
X(1,3) X(1,4) X(2,4) X(1,3) X(2,4) X(2,3)
Y(5,5) Y(1,2) Y(1,5) Y(2,5) Y(1,5) Y(1,2)
Z(1,3) Z(3,3) Z(3,4) Z(3,3) Z(1,4) Z(1,3)
```

■ affected ♂
● affected ♀
□ unaffected ♂
○ unaffected ♀

Fig. 6.17 Identifying linkage between polymorphic markers and disease genes. In these examples, three polymorphic markers are used (X, Y, and Z) that map to three different chromosomes (2, 3, and 5, respectively). (A) In this pedigree showing autosomal recessive inheritance, the disease is segregating with the "3" and "4" alleles of marker X, suggesting that the disease maps to chromosome 2. (B) In this pedigree showing autosomal dominant inheritance the disease is segregating with the "1" allele of marker Z, suggesting that the disease maps to chromosome 5.

to isolate the appropriate mRNAs and use them (or cDNAs derived from them) as probes for the gene. This approach was used to define the genes responsible for phenylketonuria and sickle-cell anemia.

Candidate gene approach

Previously isolated genes are considered as candidates for causing a specific genetic disease if they are known to have a role in the physiology of the diseased tissue. For example, when researchers interested in retinal degeneration screened patients for mutations in cloned genes known to be involved in phototransduction, they found that mutations in rhodopsin are responsible for some cases of retinitis pigmentosa.

Mutation analysis

If mutation within a particular gene is responsible for a specific genetic disease, then patients with the disorder should have mutations in the gene that are not found in unaffected individuals.

The normal structure and base sequence of the DNA (determined by the HGP) is compared to patient DNA. Screening for mutations may include methods such as:
- SSCP (single-strand conformation polymorphism) analysis.
- Heteroduplex analysis.
- Direct sequencing.

DNA diagnostics

Once a disease-causing mutation has been identified, molecular methods are developed that enable its identification in patient DNA:
- PCR-based techniques are used to detect base changes wherever possible.
- Cytogenetic techniques are used to detect microdeletions, insertions, and translocations.
- Southern blotting is used to detect some triplet repeat expansions.

Large scale mutation testing is on the horizon, promising rapid testing of hundreds or thousands of nucleotides simultaneously. Provided the technology is affordable and the technique is robust, this may lead to a revolution in mutation detection, expanding the number of genes screened exponentially.

Gene therapy

Our increased understanding of the molecular basis of disease has led to the proposal that it may be possible to treat some disease by gene therapy. Gene therapy (GT) can be defined as the treatment of a disease by addition, insertion, or replacement of a normal gene or genes. Many diseases have been identified, both genetic and acquired, that could potentially be treated in this way (Fig. 6.18).

Gene therapy trials

Several countries have established regulatory bodies whose remit is to oversee the technical, therapeutic, and safety aspects of GT trials. There are two possible strategies for GT:
- Germ-line GT—genetic changes would be introduced into every cell type, including the germ line. These changes would then be passed from generation to generation.
- Somatic cell GT—the genetic modifications are targeted specifically to the diseased tissue. Germ cells would continue to carry the mutant forms of the disease gene.

There is unanimous agreement between all regulatory bodies that only somatic cell GT strategies should be allowed. Germ-line strategies are considered unethical on the grounds that genetic changes would be transmitted to future generations. Before a gene therapy trial is commenced, the following requirements should be fulfilled:
- The gene involved should be cloned and characterized.
- The specific tissue to be targeted should be accessible and identified.
- A safe and efficient vector system for the gene should be defined.
- The scientific rationale for the gene therapy approach should be sound and the perceived risks commensurate with the potential benefits.

Vector systems

The vector system is the means by which DNA is delivered to the target cells. Achieving efficient delivery of DNA is one of the major difficulties that must be overcome. The ideal vector for GT would have the following properties:

Diseases which can potentially be treated by gene therapy	
Disorder	**Defect**
Immune deficiency	Adenosine deaminase deficiency
	Purine nucleoside phosphorylase deficiency
	Chronic granulomatous disease
Hypercholesterolemia	Low-density lipoprotein receptor abnormalities
Hemophilia	Factor VIII deficiency (A) Factor IX deficiency (B)
Gaucher disease	Glucocerebrosidase deficiency
Mucopolysaccharidosis VII	β-Glucuronidase deficiency
Emphysema	α_1-Antitrypsin deficiency
Cystic fibrosis	CFTR mutations
Phenylketonuria	Phenylalanine hydroxylase deficiency
Urea cycle abnormalities Hyperammonemia	Ornithine transcarbamylase deficiency
Citrullinemia	Argininosuccinate synthetase deficiency
Muscular dystrophy	Dystrophin mutations
Thalassemia/sickle-cell disease	α- and β-globin mutations
Cancer Malignant melanoma Ovarian cancer Brain tumors Neuroblastoma Renal cancer Lung cancer	
Acquired immune deficiency syndrome (AIDS)	
Cardiovascular diseases	
Rheumatoid arthritis	

Fig. 6.18 Diseases that can potentially be treated by gene therapy. (Adapted from Mueller and Young, 2001.)

- It would be easily produced.
- It would give sustained and regulated expression of the delivered gene.
- Immunologically, it would be inert.
- It would deliver the gene only to the required tissue.
- It would be able to deliver the largest of genes and the controlling elements required for their expression.
- It would integrate precisely into the genome in a site-specific manner, or else would be maintained as a stable episome.
- It would be able to infect both dividing and nondividing cells.

There are two main types of vector system:
- Physical (nonviral) vector systems (e.g., liposomes).
- Viral vectors, which may integrate into the genome (retroviral, lentiviral, and adenoassociated vectors) or be maintained as an episome (adenovirus).

Viral vectors are derived from viruses by replacing the genetic components essential for further propagation with the therapeutic gene. Liposomes are artificial lipid vesicles that fuse with the cell membrane to deliver their contents (DNA in the case of gene therapy).

Both types of vector system, each with its own inherent advantages and disadvantages, have been used in clinical trials—for example, the treatment of cystic fibrosis by GT (Fig. 6.19).

Tragically, Jesse Gelsinger became the first person reported to have died in a phase I gene therapy trial in 1999. He was part of a study in which patients with ornithine transcarbamylase (OTC) deficiency were given escalating doses of an adenoviral vector.

137

CFTR delivery vectors advantages and disadvantages

Vector	Advantages	Disadvantages
Recombinant adenovirus	Targets the respiratory tract epithelium; infects nonreplicating cells; in preliminary experiments 40% of respiratory epithelial cells took up the vector	Expression in target cells transient; can create an inflammatory response in recipient not known whether re-administration is safe (possibility of secondary immune response)
Liposome	Can be delivered directly to the lung (in an aerosol or by direct irrigation or intravenous infusion); re-administration is unlikely to cause an immune response	Low uptake of liposomes: only 5% of epithelial cells transfected in preliminary experiments, which is not enough to have a therapeutic effect

Fig. 6.19 Advantages and disadvantages of adenovirus and liposome vectors for cystic fibrosis gene therapy.

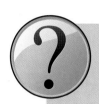

- What is a restriction enzyme? Give three examples.
- Why, when visualized on an agarose gel, does plasmid DNA digested with a six base pair cutter appear as discrete bands whereas human DNA appears as a smear?
- Suggest why PCR-based methodologies are preferred in diagnostic laboratories to Southern hybridization techniques whenever possible.
- Describe two methods used for studying gene expression.
- Describe FISH and its applications.
- What was the purpose of the Human Genome Project?
- Describe the differing approaches used in the construction of physical and genetic maps.
- Define the unit Morgan. What is the relationship between distance on genetic and physical maps?
- Define the term proteome.
- What is a polymorphic marker?
- What is a microsatellite marker? Describe the steps you would undertake to determine the genotype of a family with respect to a specific microsatellite marker.
- What is the relationship between linkage and recombination?
- Describe the different approaches of positional cloning, functional cloning, and the candidate gene approach in identifying disease genes. Give an example of a disease gene cloned by each method.
- Outline the steps involved in positional cloning.
- What is gene therapy?
- What is the difference between somatic and germ-line gene therapy?
- List five properties of the ideal gene therapy vector.

7. Genetic Disease

Single gene disorders

Terminology
Pleiotropy
Pleiotropy is the phenomenon in which a gene is responsible for several distinct and apparently unrelated phenotypic effects, which may concern the organ systems involved and the signs and symptoms that occur. Pleiotropic effects may be explainable once the disease gene has been cloned and the protein it encodes characterized.

Genotype
This is the genetic constitution of an individual, and it is also used to refer to the alleles present at one locus.

Phenotype
This is the observed biochemical, physiological, or morphological characteristics of an individual that are determined by the genotype and the environment in which it is expressed.

Homozygote
This is an individual or genotype with identical alleles at a given locus on a pair of homologous chromosomes.

Heterozygote
This is an individual or genotype with two different alleles at a given locus on a pair of homologous chromosomes.

Compound heterozygote
This is an individual with two different mutant alleles at the same locus.

Autosomes
These are any chromosomes other than the sex chromosomes.

Autosomal inheritance
This involves any chromosome other than the sex chromosomes.

Pedigree charts
These are used to illustrate inheritance (Fig. 7.1).

Introduction
Single gene disorders are caused by individual mutant genes, and frequently they show obvious and characteristic patterns of inheritance. There are approximately 11,000 single gene disorders. Individually they are rare, usually affecting from 1 in 10,000 to 1 in 100,000. However, taken all together single gene disorders are common, affecting 1% of the population. Certain single gene disorders depend on an environmental trigger before the phenotype is expressed:

- Lactose intolerance is not seen in the absence of lactose in the diet.
- Severe emphysema in individuals homozygous for α_1-antitrypsin deficiency mutations is largely confined to smokers.

Single gene disorders follow Mendelian patterns of inheritance; therefore, relatives in families in which these disorders are segregating are at a much higher risk of developing the condition than the population as a whole.

Mutations are random heritable changes in the amount or structure of genetic material. They can be inherited or occur spontaneously. At the single gene level they may result from:
- Substitution (point mutation).
- Deletion.
- Insertion.
- Triplet repeat expansion (unstable expansion).
- Inversion.

Mechanisms of mutation
Substitution
Substitution is the replacement of a single nucleotide by another with no net gain or loss of chromosomal material. Point mutations may arise as a result of mistakes in DNA replication, mistakes in repair following DNA damage, or (most commonly) as the result of the spontaneous deamination of methylated cytosine to thymine. Substitutions are classified as:
- Transition—purine to purine or pyrimidine to pyrimidine.
- Transversion—purine to pyrimidine or vice versa.

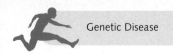

Pedigree charts

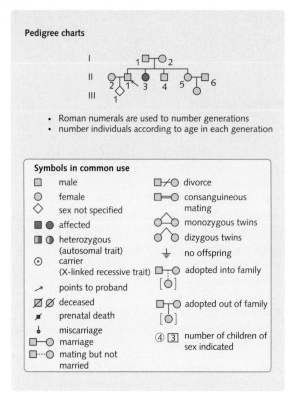

- Roman numerals are used to number generations
- number individuals according to age in each generation

Symbols in common use

□	male	□⟋○	divorce
○	female	□═○	consanguineous mating
◇	sex not specified		
■ ●	affected	△○	monozygous twins
◨ ◑	heterozygous (autosomal trait)	○ ○	dizygous twins
⊙	carrier (X-linked recessive trait)	⟂	no offspring
		□━○ [○]	adopted into family
⟋	points to proband		
▨ ⊘	deceased	□━○ [○]	adopted out of family
⚥	prenatal death		
⚬	miscarriage	④ ③	number of children of sex indicated
□━○	marriage		
□┈○	mating but not married		

Fig. 7.1 Symbols and configuration of pedigree charts.

Point mutations may be silent or deleterious depending upon the site (Fig. 7.2). Rarely, a mutation may be advantageous and favored by natural selection.

Deletion and insertion

Deletion is a loss of chromosomal material involving from one to many thousands of base pairs that may result from recombination or chromosome breakage. Sequences at the ends of deletions are often similar, as these predispose to recombination errors (Fig. 7.3).

Insertion is a gain in chromosomal material involving from just one to many thousands of base pairs. Duplication is a special type of insertion that is identical to an adjacent sequence. Runs of bases and repeated motifs predispose to duplication by replication slippage (Fig. 7.4).

The effects on the protein of deletion and insertion depend on:
- The amount of material lost.
- Whether the reading frame is affected (see Fig. 7.2).

If the mutation involves the insertion or deletion of nucleotides that are not multiples of three, a frameshift mutation will occur. Frameshift mutations concern the disruption of the open reading frame and result in a protein amino acid sequence, downstream of the mutation, that bears no resemblance to the wild-type protein.

Triplet repeat expansions

Triplet repeat expansions are a type of unstable insertion that have been associated with a variety of neurological disorders (Fig. 7.5), many of which show anticipation (Fig. 7.6). Most of these disorders are inherited dominantly, but Friedreich ataxia is an example of a recessive triplet repeat disorder.

Runs of triplet repeats are found in all members of the population, but in individuals affected with these diseases the triplet repeats generally occur in a higher copy number in the disease gene (i.e., the triplet repeat has expanded). Nearly all these repeats involve cytosine/guanine (C/G)-rich trinucleotides (CGG, CCG, CAG, CTG), and they may involve a few copies to several thousand repeats.

In the case of Huntington disease, normal individuals have 6 to 35 trinucleotide repeats, whereas Huntington disease patients have 36 repeats or more.

Triplet repeats below a certain length (which varies between the different disorders) are transmitted faithfully after meiosis and mitosis. However, if they expand above a certain size (27 repeats for Huntington disease) they become likely to expand or (rarely) contract during cell division. This phenomenon is the molecular basis of anticipation. Expansion above a certain number of repeats (36 for Huntington disease) leads to clinical symptoms.

Depending on the disorder, the repeats may arise in coding or noncoding sequence, and they may affect the protein in a variety of ways (see Fig. 7.2). However, a large proportion of triplet repeat disorders are, like Huntington disease, associated with the expansion of a polyglutamine tract within the coding region of the gene. The expanded polyglutamine tract is thought to be cytotoxic, and it is an example of "gain of function" (see below). Diseases associated with an expanded polyglutamine tract include:
- Huntington disease.
- Kennedy disease (spinobulbar muscular atrophy (SBMA)).

Mutations and their effects on protein product			
Class	**Group**	**Type**	**Effect on protein product**
Stable/fixed	Synonymous	Substitution	Silent—same amino acid
	Nonsynonymous	Substitution Missense Nonconservative	Altered amino acid Altered activity, function or stability
		Conservative Nonsense	No effect Stop codon—premature termination with loss-of-function/activity/stability
		Deletion/insertion Multiple of 3 (codon)	Deletion/insertion of one or more amino acid(s) in protein—altered activity/function/stability
		Not multiple of 3	Altered reading frame or frameshift, premature termination of protein—altered amino acid sequence, loss-of-function/activity/stability
Dynamic/unstable	Triplet repeat	Expansion	Altered gene expression, reduced transcription or translation, altered transcript—altered function/activity/stability

Fig. 7.2 The main classes, groups, and types of mutations and effects on protein products. (Adapted from Mueller and Young, 2001.)

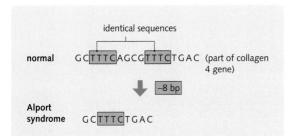

Fig. 7.3 Deletion in Alport syndrome. (A, adenine; bp, base pairs; C, cytosine; G, guanine; T, thymine.)

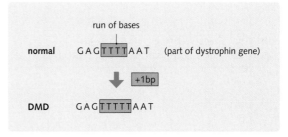

Fig. 7.4 Duplication in Duchenne muscular dystrophy (DMD). (A, adenine; bp, base pairs; C, cytosine; G, guanine; T, thymine.)

141

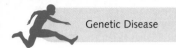
Examples of diseases caused by triplet repeat expansions

Disorder	Etiology	Features	Diagnosis	Prognosis
Fragile X syndrome	Fragile X syndrome is caused by a triplet repeat expansion at Xq27.3; this is accompanied by a visible gap in the chromatin, which can be detected on metaphase chromosomes under certain cell culture conditions. The disorder is caused by an unstable expansion of a CGG trinucleotide in the 5′ UTR (untranslated region) of the *FMR1* (fragile X mental retardation) gene. Typically, normal individuals have 6–50 repeats, those with a premutation 50–200 repeats and affected individuals >200

The defect is thought to cause hypermethylation of the *FMR1* gene, shutting down its expression (i.e., loss of function). It is proposed that *FMR1* may regulate gene expression in the nervous system | The incidence of fragile X syndrome is 1 in 2250 males. It is X-linked, but one-third of carrier females have mild learning difficulties. One-fifth of affected males inheriting the defect are normal, but may pass the disease on to their grandsons. This is called Sherman's paradox, where the grandsons of 20% of males (carrying the FRAXA mutation, who are phenotypically normal) exhibit the full clinical phenotype. Fragile X syndrome is the commonest inherited cause of learning difficulties.

The clinical features of fragile X syndrome are:
• Male sex
• Moderate learning difficulties
• Macrocephaly
• Macroorchidism (usually post-puberty)
• Characteristic facies with a long face, prominent jaw, high forehead, and large everted ears

A clinical phenotype has recently emerged for the *premutation* carrier as well: increased risk for premature ovarian failure among females and a tremor/ataxia syndrome among males | Diagnosis is by DNA analysis (PCR or Southern analysis) which can detect both the repeat expansion and methylation changes. Males carrying the full mutation have either:
• A single larger band
• A smear representing somatic instability

Individuals carrying a premutation have an intermediate sized band | A normal lifespan can be expected, but lifestyle will be somewhat restricted because of the learning difficulties |
| Huntington disease | Huntington disease is caused by a triplet repeat expansion in the *huntingtin* gene on 4p 16.3. This results in an expanded | The incidence of Huntington disease is 1 in 10,000 Northern Europeans. The onset is usually in the fourth or fifth decades | Diagnosis is by genetic testing, usually restriction fragment analysis or polymerase chain reaction (PCR) | The prognosis is poor, with death within 15–20 years of disease onset |

		Diagnosis	Prognosis
	polyglutamine tract that is thought to result in cytotoxicity (i.e., gain of function). The normal gene has 10–29 copies of the CAG repeat. In Huntington disease there can be up to 120 copies (but usually there are 40–55). The severity of the disease and age of onset are related to the size of the triplet repeat expansion. The symptoms of Huntington disease are associated with changes in the caudate nucleus due to loss of neurons that connect to the caudate nucleus from their origin in the corpus striatum	with increasing chorea and behavioral disturbances. It progresses to include: • Personality changes • Psychiatric disorders such as severe depression • Progressive chorea • Dystonia • Dementia Juvenile onset of Huntington disease is rare, and it is associated with a severe form of the disease and early death		
Myotonic dystrophy	Myotonic dystrophy is thought to be a result of a faulty kinase enzyme, dystrophica myotonica kinase (DM kinase), which occurs at neuromuscular junctions. Triplet repeat expansion of CTG occurs on chromosome 19q13.3 at the 3′ end of the DM kinase gene. There tend to be: • 5–35 repeats in the normal population • 50–99 repeats in mild disease • 100–1000 repeats in moderate disease • 1000–2000 repeats in severe disease Expansion appears to occur most readily after maternal transmission and occurs during early embryogenesis, but expansion or reduction can occur during transmission	The incidence of myotonic dystrophy is 1 in 8000. It is an autosomal dominant disorder with pronounced anticipation (i.e., increasing disease severity through generations). The clinical features of myotonic dystrophy are: • Myotonia • Progressive muscle weakness and wasting • Associated symptoms of cardiac conduction defects, smooth muscle involvement, hypersomnia, cataracts, and an abnormal glucose response • In males, premature balding and testicular atrophy There are three forms of myotonic dystrophy with differing ages of onset: • Mild—there is no muscle involvement and cataracts develop in middle or old age: the diagnosis is usually made	Diagnosis is based on the family history or molecular techniques	Those with the mild disease have a life span ranging from 60 to normal. The moderate disease is associated with a reduced lifespan (death age 48–55). Those with the congenital form of the disease that survive the neonatal period generally survive to age 45

Fig. 7.5 Examples of diseases caused by triplet repeat expansions. (A, adenine; C, cytosine; G, guanine; T, thymine.)

		because of family history of myotonic dystrophy • Moderate—myotonia and muscle weakness develop in adolescence or early adult life • Severe—this is characterized by congenital muscular hyperplasia, mental retardation, and a high neonatal mortality. The survivors develop the adult form of myotonic dystrophy before puberty	The diagnosis is made by genetic analysis, usually PCR	After 1–2 decades of symptoms most patients have difficulty climbing stairs. One-third require wheelchairs after 2 decades. Lifespan is normal
Spinobulbar muscular atrophy (SBMA) (Kennedy disease)	SBMA is caused by a CAG expansion in the coding region of the androgen receptor gene on Xq11–12. There tend to be: • 17–24 repeats in the normal population • 40–55 repeats in individuals with the disease Clinically, there are signs of androgen insensitivity and a characteristic degeneration of spinal and bulbar motor neurons	This X-linked recessive neurodegenerative disorder has an incidence of approximately 1 in 50,000 and an age of onset of 20–50. Female carriers can have symptoms (muscle cramps). The clinical features are: • Usually male • Progressive muscle weakness and atrophy • Features of androgen insensitivity (i.e., gynecomastia and reduced fertility)		
Friedreich ataxia (FA)	FA is generally caused by a GAA triplet repeat expansion in intron 1 of the *frataxin* gene. There tend to be: • 17–22 repeats in the normal population • 200–900 repeats in individuals with the disease The expansion is thought to interfere with RNA processing leading to reduced frataxin expression. Frataxin is a protein that is involved in mitochondrial iron metabolism. A minority of cases are due to inactivating point mutations	FA is an autosomal recessively inherited form of spinocerebellar ataxia. It usually presents before adolescence with: • Incoordination of limb movements • Speech difficulties • Foot deformities	Diagnosis is based on clinical and molecular findings. The expansion is detected by PCR or Southern analysis. 25% of patients homozygous for the expansion exhibit atypical clinical findings. 1% of patients meeting clinical criteria do not have mutations within the *frataxin* gene	The rate of progression is highly variable. The mean age of loss of ambulation is 25. Death is usually in the mid-thirties

Fig. 7.5—cont'd.

Genetics of some trinucleotide repeat disorders						
	FRAX	**HD**	**MD**	**SBMA**	**SCA-1**	**DRPLA**
Triplet repeat	CGG	CAG	CTG	CAG	CAG	CAG
Position	Xq27.3	4p16.3	19q13.3	xq11.12	6p22–23	12
Increased repeat associated with greater disease severity?	No	Yes	Yes	Yes	Yes	Yes
Inheritance	X-linked	AD	AD	X-linked	AD	AD
Severe juvenile onset?	No	Yes	Yes	No	Yes	Yes
Anticipation?	Yes	Yes	Yes	No	Yes	Yes
Most likely stage of repeat expansion	Early embryogenesis	Greatest instability during spermatogenesis	Early embryogenesis	Spermatogenesis	Spermatogenesis	Not known

Fig. 7.6 Summary of the genetics of the trinucleotide repeat disorders. (FRAX, fragile X syndrome; HD, Huntington disease; SBMA, spinobulbar muscular atrophy; SCA-1, spinocerebellar atrophy type 1; MD, myotonic dystrophy; DRPLA, dentatorubral-pallidoluysian atrophy; AD, autosomal dominant.)

- Spinocerebellar ataxia types 1, 2, 3, 6, and 7 (SCA1, etc.).
- Dentatorubral-pallidoluysian atrophy (DRPLA).

Shake hands with the patient—patients with myotonic dystrophy characteristically have trouble relaxing their grip.

Inversion

Inversions involve from just two to many thousands of base pairs. Sequences at each end of the inverted segment often resemble each other. In hemophilia A, 40% of mutations result from an inversion of several hundred thousand base pairs within the factor VIII gene.

Functional effects of mutation on protein

With the exception of imprinted genes, genes on both the maternal and paternal chromosomes are expressed. If either the maternal or the paternal gene contains a mutation, the cell will express two different protein products. Mutations exert their phenotypic effects by one of two mechanisms: loss of function, or gain of function.

Loss of function mutations

These mutations result in either reduction in activity or loss of the gene product. In the heterozygous state such mutations would, typically, be associated with levels of the functional protein that are half the normal level. They may be dominantly or recessively inherited.

Gain of function mutations

These are inherited dominantly and result in either:
- Increased levels of normal protein expression (simple gain of function).
- The development of new protein functions (dominant negative mutations).

Mendelian inheritance of single gene disorders

On average, Mendelian traits occur in predictable proportions among the offspring of parents with

145

the trait. The pattern of inheritance of a trait shown in pedigrees depends on the chromosomal location of the gene (X-linked or autosomal) and whether the phenotype is dominant or recessive. Therefore, there are four patterns of single gene inheritance:

- Autosomal dominant.
- Autosomal recessive.
- X-linked dominant.
- X-linked recessive.

In medical genetics, a dominant phenotype is one that is expressed in heterozygotes, whereas a recessive trait is expressed only in homozygotes. If the expression of each allele can be detected in the presence of the other, the two alleles are termed codominant.

Dominant and recessive inheritance is defined according to clinical phenotypes, which may not always reflect the behavior of the allele at the molecular level. Mutations in the retinablastoma protein are recessive at the cellular level because one allele expresses enough protein for biological function. However, at the phenotypic level the predisposition to cancer is inherited dominantly because random loss of the compensating allele always occurs in at least one cell.

Autosomal dominant disorders
Autosomal dominant inheritance
A dominant mutation is phenotypically expressed in homozygotes and heterozygotes for that gene (Fig. 7.7). In this pattern of inheritance:

- There is vertical inheritance (affected child usually has an affected parent).
- Unaffected family members usually have unaffected partners, and they produce normal children.
- Affected family members usually have unaffected partners, and they produce a 1 : 1 ratio of normal and affected children.
- Usually both sexes are equally affected, and they are equally likely to pass on the disease.

Homozygotes for the trait are rare. In some autosomal dominant (AD) conditions, new mutations account for a substantial proportion of cases (e.g., achondroplasia, familial adenomatous polyposis). AD genes can show:

- Sex limitation (e.g., balding, gout, male-limited precocious puberty, familial breast/ovarian cancer).

- Reduced penetrance (e.g., retinoblastoma).
- Variable expressivity (e.g., tuberous sclerosis).
- Imprinting (see below).
- Anticipation (see below).

Molecular basis of dominant inheritance
In AD disorders, the disease occurs despite the presence of the normal gene product expressed from the wild-type allele. This may arise as a result of:

- Haploinsufficiency—loss of half of normal protein activity is sufficient for disease to occur (e.g., familial hypercholesterolemia; Fig 7.8).
- Dominant negative effect—the mutant gene product interferes with the function of the normal gene product expressed from the corresponding allele (e.g., osteogenesis imperfecta; Fig. 7.9).
- Simple gain of function—disease arises from increased expression of the normal protein (e.g., Charcot–Marie–Tooth disease type 1a) or expression of an abnormal protein with novel properties that may cause cell toxicity (e.g., Huntington disease).

Examples of autosomal dominant disorders
Fig. 7.10 summarizes the features of the following examples of AD inherited disorders:

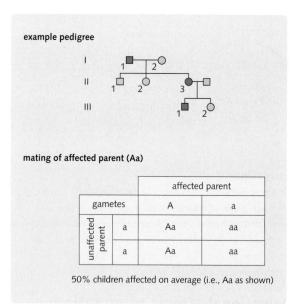

Fig. 7.7 Example pedigree and typical offspring of mating in autosomal dominant inheritance. (A, disease allele.)

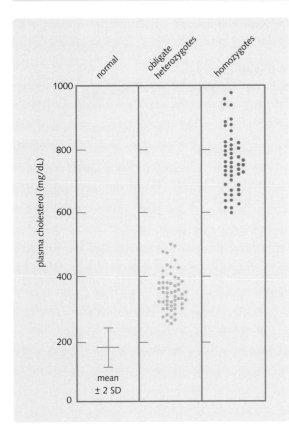

Fig. 7.8 Gene dosage in familial hypercholesterolemia. This disease results from mutations in the gene that codes for the low-density lipoprotein (LDL) receptor, a cell surface protein that binds extracellular LDL and delivers it to the cell interior. Heterozygotes show levels of plasma cholesterol intermediate between normal and homozygotes for the mutation. However, plasma cholesterol level in heterozygotes is sufficient for the development of premature heart disease, so the condition shows an AD pattern of inheritance. (Adapted from Nussbaum, McInnes, and Willard, 2001.)

- Achondroplasia.
- Acute intermittent porphyria.
- Gilles de la Tourette syndrome.
- Familial hypercholesterolemia.
- Marfan syndrome.
- von Willebrand disease.

Autosomal recessive disorders
Autosomal recessive inheritance

A recessive gene or trait is expressed only in homozygotes for the abnormal gene (Fig. 7.11). In autosomal recessive inheritance:

- There is horizontal inheritance (normal parents often have more than one affected child).
- Affected individuals have phenotypically normal parents.
- Affected individuals usually have unaffected partners and all their children will be carriers.
- If a carrier has an unaffected partner, there is a 50% chance of the children being carriers.
- Only matings between heterozygotes will produce affected individuals, with an expected frequency of 1 in 4.
- There is an association with consanguinity due to sharing of genes in families (rare recessive genetic disorders are more likely to arise through consanguinity).
- Both sexes are equally affected and equally likely to pass the mutation to the next generation.

Consanguinity is where there is a mating between two people who have a familial relationship closer than that of second cousins.

Autosomal recessive (AR) genes may show a sex influence: for example, hemochromatosis (see Fig. 7.13) is autosomal recessive, but it has a higher incidence in males due to lower dietary iron intake and menstruation in females.

Complementation

In recessive conditions, affected individuals are homozygous for mutations in a particular gene, so it is expected that two parents with the same phenotype will always have affected children. However, occasionally two such parents will have an unaffected child as a result of complementation. Complementation arises if parents who have the same disorder are homozygous for mutations in different genes in the same pathway (Fig. 7.12). It is defined as the ability of two different genetic defects to correct for one another.

Molecular basis of recessive inheritance

AR disorders are frequently (though not exclusively) attributed to enzyme defects, where expression from the wild-type allele in the heterozygote provides sufficient functional protein to prevent disease. However, homozygotes that express no functional protein develop the associated disorder.

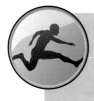

It is believed from studies of the offspring of incestuous matings that everyone carries at least eight to ten mutant alleles for known autosomal recessive disorders.

Examples of autosomal recessive disorders

Fig. 7.13 summarizes the features of the following examples of autosomal recessive disorders:

- α-thalassemia.
- β-thalassemia.
- Congenital adrenal hyperplasia.
- Cystic fibrosis.
- Friedreich ataxia.
- Gaucher disease.
- Hemochromatosis.
- Phenylketonuria.
- Sickle-cell disease.
- Tay–Sachs disease.

X-linked disorders
X-linked recessive inheritance

For X-linked recessive genes the inheritance pattern (Fig. 7.14) is as follows:

- Many more males than females show the recessive phenotype.
- The disease is transmitted by a carrier female, who is usually asymptomatic.
- If a mother is a carrier, her sons have a 50% chance of being affected and her daughters a 50% chance of being carriers.
- An affected male will usually have no affected offspring, but all his daughters will be carriers and, in turn, 50% of their sons will be affected.
- No sons of the affected male will inherit the gene (i.e., there is no male-to-male transmission).

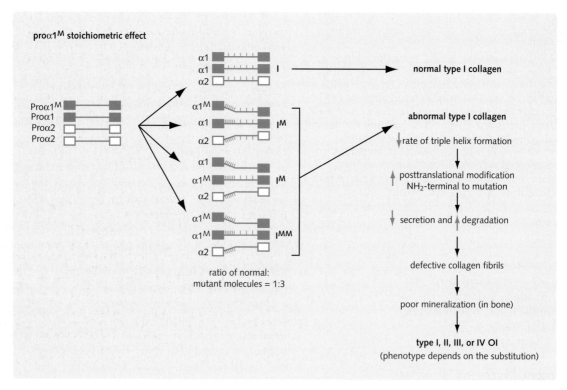

Fig. 7.9 Dominant negative effect. Normal collagen is formed by a triple helix that consists of two molecules of proα1 and one molecule of proα2. Procollagen containing a missense mutation (proα1^M) destabilizes the triple helix, resulting in increased degradation and reduced secretion of the mature protein, which ultimately results in osteogenesis imperfecta (OI). (Adapted from Nussbaum, McInnes, and Willard, 2001.)

A	Autosomal dominant disorders and their features		
Disorder	Etiology	Symptoms	Diagnosis, prognosis, and treatment
Achondroplasia; prevalence 1 in 10,000	Mutation of the FGF receptor encoded on chromosome 3; causes decreased growth of cartilaginous bone; membranous bone is unaffected; 80% new mutation rate (i.e., 80% of cases are due to a mutation arising *de novo* in that individual, not inherited); increased incidence with paternal age; same gene with a different mutation causes a different phenotype (e.g., thanatophoric dwarfism, which is more severe, and hypochondroplasia, which is less severe)	Large head, prominent forehead, short limbs, normal trunk size, lumbar lordosis	Normal IQ and life expectancy
Acute intermittent porphyria	Mutation in porphobilinogen deaminase on chromosome 11; 80% are asymptomatic; environmental factors (e.g., drugs, alcohol, infection, or starvation) may trigger an attack	Colicky abdominal pain, vomiting, constipation, fever, peripheral neuritis (may cause respiratory paralysis), psychosis	Diagnosis—erythrocyte porphobilinogen deaminase assay; treatment—avoid environmental triggers and treat acute attacks with sedation, pain relief, electrolyte balance, carbohydrate, anticonvulsant, antiemetic, propranolol and physiotherapy; prognosis—fatal in 5%
Gilles de la Tourette syndrome; prevalence 1 in 2000	Unknown	Motor and verbal tics (often obscene or animal noises), obsessive–compulsive behavior, attention deficit, learning difficulties	Diagnosis—tics for over 1 year; treatment—haloperidol or clonidine; prognosis—often improves with age
Familial hyper-cholesterolemia	Mutation in LDL receptor gene on chromosome 19	At 30–40 years—xanthoma, xanthelasma, corneal arcus, ischemic heart disease	Diagnosis—family history, increased fasting LDL and cholesterol; definitive diagnosis by DNA pedigree analysis of RFLPs or specific mutations

B	Etiology, symptoms and treatment of Marfan syndrome and von Willebrand disease		
Disorder	Etiology	Symptoms	Diagnosis, prognosis, and treatment
Marfan syndrome	Mutation in gene coding for connective tissue factors	Arachnodactyly (long spidery limbs and fingers); armspan > height; upper to lower segment ratio ↓; high-arched palate, lens dislocation, aortic incompetence	Diagnosis—clinical, combined with ECG; treatment—β blockers may slow aortic dilatation; prognosis—life expectancy 40–50 years due to CVS complications
von Willebrand disease	Deficiency of von Willebrand factor (vWF) which adheres to platelets and binds to factor VIII, preventing its breakdown	Hemorrhage from mucosal sites and postoperatively	Diagnosis—vWF low, factor VIII activity low, prolonged bleeding time, normal platelet count and whole-blood clotting time; treatment—vasopressin, factor VIII, cryoprecipitate

Fig. 7.10 (A) Features of examples of autosomal dominant disorders. (LDL, low-density lipoproteins; RFLPs, restriction fragment length polymorphisms.) (B) Marfan syndrome and von Willebrand disease. (CVS, cardiovascular system; ECG, electrocardiogram; FGF, fibroblast growth factor; LDL, low-density lipoprotein; RFLPs, restriction fragment length polymorphisms.)

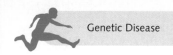

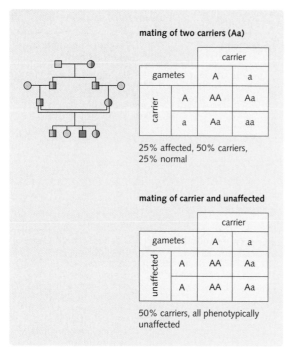

mating of two carriers (Aa)

gametes	carrier	
	A	a
carrier A	AA	Aa
carrier a	Aa	aa

25% affected, 50% carriers, 25% normal

mating of carrier and unaffected

gametes	carrier	
	A	a
unaffected A	AA	Aa
unaffected A	AA	Aa

50% carriers, all phenotypically unaffected

Fig. 7.11 Example pedigree and typical offspring of matings in autosomal recessive inheritance. (a, disease allele.)

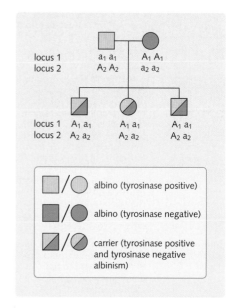

locus 1   a₁ a₁   A₁ A₁
locus 2   A₂ A₂   a₂ a₂

locus 1   A₁ a₁   A₁ a₁   A₁ a₁
locus 2   A₂ a₂   A₂ a₂   A₂ a₂

■/● albino (tyrosinase positive)

■/● albino (tyrosinase negative)

▨/◐ carrier (tyrosinase positive and tyrosinase negative albinism)

Fig. 7.12 Pedigree showing complementation. Both parents are albino, but all their children are normal. Given that albinism is an autosomal recessive condition, this observation can be explained if the parents are homozygous for mutations in different genes in the same pathway. The children are thus unaffected carriers of both mutations. (A_1, wild-type at locus 1, a_1, mutant at locus 1, A_2, wild-type at locus 2, a_2, mutant at locus 2.)

- Affected males may have unaffected parents, but they will often have an affected maternal uncle or cousin.

X-linked dominant inheritance

The X-linked dominant inheritance pattern is rare and difficult to distinguish from AD except that affected males have normal sons, but all daughters are affected. Examples include Xg blood group, X-linked hypophosphatemic rickets, Rett syndrome (usually sporadic, but X-linked dominant familial forms exist that are only seen in females because the condition is lethal in males).

Molecular basis of X-linked inheritance

Males (XY) have only one X chromosome, and they are, therefore, said to be hemizygous. Since males receive only one copy of X-linked genes (except for those in the pseudo-autosomal region) they will express any X-linked recessive traits because they do not have a compensating wild-type allele.

To compensate for the double complement in females, X chromosome inactivation ensures that

X-linked genes are only expressed from one of the two X chromosomes in any given cell. The selection of an X chromosome for inactivation within a specific cell is random, but once established early in development inactivation is transmitted to daughter cells. Females do not tend to show X-linked recessive disease because many of their cells will be expressing the wild-type allele. However, women can be affected with X-linked recessive conditions in the following situations:

- If she is the daughter of an affected male and a carrier female.
- If there is lyonization (inactivation) of a normal X chromosome in a skewed pattern, so that a greater proportion of normal X chromosomes are inactivated.
- If there is X chromosome–autosome translocation.
- If 45,X (Turner syndrome) is present.

Examples of X-linked recessive disorders

Figure 7.15 summarizes the features of the following examples of X-linked recessive disorders:

Autosomal recessive disorders and their features			
Disorder	Etiology	Symptoms	Diagnosis, prognosis and treatment
Gaucher disease; incidence 1 in 25,000; carriers 1 in 15 Ashkenazi Jews	Mutation in β-glucosidase, encoded on chromosome 1; causes glucocerebrosidase accumulation	Type I (adult)—no neurological features, onset 2–70 years, bone pain, splenomegaly; type II (infantile)—marked neurological symptoms, onset 1–2 months, hepatosplenomegaly, death by 2 years of age; type III (juvenile)—neurological symptoms present, onset at 5 years	Diagnosis—biochemical assay of β-glucosidase activity; treatment—enzyme replacement therapy, bone marrow transplant (only if severe) and gene therapy in the future; prognosis—assay does not predict prognosis, which depends on phenotype I, II, or III
Hemochromatosis	Primary is inherited via a gene on chromosome 6; secondary is caused by another disease or transfusion	Excess iron accumulates in tissues, especially liver, causing cirrhosis, cardiomyopathy, and diabetes mellitus	Diagnosis—high transferrin saturation, high serum iron, high serum ferritin; liver biopsy is definitive; treatment—phlebotomy
Phenylketonuria	Mutation of phenylalanine hydroxylase encoded on chromosome 12	Decreased IQ, fair hair, fits, eczema, musty urine; untreated affected females have malformed offspring	Treatment—diet low in phenylalanine, with tyrosine supplements for entire life; diagnosis—elevated blood or urine phenylalanine; mandatory test in all neonates by Guthrie heel-prick test
Sickle-cell disease	Point mutation Glu-6 to Val on position 6 of β-globin gene encoded on chromosome 11p (HbA to HbS); distorted sickle-shaped cells by polymerization of deoxygenated HbS; sickle cells can block vessels or hemolyze; electrophoresis—majority HbS, some HbA2, persistence of HbF; common in Africans	Homozygotes (SS)—hemolytic anemia, infarction (e.g., hand and foot syndrome), splenomegaly early, then splenic infarction after more than 10 years, respiratory infections, osteomyelitis (especially *Salmonella*), crises (painful bone marrow aplasia, sequestration, or hemolytic) often triggered by infections; heterozygote (AS)—has an advantage against cerebral malaria; hypoxia may precipitate an occlusive crisis	Diagnosis—prenatal diagnosis by direct assay involves PCR amplification of the relevant β-globin region, followed by digestion with a restriction enzyme as *Mst*II restriction site lost; carrier detection by hematologic assay (e.g., Hb electrophoresis); treatment—pneumococcal vaccine and support during crises; prognosis—decreased life expectancy in HbSS
Tay–Sachs disease; carrier 1 in 250 in general population; 1 in 25 in Ashkenazi Jews	Lysosomal storage disorder; mutation in hexosaminidase A α-chain encoded on chromosome 15 causes ganglioside GM2 accumulation	Progressive neurological abnormalities begin in late infancy; cherry red macular spot in 90% (not pathognomonic); decreased serum β N-acetyl hexosaminidase activity; death at 3–4 years of age	Diagnosis—carrier screening in Jewish population; carrier detection by decreased hexosaminidase levels on assay; prenatal diagnosis by assay on fetal samples; treatment—no specific treatment, just supportive
α-thalassemia	The fetus normally has HbF (α_2, γ_2); normal adults have 95% HbA (α_2, β_2) and a small amount of HbA2 (α_2, δ_2); mutation occurs in the two α-globin genes encoded on chromosome 16p; each person has two	α-thalassemia type I homozygotes (––/––) have no functional α-globin genes, resulting in hydrops fetalis; in hemoglobin H disease (––/–α) there is a single α-globin gene and a good prognosis; the following have absence of one	Diagnosis—Hb electrophoresis, FBC, MCV; α-thalassemia type I homozygote—80% hemoglobin Barts (four γ-chains), persistent fetal hemoglobin; hemoglobin H disease—some hemoglobin Barts, 5–30% HbH (four

Fig. 7.13 Features of examples of autosomal recessive disorders. (ACTH, adrenocorticotrophic hormone; FBC, full blood count; HbA, hemoglobin A; HbF, hemoglobin F; HbS, hemoglobin S; MCV, mean red cell volume; MCHC, mean red cell hemoglobin concentration; PCR, polymerase chain reaction.)

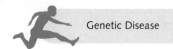

	chromosome 16s, so four α-globin genes (αα, αα); severity depends on the number of functional α-genes; this disorder is more common in Black populations	or two genes, resulting in mild anemia—α-thalassemia type 2 homozygote (−α/−α), α-thalassemia type γ heterozygote (−−/αα), α-thalassemia type 2 heterozygote (−α/αα)	β-chains), reduced MCHC and MCV; treatment—transfusion, iron chelation, folate, ascorbic acid, and splenectomy in hypersplenism
β-thalassemia	Mutation in β-globin gene encoded on 11p; common in Mediterranean populations, Chinese, Indians, and American Blacks	Severe chronic hemolytic anemia; iron overload (despite chelation) causes endocrine, liver, and heart failure	Diagnosis and treatment—as in α-thalassemia, β-thalassemia major—blood film (hypochromic microcytic cells and target cells), HbF increases, HbA2 variable, HbA absent; β-thalassemia minor—HbA2 > 3.5%, mild anemia and decreased MCV; moderate mutational heterogeneity but each population has a prevalent set of mutations; mutations are detected by using the indirect method of a bank of related assays (the reverse dot-blot method); prenatal diagnosis is available; prognosis—minor has good prognosis, major results in death within 1 year if not treated with transfusions; with transfusions death occurs at 20–40 years of age due to iron overload
Congenital adrenal hyperplasia	Mutation usually in 21-hydroxylase gene on chromosome 6 which produces aldosterone and cortisone; absence of enzyme causes procursor conversion into testosterone	Masculinization of female genitalia, precocious puberty in male, salt-losing crises may occur owing to deficiency of mineralocorticoid (mainly aldosterone)	Diagnosis—low cortisol and aldosterone, high ACTH levels (no negative feedback)
Cystic fibrosis	Incidence 1 in 2000 Caucasians; carrier rate is 1 in 25 of the US population. Gene on 7q31 encodes chloride channel transmembrane conductance regulator; defective regulation of chloride transport results in accumulation of thick viscid secretions in pancreas, respiratory, gastrointestinal, and genitourinary tracts; in the US 58% of CF mutations are deletion of phenylalanine at codon 508 (Δ508); rare in African or Asian population	Chronic obstructive airways disease, shortness of breath, pancreatic insufficiency, failure to thrive, malabsorption, meconium ileus; male infertility (some mild forms present with this), fatal heat prostration	Diagnosis—sweat test [Na⁺] + [Cl⁻] > 70 mM; prenatal diagnosis—Brock test (microvillar enzymes in amniotic fluid); treatment—pancreatic enzyme supplements, diet, physiotherapy clears lungs, inhalers, nebulizers, antibiotics for infections, heart/lung transplant and gene therapy (currently trials with nasal spray); prognosis—until recently death in infancy or childhood, now many live into 40s
Friedreich ataxia	Gene located on 7q, encodes *frataxin*; spinocerebellar degeneration with cerebellar ataxia and degeneration of posteric; columns and cortico-spinal and spinocerebellar tract	At 6–8 years develop ataxia, pigeon chest, loss of deep tendon reflexes in legs, extensor plantars; need wheelchair in 20s	Prognosis—life expectancy into 5th or 6th decade

Fig. 7.13—cont'd.

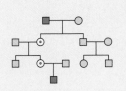

mating of affected male		
	affected male	
gametes	X^D	Y
unaffected female — X	X^D X	XY
unaffected female — X	X^D X	XY

all daughters carriers, all sons normal

mating of carrier female		
	unaffected male	
gametes	X	Y
carrier female — X^D	X^D X	X^D Y
carrier female — X	XX	XY

half of children inherit gene regardless of sex, 50% daughters carriers, 50% sons affected, 50% children normal

Fig. 7.14 Example pedigree and typical offspring of mating in X-linked recessive inheritance. (X^D, disease allele.)

- Adrenoleucodystrophy.
- Duchenne muscular dystrophy.
- Becker muscular dystrophy.
- Fabry disease.
- Glucose-6-phosphate dehydrogenase (G6PD) deficiency.
- Hemophilia A.
- Hemophila B (Christmas disease).
- Lesch–Nyhan syndrome.

Heterogeneity in Mendelian disorders
Genetic heterogeneity
This is the phenomenon by which a disorder can be caused by different allelic mutations, or mutations in different loci. Such disorders might (but will not necessarily) show more than one mode of inheritance (Fig. 7.16).

Alleleic heterogeneity
This is an important cause of clinical variation. Different mutations in the same gene may result in different phenotypes. For example, specific mutations within the *CFTR* gene are associated with pancreatic sufficient as opposed to pancreatic insufficient forms of cystic fibrosis.

Locus heterogeneity
This is the situation in which mutations at two or more distinct loci can produce the same or similar phenotype. For example, retinitis pigmentosa may result from mutations in many different genes, including the rhodopsin gene on chromosome 3 and a GTPase regulator gene on the X chromosome.

Molecular genetic research moves at a frantic pace and disease genes are being cloned and characterized all the time. The Online Mendelian Inheritance in Man (OMIM) webpage [http://www.ncbi.nlm.nih. gov/omim/] is a regularly updated source of information, as are the data at GeneTests [http://www. genetests.org], which also includes links to the laboratories that offer diagnostic testing for individual disorders.

Non-Mendelian inheritance of single gene disorders
A number of disorders have been identified that do not follow classic patterns of Mendelian inheritance. The molecular mechanisms underlying these observations are now beginning to be understood.

Terminology
Penetrance
This is the proportion of individuals with a specified genotype that show the expected phenotype under defined environmental conditions. The term is usually used in association with dominant disorders.
- If a genetic lesion is completely penetrant (100%), all the individuals with that altered gene express it (e.g., Huntington disease).
- About 75% of women with certain mutations in the *BRCA1* gene develop breast or ovarian cancer (i.e., the mutations have a penetrance of 75%).

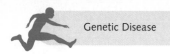

X-linked recessive disorders and their features

Disorder	Etiology	Symptoms	Diagnosis, prognosis, and treatment
Glucose-6-phosphate dehydrogenase (G6PD) deficiency	G6PD enzyme defect on Xq28; erythrocytes susceptible to oxidative damage, which is often precipitated by drugs, illness, or fava beans	Hemolytic anemia; variable phenotype, most severe resulting in neonatal jaundice	Diagnosis—enzyme assay; treatment includes avoiding precipitating factors
Hemophilia A; incidence 1 in 5000 liveborn males	Mutation in factor VIII locus, on Xq28; gene product is involved in intrinsic blood coagulation pathway	Recurrent hemorrhage into soft tissues and joints when levels less than 30% (severity varies)	Diagnosis—prenatal diagnosis by fetal sampling and DNA analysis, direct and definitive; carrier detection by pedigree studies; less accurate carrier detection possible by factor VIII coagulation (but result may be spuriously normal due to random X inactivation); treatment—administer coagulation factor; risk of producing inhibitor complication where antibodies are produced against "foreign therapeutic coagulation factors"—this complication may arise if the mutation results in no factor VIII being produced so the immune system is not primed; prognosis—blood transfusions during the 1980s inadvertently transmitted bloodborne viruses (e.g., HIV, hepatitis B, C, and D), which have decreased the life expectancy of many patients transfused over this period, so now synthetic (recombinant) factor VIII is preferred
Hemophilia B (Christmas disease); incidence 1 in 30,000 liveborn males	Mutation of factor IX gene on Xq27.1; factor IX is involved in the coagulation cascade	Hemorrhage usually less severe than in hemophilia A	Diagnosis—highly heterogenous mutation, so needs direct diagnosis by sequencing the mutation in the family under investigation, as in hemophilia A; treatment—administer coagulation factor; risk of inhibitor complication but less than for hemophilia A; prognosis—decreased life expectancy in those that have acquired bloodborne infections through transfusion but HIV rarely contaminated factor IX preparation
Lesch–Nyhan syndrome	Disorder of purine synthesis causing hyperuricemia and reduced erythrocyte hypexanthine-guanine phosphoribosyltransferase (HPRT)	Spasticity, mental retardation, self-harm, renal stones, gouty arthritis	Diagnosis—enzyme assay of HPRT; treatment—allopurinol (does not affect neurological signs)
Adrenoleucodystrophy	Type 3 peroxisomal disorder, due to a single enzyme defect; enzyme affected is involved in β oxidation	Onset is at 4–5 years, with behavioral, visual, and neurological abnormalities	Diagnosis—first made by measuring metabolites, then confirmed by enzyme assay

Disorder	Pathology/genetics	Clinical features	Diagnosis/treatment/prognosis
Duchenne muscular dystrophy (DMD); incidence 1 in 3500 liveborn males	Most common severe X-linked disease; mutation in Xp21 coding for cytoskeletal protein dystrophin, causes protein to lose its C-terminal proteins; one-third are new mutations; 2–3 Mb, largest known gene, *dystrophin*; prevents the muscle from tearing during contraction and prevents degeneration of muscle fibers; fiber appearance—variation in fiber size, eosinophilic fibers (with intracellular calcium), increased connective tissue between fibers and lipid droplet accumulations	30% have decreased IQ; electroretinopathy (form of night blindness), increased phospho-fructokinase; newborn appears normal; at 3–4 years of age there is difficulty rising from sitting (Gower's manouver—climbing up legs), pseudohypertrophy of calf muscles, deltoid, scapula, and quadriceps (muscle replaced by fat and connective tissue) and cardiomyopathy; at 6 years of age ambulation is difficult (require callipers), symmetrical wasting; at 12 years of age most are wheelchair bound and have scoliosis; die at 17–20 years of age due to respiratory insufficiency	Diagnosis—creatine kinase grossly elevated; EMG myopathic; DNA analysis—many mutations possible, need to isolate family-specific mutation and set up an assay for clinical diagnosis (60% are deletions or duplications, 40% are point mutations); stain for dystrophin on muscle biopsy—absent; carrier detection by creatine kinase assay and definitive DNA analysis (risks only lowered to 5–10% due to germ-line mosaicism); treatment—physiotherapy, prednisolone (a catabolic steroid which helps to preserve muscle strength), minimal bed rest when ill or may never walk again; ambulation aids—callipers, percutaneous tenotomy, foot orthosis, etc., early spinal fusion; monitor heart (protected to a degree by lack of mobility; do not fuse spine if severe cardiomyopathy as anesthetics cannot be given; nasal ventilation at night (decreases somnolence); gene therapy awaited; prognosis—death in early twenties
Becker muscular dystrophy; incidence 1 in 30,000 liveborn males	Caused by in-frame deletions in the Xp21 *dystrophin* gene, which remove amino acids but preserve the translational reading frame	At 16 years of age some are wheelchair bound; some have cardiomyopathy; there is an intermediate phenotype to DMD with loss of ambulation at 12–16 years of age	Diagnosis—creatine kinase increased, EMG myopathic; DNA deletion screen; stain for dystrophin on muscle biopsy—present; ECG and echocardiogram show cardiomyopathy; treatment—prednisolone; prognosis— near-normal life expectancy
Fabry disease	Deficiency of galactosidase A, causes accumulation of ceramide in skin, kidneys, and cardiovascular system	Angiokeratoma; cardiovascular system—infarction, angina, valve lesions, cardiomyopathy	Enzyme replacement therapy now available; prognosis— live into fifties

Fig. 7.15 Features of examples of X-linked recessive disorders. (ECG, electrocardiogram; EMG, electromyography; RFLPs, restriction fragment length polymorphisms.)

Single gene disorders with more than one mode of inheritance

Disorder	Etiology	Symptoms	Diagnosis, prognosis, and treatment
Alport syndrome; carrier frequency 1 in 5000	X-linked or autosomal recessive glomerulonephritis; associated with sensorineural deafness and eye lesions; genes affected each code for different α chains of type IV collagen—chains of type IV collagen—α_1 (COL4A1) on chromosome 13, α_2 (COL4A2) on chromosome 13, α_3 (COL4A3) on chromosome 2, α_4 (COL4A4) on chromosome 2, α_5 (COL4A5) on Xq22; type IV collagen is the major structural protein in the basement membrane; type COL4A5 is important in the basement membrane of glomeruli, lens, and organ of Corti	By 5 years of age—microscopic hematuria; by 10 years—high-tone deafness; mid-teens—increased blood pressure; by 20 years—increased plasma creatinine; by 25 years—end-stage renal failure; associated with leiomyomatosis; course due to random X inactivation	Renal failure
Charcot–Marie–Tooth syndrome (peroneal muscular atrophy)	Also known as hereditary motor and sensory neuropathy type I; inheritance usually AD (chromosome 17) but can be AR or X-linked dominant; genetically determined polyneuropathies, classified according to inheritance	Progressive from puberty—foot drop, leg weakness, "inverted champagne bottle" legs (ankles are the corks), general limb weakness, diminished sensation and reflexes	Diagnosis—nerve biopsy shows demyelination
Ehlers–Danlos syndrome	Abnormal collagen affects skin, joints, and vasculature; inheritance usually AD but may be AR or X-linked	Lax skin, hypermobile joints, scoliosis, purpura (skin bruising), bleeding of internal organs, fragile eyes	Prognosis—decreased if vasculature is affected
Mucopoly-saccharidoses; incidence 7 in 100,000 live births	Lysosomal storage disorders; uronic acid alternates with an amino sugar in a mucopolysaccharide; degradation occurs in a stepwise manner, with any deficient enzyme resulting in a disease; AR inheritance except for the following X-linked disease (Hunter syndrome)	Progressive neurological degeneration, hepato/splenomegaly, skeletal dysplasia, short stature, bone pain, coarse facies, eyes—cherry red spots, corneal clouding	Diagnosis—biochemical identification of mucopolysaccharides in urine and amniotic fluid
Polycystic kidney disease; incidence AD 1 in 1000, AR 1 in 40,000; carrier frequency 1 in 100	Primary polycystic kidney disease (PKD) is either adult (AD) or infantile (AR); secondary PKD may have no genetic link (e.g., due to obstructive anomalies in utero); AD PKD type 1 due to mutation on chromosome 16; type II due to mutation on chromosome 4; AR PKD—gene affected is on chromosome 6, causing disease with four distinct levels of severity	Normally fatal in infants; adult type symptoms—loin pain, renal colic, hypertension, hematuria (blood in urine), urinary tract infection, uremia	AD PKD type II has a more benign course than type I; AR PKD—perinatal rapidly die at birth, neonatal (onset neonatal) die by 3 months; infantile (onset in first 6 months)—liver cysts prominent; juvenile (onset at 1–5 years of age)—severe liver involvement
Retinitis pigmentosa	AD, AR, or X-linked variants; macrophages around retinal vessels accumulate melanin from the choroid	Progressive night blindness and tunnel vision	Diagnosis—visualize retinal pigment particles; prognosis—progressive blindness
Severe combined immuno deficiency	Many AR and X-linked variants; adenosine deaminase deficiency; purine nucleoside phosphorylase deficiency	Recurrent viral, fungal, and bacterial infections; failure to thrive	Treatment—traditionally by marrow transplant; first disease to be treated by gene therapy (1990); prognosis—death in infancy if untreated

Fig. 7.16 Features of examples of single gene disorders with more than one mode of inheritance. (AD, autosomal dominant; AR, autosomal recessive; COL4 An, collagen type IV of n type α-chain.)

Variable expressivity

This occurs when a genetic lesion produces a range of phenotypes: for example, tuberous sclerosis can be asymptomatic with harmless kidney cysts, but in the next generation it may be fatal, owing to the development of brain malformations.

Mechanisms underlying non-Mendelian inheritance

Anticipation

Anticipation is the occurrence of a heredity disease with a progressively earlier age of onset, progressively more serious clinical symptoms, or an increase in frequency in successive generations. The mutations in genes associated with anticipation are trinucleotide repeat expansions, which have a tendency to get larger in successive generations (e.g., Huntington chorea, myotonic dystrophy). Large expansions of the triplet repeat are associated with early age of onset (Fig. 7.17).

Imprinting

This is differential expression of genetic material at chromosomal or allelic level, depending upon which parent (male or female) it has been inherited from. It is thought to result from the selective inactivation of genes (probably through methylation) in different patterns in the course of male and female gametogenesis. Hydatidiform moles illustrate the different roles of paternal and maternal genomes:

- A complete mole (46,XX) has chromosomes that are all paternal in origin (both X chromosomes being of paternal origin, i.e., extra paternal set, but no maternal set), and it results in either no fetus or a normal placenta with severe hyperplasia of the cytotrophoblast.
- A partial mole (69) is a triploid with an extra set of chromosomes of maternal or paternal origin. An extra paternal set (diandric) results in abundant trophoblast, but poor embryonic development. An extra maternal set (digynic) results in severely retarded embryonic development with a small fibrotic placenta.

Imprinting is important in the etiology of Prader–Willi and Angelman syndromes, which both arise from the same microdeletion of chromosome 15 (q11–13). The phenotype varies between Prader–Willi (PWS) and Angelman syndromes (AS) according to whether the deleted chromosome is

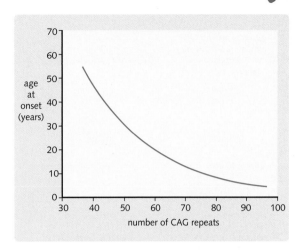

Fig. 7.17 The relationship between the size of triplet repeat expansion and age of onset of Huntington disease. (Adapted from Squitieri *et al.*, *Am J Med Genet* 95(4): 366–373, 2000.)

paternally or maternally inherited (Fig. 7.18). Several genes map to this area, and are expressed in the normal individual. However, the genes associated with PWS are only expressed on the paternally derived chromosome, while the *UBE3A* gene associated with AS is only expressed on the maternally inherited chromosome. Imprinting has switched off the PWS genes on the maternally derived chromosome and switched off the *UBE3A* gene on the paternally derived copy. When a child inherits a chromosome 15 with the microdeletion:

- Prader–Willi syndrome is due to paternal deletion (the PWS genes are not expressed from either chromosome).
- Angelman syndrome is due to maternal deletion (the AS associated *UBE3A* gene is not expressed from either chromosome).

The imprinting patterns at this region are controlled by an "imprinting center," located within 15q11–13. Mutations in the imprinting center can permanently "fix" the imprint of a chromosome, also leading to AS or PWS.

Uniparental disomy

This is caused by duplication of a chromosome from one parent with loss of the corresponding homolog from the other parent (Fig. 7.19). For example, uniparental disomy of maternal chromosome 15 can result in the same phenotype as Prader–Willi, but with no deletion because there

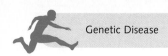

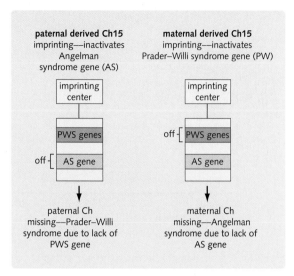

Fig. 7.18 How deletion of one parental chromosome 15 with imprinting of the present chromosome 15 can lead to Prader–Willi or Angelman syndrome. Normal development requires both maternally and paternally derived genes to be expressed (see Fig. 7.27).

is no paternally contributed chromosome 15. A few cases of cystic fibrosis with severe growth retardation have two homologous chromosomes 7 of maternal origin, and probably growth retardation reflects imprinting of a growth function gene. Beckwith–Wiedemann syndrome can be due to paternal duplication of 11p15.

Mitochondrial inheritance

Mitochondrial growth and division are dependent on genes expressed from both the mitochondrial and the nuclear chromosomes. Mitochondrial DNA is maternally inherited because sperm contributes no mitochondria to the zygote. Thus, diseases that result from mutations in mitochondrial DNA (Fig. 7.20) are maternally inherited, and affected males cannot transmit the disease.

Mitochondria are distributed randomly in daughter cells, so these may contain entirely normal mitochondrial DNA or entirely mutant DNA (homoplasmy), or else a mixture of both (heteroplasmy). There is, therefore, variable expression of disease due to mutation in mitochondrial DNA, depending upon the relative proportion of normal to mutant DNA.

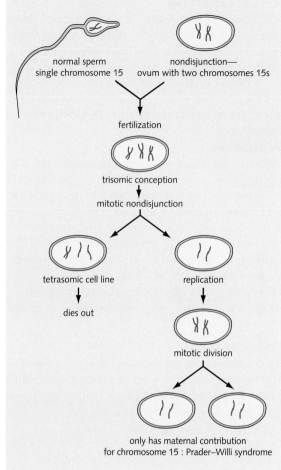

Fig. 7.19 Mechanism of uniparental disomy (here for chromosome 15).

Mosaicism

A mosaic is an individual with multiple cell lines (which exhibit different genotypes) that arise from a single zygote. Mosaics arise when a genetic mutation occurs in postzygotic mitotic division. All progeny of the mutant cell and, therefore, the cell types derived from it will exhibit the new mutation. Mosaicism can be an important clinical factor in some instances of chromosomal disorders (e.g., mild cases of Down syndrome may be mosaics (46,XX and 47,XX+21)) during the early stages of division of a normal (46,XX) zygote and in tumor development.

Germ-line mosaicism occurs when an abnormal cell line is confined to the gonads, and it may

Examples of mitochondrial disorders	
Disease	Phenotype
Leber's hereditary optic neuropathy	Rapid optic nerve death, leading to blindness in young adult life
NARP, Leigh disease	Neuropathy ataxia, retinitis pigmentosa, developmental delay, mental retardation, lactic acidemia
MELAS	Mitochondrial encephalomyopathy, lactic acidosis, and strokelike episodes; may manifest only as diabetes mellitus
MERRF	Myoclonic epilepsy, ragged red fibers in muscle, ataxia, sensorineural deafness
Deafness	Progressive sensorineural deafness, often induced by aminoglycoside antibiotics Nonsyndromic sensorineural deafness
Chronic progressive external ophthalmoplegia (CPEO)	Progressive weakness of extraocular muscles
Pearson syndrome	Pancreatic insufficiency, pancytopenia, lactic acidosis
Kearns–Sayre syndrome (KSS)	Progressive external ophthalmoplegia of early onset with heart-block, retinal pigmentation

Fig. 7.20 Examples of mitochondrial disorders. (Adapted from Nussbaum, McInnes, and Willard, 2001.)

account for apparently unaffected parents producing more than one child with an AD condition.

Somatic mosaicism is where either the paternal or maternal representative of a chromosome is randomly inactivated in each somatic cell. Cells differ with respect to which chromosome is inactivated, but once inactivation is established all the cells progeny will retain the same pattern of inactivation. It may account for:

• Unusually mild symptoms in AD metabolic conditions, if there is disproportionate inactivation of the aberrant gene.
• Expression of X-linked disease alleles in female carriers if there is disproportionate inactivation of the normal gene.

Chromosomal disorders

Terminology
Karyotype
The chromosome constitution of an individual. The normal human karyotype is 46,XY (male) or 46,XX (female).

Polyploidy and triploidy
Polyploidy occurs when the number of haploid chromosome sets is greater than two (triploidy, tetraploidy, etc.). Triploidy is having three haploid sets of chromosomes in the cell nucleus (i.e., three copies of each chromosome). In humans, this condition is not compatible with life, but it is common in plants.

Aneuploidy
The condition in which the chromosome number of the cell is not an exact multiple of the haploid number. Monosomies and trisomies are examples of aneuploidy.

Trisomy
The state of having three representatives of a given chromosome instead of the usual pair (e.g., as in trisomy 21—Down syndrome).

Monosomy
A chromosome constitution in which one member of a chromosome pair is missing (e.g., Turner syndrome (45,X)).

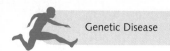
Translocation

The transfer of one segment of a chromosome to another.

Introduction

Chromosomal disorders occur in at least 10% of all spermatozoa and up to 25% of mature oocytes, but live-birth incidence is only 6 in 1000 since most end in spontaneous abortion. Chromosomal disorders may be numerical or structural. Numerical disorders concern:

- Extra single chromosomes (e.g., trisomy).
- Missing single chromosomes (e.g., monosomy—lethal except for 45,X).
- Extra haploid sets (e.g., tetraploids or triploids).

These disorders result in gene-dosage effects. In the case of polyploidy and trisomy, disease results from overexpression of the chromosomal genes (simple gain of function). In monosomies disease results from haploinsufficiency (loss of function) of the genes that are expressed from the missing chromosome.

Structural disorders include conditions resulting from:

- Translocation.
- Inversion.
- Isochromosome.
- Duplication and deletion of chromosomal segments involving many genes.
- Ring chromosomes.

Disease arising from these disorders may result from gene dosage effects or misexpression of critical genes due to disruption of the regulatory regions.

Nomenclature used for chromosome disorders

All chromosomal disorders are individually rare, with no clear patterns of inheritance and minimal risk to relatives. International Standard Chromosome Nomenclature (ISCN) is as follows:

- Numerical disorders are described as follows—number of chromosomes, sex chromosomes, + or – chromosome number, for example, boy with trisomy 21 is [47,XY,+21], Turner syndrome is [45,X].
- Structural disorders are described as follows—number of chromosomes, sex chromosomes, mutation (chromosomes involved), (break points, margins or region) (p, short arm; q, long arm).

Examples of ISCN for structural disorders are as follows:

- Translocation (t)—[46,XY, t(14;21) (q11,p10)].
- Inversion (inv)—[46,XY, inv(9)(p12,q14)] pericentric inversion.
- Isochromosome (I)—[46,X, I(Xq)] long chromosome arm of X duplicated.
- Duplication (dup)—[46,XY, dup(5) (q20–q30)].
- Deletion (del) and ring chromosome (r)—[46,XY, del(15)(q11–q13)] in Prader–Willi syndrome; [46,XX, r(X)(p12,q14)].

Mechanisms leading to numerical chromosomal disorders

Polyploidy

Polyploids arise as a result of:

- Fertilization by two sperm.
- A diploid sperm due to failure in meiosis.
- A diploid ovum due to a failure in meiosis.

Trisomies

Trisomies may result from the failure of separation (nondisjunction) of homologous chromosomes at meiosis I or from the failure of separation of chromatids in meiosis II (Fig. 7.21).

The cause of nondisjunction is not fully understood. There is a well-documented association between advancing maternal age and increased incidence of trisomy. It is believed that there is an aging effect on the oocyte, which remains in a state of suspended arrest (dictyotene) from before birth until the time of ovulation—up to 50 years. Research has also shown an association between absent or aberrant meiotic recombination during meiosis I prophase and subsequent nondisjunction.

Most cases of autosomal trisomy result from nondisjunction at meiosis I in the female germ line.

Monosomies

Monosomies may result from nondisjunction (Fig. 7.21) or from "anaphase lag". Anaphase lag occurs

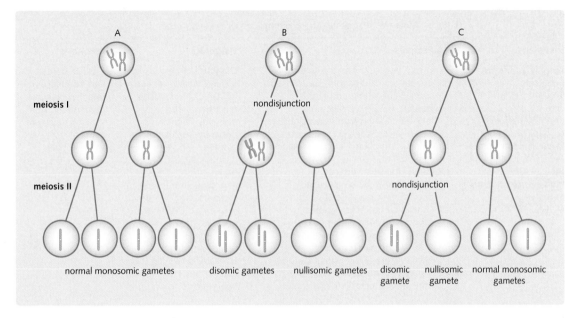

Fig. 7.21 Segregation at meiosis of a single pair of chromosomes. (A) Normal meiosis. (B) Nondisjunction in meiosis I. (C) Nondisjunction in meiosis II. Note that nondisjunction results in disomic and nullisomic gametes, which following fertilization would result in trisomy and monosomy, respectively. (Adapted from Mueller and Young, 2001.)

when there is a delay in the movement of one chromosome from the metaphase plate during anaphase. This may result in the loss of a chromosome if it fails to reach the pole of the cell before the nuclear membrane reforms.

Examples of numerical chromosomal disorders
Autosomal disorders
There are only three well-defined autosomal trisomies that are compatible with postnatal survival:
- Trisomy 21—Down syndrome (Fig. 7.22).
- Trisomy 18—Edwards syndrome (Fig. 7.23).
- Trisomy 13—Patau syndrome (see Fig. 7.23).

Sex chromosome disorders
Examples of sex chromosome abnormalities are:
- Klinefelter syndrome (Fig. 7.24).
- Turner syndrome (see Fig. 7.24).

XXX
This is a female with an extra X chromosome. The incidence is 1 in 1500 females; 25% are infertile and some have mild mental retardation, otherwise there are no distinguishing features.

XYY
This male has an extra Y chromosome; the incidence is 1 in 1000 males. XYY males are often tall but have normal body proportions. Although often asymptomatic, there may be subtle motor incoordination and behavior problems, with aggression in childhood. It is debatable whether an increase in criminal behavior is seen among XYY adults, although it is important to stress that most 47,XYY men have neither learning disabilities nor a criminal record.

XX male
Y sequences are transferred to the X chromosome, with an incidence of 1 in 20,000 males. These males have a similar appearance to males with Klinefelter syndrome, but:
- Are sterile.
- Show no skeletal disproportion.
- Have a normal IQ.

XX males usually present at the infertility clinic or when a prenatally predicted female appears to be male. Confirmation is by banding studies, DNA analysis, and *in situ* hybridization, which identify Y-specific sequences.

161

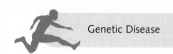

Features, diagnosis, and prognosis of Down syndrome

Disorder	Features	Diagnosis	Prognosis
Trisomy 21 (Down syndrome); 1 in 650 liveborns: extra chromosome 21; age of mother affects probability of having Down syndrome baby —1 in 1000 probability for 25–30-year-old mothers, but 1 in 40 probability for 45-year-old mothers	Facial: upward sloping palpebral fissures, epicanthic folds, Brushfi eld spots on iris, flat round face, flat occiput, brachycephalic skull, low-set ears, protruding tongue: other—dermatoglyphics (abnormal palmar and plantar creases, including single palmar (simian) crease); congenital heart disease in 46% (lack endocardial cushion); duodenal alresia (bile-stained vomit); mental retardation IQ < 50 (but highly variable); later—lymphoblastic leukemia (1%), Alzheimer disease by 30–40 years of age, small stature, respiratory infections, secretory otitis media, cataracts and squints (2%), hypothyroid (3%), epilepsy (10%), diabetic risk increased, early onset atheromatous degeneration of the CVS	Diagnosis is obvious by facial appearance alone in 90%; chromosome analysis is definitive; prenatal diagnosis is available—screening of women > 35 years only includes 10% of the pregnant population; improved strategy combines age, maternal serum AFP (MSAFP), unconjugated estradiol and HCG to give a composite risk; first-trimester screening markers are currently being tested	Cardiac defects can lead to death in infancy; presenile dementia > 40 years; usually life expectancy is less than 50 years

Fig. 7.22 Features, diagnosis, and prognosis of Down syndrome.

Features of trisomy 18 and trisomy 13

Disorder	Features	Diagnosis	Prognosis
Trisomy 18 (Edwards syndrome);incidence 1 in 8000 live births; etiology—extra chromosome 18	Elongated skull, small jaw, low-set malformed ears with large lobes, congenital heart disease, malformed kidneys, clenched hands, rockerbottom feet, developmental delay	Suspected clinically confirmed by chromosome analysis	90% die within the first years, most in first few weeks
Trisomy 13 (Patau syndrome); incidence 1 in 14,000 live births; etiology—extra chromosome 13	Severe bilateral cleft lip (+/− cleft palate), narrow temples, deformed ears and deafness, structural brain defect, congenital heart disease, malformed kidneys, polydactyly (extra digits), malformed small widely set eyes (eyes may be absent)	Clinical suspicion confirmed by chromosomal analysis	Most die within hours to days

Fig. 7.23 Features of trisomy 18 and trisomy 13.

Mechanisms leading to structural chromosomal disorders

All structural disorders result from breakage (Fig. 7.25). Chromosomal damage is increased by some environmental conditions (e.g., mutagenic chemicals, radiation) and by genetic chromosome instability disorders (e.g., ataxia telangiectasia and Fanconi syndrome).

Translocation

A reciprocal translocation involves breakage of at least two chromosomes, followed by an exchange

Features of some sex chromosome abnormalities

Disorder	Etiology	Features	Diagnosis	Prognosis
Klinefelter syndrome; incidence 1 in 500 liveborn males	Male XXY (47 chromosomes); extra maternal or paternal chromosome; incidence is increased in infertile male populations	Female body shape with gynecomastia in adolescence, female distribution of body hair, enter puberty but sterile (adequate quantities of sperm not produced), hypogonadism (testes < 2 cm), upper to lower body segment ratio is low (limbs are elongated but not tall), breast cancer approaches frequency in female population, scoliosis, emphysema, diabetes mellitus, osteoporosis, varicose veins	Usually presents due to sterility, suspicions confirmed by chromosomal analysis	Same as normal adult population; testosterone treatment by long-term implants—improves sperm production and body hair
Turner syndrome; incidence 1 in 2500 liveborn females	Female 45,X; female with a single X chromosome; may be deletion of Xp isochromosome (has two long arms but no short arm and other defects affecting Xp), high frequency of mosaicism	Lymphoedema of neonate (cystic hygroma and swollen extremities), short stature, loose skin at neck (webbing), cubitus valgus (large carrying angle), short fingers and toes (especially fourth metatarsal), frail nails, many nevi, gastrointestinal bleeding, widely spaced nipples, no secondary sexual characteristics, sterile (gonads degenerate to connective tissue streaks at birth), congenital heart disease (20%), unexplained hypertension (27%), kidney malformations, thyroiditis, Crohn's disease, occult aneurysms of cerebral arteries	Nonmosaic 45,X is detected on detail ultrasound by the presence of cystic hygroma, increased nuchal thickening and cardiac abnormalities; usually presents with primary amenorrhea or decreased growth; clinical suspicion is confirmed by chromosomal analysis	This syndrome has only mild mental retardation; life expectancy is below normal; administration of hormones at an appropriate age allows entry into puberty

Fig. 7.24 Features of some sex chromosome abnormalities.

of the fragments (Fig. 7.26). A Robertsonian translocation results from the breakage of two acrocentric chromosomes at their centromeres, followed by a fusion of their long arms. The total chromosome number is reduced to 45. As the short arms contain multiple copies of ribosomal RNAs (present on many acrocentric chromosomes), their loss is of no clinical significance.

In balanced translocations there is usually no loss of genetic material, so the individual is phenotypically normal. However, depending on the segregation of chromosomes in meiosis, gametes may result that do not contain a single complete copy of the genome (see Fig. 7.26). For this reason, prenatal diagnosis may be offered to known balanced carriers.

Inversion

This arises when two breaks occur in the chromosome and the intervening DNA rotates through 180 degrees. Paracentric inversions occur if the breaks occur in one arm, whereas pericentric inversions involve the centromere. In meiosis, homologous chromosomes can pair only if a loop is formed in the region of the inversion. Meitoic recombination within the loop structure can lead to duplicated and deleted segments in a pericentric inversion, and unstable chromosome fragments

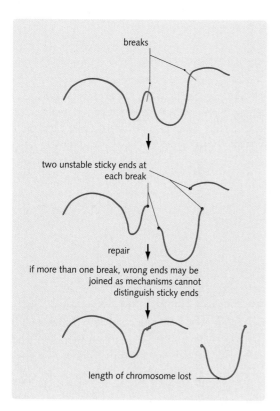

Fig. 7.25 Mechanism of structural chromosome damage, due to the limitations of DNA repair systems.

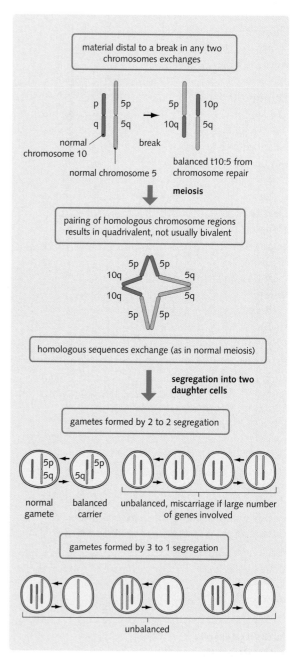

Fig. 7.26 Mechanism of reciprocal translocation (highly simplified).

lacking a centromere or containing two centromeres in paracentric inversions. As all of these options are often incompatible with life, a carrier of a balanced inversion has a relatively low risk of having a child with a viable imbalance.

Isochromosome

This chromosome has a duplication of one arm, but lacks the other. It results from breakage of a chromatid with fusion above the centromere or transverse division. It occurs in 17% of cases of Turner syndrome.

Duplication

This implies an extra copy of a chromosome region. Causes include inheritance from parents with balanced structural disorders and *de novo* duplication from unequal crossing-over in meiosis, translocation, or inversion.

Deletion and ring chromosome

Deletion results in a loss of genetic material. The telomere is important in chromosome function, so interstitial deletions are more common. If a deleted fragment has no centromere it will be lost during mitosis.

Ring chromosomes result from breaks near both telomeres of a chromosome, which aberrantly repair to form a ring, with the regions distal to the breaks being lost. If the ring has a centromere, it will be passed through generations.

Visible structural deletions are large, with the smallest microdeletion being at least 3 million base pairs (3 Mb). Single gene disorders may be caused by deletions, but if the deletions are not visible by light microscopy they are not considered structural. Structural deletions may cause deletion syndromes with more than one single gene disorder occurring concurrently. Subtelomeric microdeletions, frequently involving several genes, account for a proportion of children with multiple developmental and skeletal disorders. Modern molecular techniques such as fluorescence *in situ* hybridization (FISH), array CGH, or DNA analysis may reveal the underlying lesions (see Chapter 6).

Examples of structural chromosomal disorders

These contiguous gene disorders are diagnosed with the light microscope by high-resolution banding.

Deletion must involve at least 3 Mb to be detected by this technique. It is important to find out whether the deletion has arisen *de novo* in the proband or from a balanced translocation in the parents if the risk of recurrence is to be calculated. Recurrence is:
- Negligible with *de novo* mutations.
- Considerable with a balanced translocation.

Fig. 7.27 shows the features of some structural chromosomal disorders.

Polygenic inheritance and multifactorial disorders

Terminology
Polygenic inheritance
This is a term used to describe the inheritance of traits that are influenced by many genes at different loci.

Multifactorial disorder
This is a term used to describe disorders in which both environmental and genetic factors are important.

Phenocopy
This is the alteration of the phenotype by environmental factors during development to produce a phenotype that is characteristically produced by a specific gene (e.g., rickets due to a lack of vitamin D would be a phenocopy of vitamin D-resistant rickets).

Introduction
Multifactorial disorders result when a combination of small variations in genes, in combination with environmental factors, predispose to or produce the condition. Although multifactorial disorders tend to recur in families they do not show Mendelian patterns of inheritance (Fig. 7.28).

Multifactorial inheritance is implicated in the etiology of many common conditions including:
- Congenital malformations—for example, neural tube defects, congenital dislocation of the hip (CDH), pyloric stenosis, cleft lip and palate, and congenital heart disease.
- Common disorders of adult life—for example, diabetes mellitus, peptic ulcers, coronary artery disease, and schizophrenia.

165

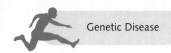
Features of some structural chromosome abnormalities

Disorder	Etiology	Features
Prader–Willi syndrome and Angelman syndrome; incidence 1 in 25,000 live births	Both result from deletion in the same region on 15q11–13; syndromes differ due to genomic imprinting, so depend on which parent the deleted gene is inherited from—Prader–Willi syndrome results from inheritance of the deletion from the father (so only have maternal contribution to the critical area), Angelman syndrome results from inheritance of the deletion from the mother; uniparental disomy can result in these syndromes but does not involve deletions	Prader–Willi syndrome—neonatal hypotonia, initial feeding difficulties, obesity of face, trunk, and limbs (after first year of life), prominent forehead, almond-shaped eyes, triangular upper lips, IQ 20–80, short stature, small hands and feet, hypoplasia of external genitalia, tendency to diabetes mellitus. Angelman syndrome—hypertonia, ataxic gait, characteristic arm posture, prominent jaw, deep set eyes, happy appearance, laughter, absent speech, mental retardation
Wolf–Hirschhorn syndrome	Partial deletion of the short arm of chromosome 4 (4p16.1); male to female ratio is 3:4	"Greek helmet" shaped head, cleft lip and palate, abnormal low-set ears, large beaked nose, hypertelorism (widely spaced eyes), epicanthic folds, microcephaly and mental retardation, failure to thrive, heart defects, convulsions, hypospadias
Cri du chat syndrome	Deletion of region on 5p15.2 or the whole short arm of chromosome 5	Round face (in adults the face elongates), cat-like cry (*cri du chat*), hypertelorism, epicanthic folds, strabismus, low-set ears, low birth weight, mental retardation (variable degree), appear normal at birth

Fig. 7.27 Features of some structural chromosome abnormalities.

- Normal human characteristics—for example, blood pressure, height, finger ridges, and intelligence.

 A genetic disorder is one that is determined by genes, whereas a congenital disorder is one that is present at birth and it may or may not have a genetic basis.

Differences between Mendelian and multifactorial inheritance

Mendelian	Multifactorial
All or nothing	Additive with a varying phenotype
If you have the gene, you have the disease	Possible to have lots of contributing genes, but if less than the threshold, do not have the disease
Risk does not increase through life	Can acquire more liability through life

Fig. 7.28 Differences between Mendelian and multifactorial inheritance.

Multifactorial disorders

A continuous (Gaussian) normal distribution curve of the trait within the population as a whole is typical, but not diagnostic, of multifactorial disorders. Abnormalities do not usually have a distinct phenotype but are extremes of the curve (although exceptions with distinct phenotypes do arise, e.g., peptic ulcer). The number of genes involved may be very few, because, even when a single locus is implicated, variation in the environment can ensure normal distribution of the trait.

Twin studies highlight the relative importance of genes and the environment. For example, cleft lip and palate has a population incidence of 1 in 1000, but:

- Concordance in monozygotic twins is 40%—if due only to genes there would be 100% concordance, so genes are important but other factors are also involved.
- Concordance in dizygotic twins is 4%—these twins are not genetically identical (having on average, like all siblings, 50% of their genes in common) but they share the same environment, showing the importance of environmental factors.

Congenital dislocation of the hip (CDH) is an example of multifactorial inheritance:
- The genetic factors are acetabular dysplasia, familial general joint laxity, and transient joint laxity at pregnancy term.
- The environmental factors are position of the legs *in utero* and after birth.

Cancer is an example of a very common multifactorial disorder (see below).

Threshold model of multifactorial disorders

Figure 7.29 shows the threshold model of multifactorial disorders. The liability of a population to a particular disease follows a normal distribution curve, with both genetic susceptibility and environmental factors defining the personal liability for any individual in the population:
- The disorder is manifested in an individual when a certain threshold of liability is exceeded.
- The liability of the majority of the population lies below the threshold level.

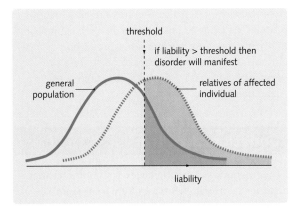

Fig. 7.29 Threshold model of multifactorial inheritance.

- Population incidence is equivalent to the proportion whose liability is greater than the threshold.

The liability curve is shifted to the right for relatives of an affected individual, such that more members of the family are likely to be above the threshold required for the disease to be manifested.

Heritability

Heritability is a statistical measure of the degree to which a trait is genetically determined. It is expressed as a percentage, with higher values denoting that the genetic contribution is more important (e.g., heritability of schizophrenia is 85% and that of peptic ulcer is 37%).

If heritability is high, there is a high correlation in relatives (e.g., finger ridge correlation in first degree relatives is 49%). Usually heritability is low, so the incidence in relatives falls off sharply (e.g., cleft lip and palate—Fig. 7.30). Empirical risks, calculated from relatives, are used in genetic counseling as there is no predictable pattern of inheritance.

Risk of recurrence rates are influenced by:
- Severity of the disorder in the affected person (e.g., severe bilateral cleft lip is more likely to recur in siblings than unilateral cleft lip).
- Number of affected individuals in a family.
- Proband being of the sex not usually affected.

There may be a sex difference in population incidence. For example, pyloric stenosis is more common in boys, so children of an affected female will be more likely to develop the condition than children of an affected male, as the female needs a high number of risk genes to manifest the condition.

Environmental factors

Multifactorial disorders result when environmental and genetic risk factors combine to bring the susceptibility of an individual to the disease above a threshold value. The liability that can be attributed to genetic factors is fixed. However, the judicious manipulation of environmental factors may enable the reduction in an individual's susceptibility to be below the threshold value.

For example, atherosclerosis has a heritability of 65%, so the environmental contribution to the etiology of the disorder is 45%. Consequently, not smoking, healthy eating, and exercise can

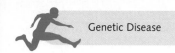

Risk to relatives for multifactorial disorders				
Disorder	Relative risk disorder			
	1° relative	2° relative	3° relative	General population
Cleft lip and palate	4	0.6	0.3	0.1
Neural tube defects	4	1.5	0.6	0.3
Epilepsy	5	2.5	1.5	1.0

Fig. 7.30 Risk to relatives for multifactorial disorders. First-degree relatives are parents, siblings, and offspring (share 50% of genome); second-degree relatives are grandparents, aunts and uncles, grandchildren (share 25% of genome); third-degree relatives include cousins and great-grandchildren (share 12.5% of genome).

significantly reduce an individual's risk of developing heart disease.

It is possible that in the future genetic analysis will allow the identification of individuals whose genetic profile puts them most at risk of developing specific multifactorial diseases, so that they can be given lifestyle advice that will minimize their risk before the disease develops. This is the goal of "personalized or predictive medicine." It is important to note that the ethics of such a public health strategy need to be considered carefully before it could be implemented.

Examples of multifactorial disorders

Diabetes mellitus, type I (insulin-dependent)

There is 40% concordance for insulin-dependent diabetes mellitus (IDDM) in monozygotic twins. Interestingly, 98% of these affected individuals have major histocompatibility complex (MHC) alleles DR3 or DR4 and B8 (this relates to a particular position in the DQ locus antigen—position 57 on the DQβ chain). Only 50% of non-diabetics have these MHC alleles. Aspartate at the DQ locus is protective—19% of the general population and 95% of the IDDM population are aspartate negative. Although a large number of other potential associations have been reported, these have been confirmed in multiple studies.

Essential hypertension

The heritability of essential hypertension is 62%. Genes are important in the cause of hypertension and the response to treatment.

Atherosclerosis

The heritability of atherosclerosis is about 65%. Heritable factors are hypertension, diabetes mellitus, premature ischemic heart disease, and abnormal lipoprotein profiles—elevated low-density lipoprotein (LDL) and reduced high-density lipoprotein (HDL).

Lipoprotein profile has been associated with single gene disorders and the polygenic inheritance of some genes such as those encoding apolipoproteins Apo AI and Apo CIII.

Peptic ulcer

The heritability of peptic ulcers is 37%, and 50% of affected families have increased pepsinogen I, which is inherited in an autosomal dominant fashion.

Schizophrenia

The heritability of schizophrenia is 85%. It may be associated with a locus on 5q, though other studies suggest alternative loci.

Asthma

The heritability of asthma is 80%, and it is associated with HLA A23.

Alzheimer disease

About 10% of patients inherit Alzheimer disease as a monogenic AD condition. Of these, a proportion arises from mutations in the amyloid precursor protein (APP) gene on chromosome 21. Mutations in other genes (e.g., presenilin 1 and 2 on chromosomes 14 and 1 respectively) are also associated with an inherited susceptibility to Alzheimer disease.

Genetics of cancer

In the majority of cases cancer is a multifactorial disorder in which genetic and environmental factors interact to initiate carcinogenesis. However, in a minority (about 5%) the disease follows a

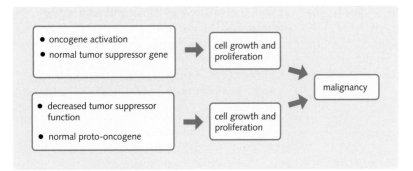

Fig. 7.31 Pathways to malignancy.

Differences between oncogenes and tumor suppressor genes	
Oncogene	**Tumor suppressor gene**
Gene active in tumor	Gene inactive in tumor
Specific translocations/point mutations	Deletions or mutations
Mutations rarely hereditary	Mutations can be inherited
Dominant at cell level	Recessive at cell level
Broad tissue specificity	Considerable tumor specificity
Especially leukemia and lymphoma	Solid tumors

Fig. 7.32 Differences between oncogenes and tumor suppressor genes.

familial pattern of transmission, suggesting a genetic cancer syndrome. Characterization of the genetic lesions segregating in such families has helped elucidate the molecular events that underline tumor genesis in the more common multifactorial form of the disease.

Cancer is characterized by abnormal growth and proliferation. Normal cell proliferation and survival is controlled by growth promoting proto-oncogenes and growth inhibiting tumor suppressor genes (see Chapter 5). Lesions in these genes, either somatically acquired, inherited or both, may result in cancer (Figs 7.31 and 7.32).

Multistage process of carcinogenesis

Carcinogenesis requires the accumulation of many mutations in both oncogenes and tumor suppressor genes. Tumors evolve from benign to malignant as subpopulations of cells acquire further mutations (Fig. 7.33). Given that mutations may arise in any tumor cell, tumors tend to be mosaics. However, when a cell acquires a mutation that is associated with a further loss of growth inhibition this cell type will tend to divide rapidly compared with the other cell types.

Oncogenes

Proto-oncogenes are normal genes that act to promote normal cell growth. Activation of oncogenes from proto-oncogenes leads to abnormal cell growth. Oncogenes tend to be dominant at the cellular level, with most mutations being gain of function mutations that result in increased expression of the gene (Fig. 7.34). They can be classified according to their position in the normal signal transduction pathway (Fig. 7.35).

Activation of oncogenes occurs by:
- Translocation (e.g., Burkitt lymphoma t(8;14) or t(8;2) activates c-*myc* on 8q).
- Amplification, (e.g., n-*myc* amplified in neuroblastoma).
- Point mutation in oncogene (e.g., Ha-*ras* mutation in bladder cancer).

No single oncogene has been found that is altered in 100% of tumors.

Tumor suppressor genes

Tumor suppressor genes (Fig. 7.36) are also known as antioncogenes, since they normally inhibit tumorigenesis. Tumors develop if there is loss of both wild-type alleles (Fig. 7.37), so tumor

169

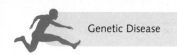

suppressor genes are recessive at the cellular level. Loss of activity can be through damage to the genome (e.g., mutation, rearrangement, nondisjunction, gene conversion, imprinting, mitotic recombination), or interaction with cellular or viral proteins (e.g., MDM2, HPV E6 antigen, adenovirus E1b protein).

Tumor suppressor genes are important in:

- Inherited predisposition to cancer.
- Early events in tumorigenesis (they cooperate with dominant transforming genes to cause neoplasia).

The detection of mutations in tumor suppressor genes can be used for presymptomatic diagnosis (e.g., of adenomatous polyposis coli by demonstrating mutations in the APC (adenomatous polyposis coli) gene).

normal colon cell
APC (chromosome 5q loss)
↑ cell growth
(DNA loses methyl groups)
early adenoma
K–ras (12p activation)
intermediate adenoma
DCC (18q loss)
late adenoma
p53 (17p loss)
carcinoma
other chromosome losses
metastasis

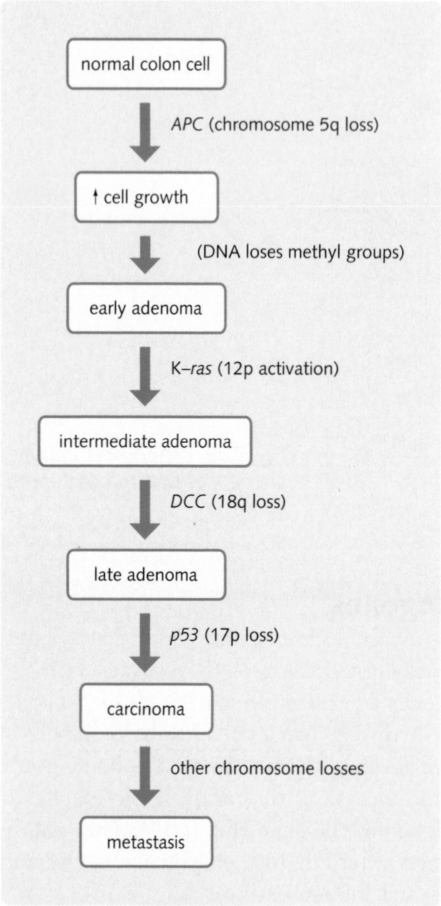

Fig. 7.33 Stages in the evolution of colorectal cancer.

extracellular matrix
cell membrane
cytoplasm
nucleus
1
2
3
4
5
6
cell division↑

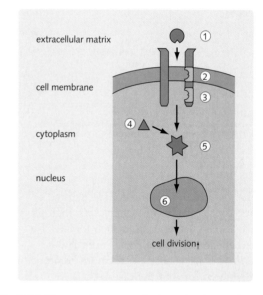

Fig. 7.35 Classes of oncogene by transduction position. (1) Growth factors (e.g., platelet-derived growth factor (PPGF)—*sis*). (2) Growth factor receptors (e.g., EGFR—*Gb*). (3) Postreceptor proteins (e.g., *ras*). (4) Postreceptor tyrosine kinase (e.g., *abl*, *src*). (5) Cytoplasmic proteins (e.g., *raf*). (6) Nuclear proteins (e.g., *myc*).

Categories of genes involved in the development of carcinoma

	Function	Mutation	Examples
Category I (growth and proliferation genes—oncogenes	I. transcription factors II. cyclins III. mediate signal transduction	Gain of function	*myc* *cyclin D1* *ras, abl*
Category II (tumor suppressor genes)	I. inhibit growth and proliferation	Loss of function	*Rb, p16*
Category III (programmed cell death genes)	I. abrogate cell death II. promote cell death	Gain of function Loss of function	*bcl-2* *p53*

Fig. 7.34 Categories of genes involved in the development of carcinoma.

Tumor suppressor genes			
Gene	**Locus**	**Function**	**Tumor**
Rb	13q14	Substrate of CDK (cell cycle regulation)	Retinoblastoma, osteosarcoma
p53	17p13	Growth arrest and apoptosis	Mutated in 70% of all human tumors
WT-1	11p13	Zinc finger	Wilms tumor
NF-1	17q	Transcription factor	Neurofibromatosis
APC	5q21	Cell adhesion	Adenomatous polyposis
DCC	18q21	Cell adhesion	Colorectal cancer, pancreatic cancer, esophageal cancer

Fig. 7.36 Examples of tumor suppressor genes.

Tumor suppressor genes in inherited cancers

Tumor suppressor genes are recessive at the cellular level. Therefore, if an individual inherits a mutation in one allele, every cell in the body will be relying on the product of the wild-type allele to regulate cell growth. Given the number of cells in the body, it is statistically likely that the wild-type allele will undergo somatic mutation in at least one cell. Thus, inherited mutations in tumor suppressor genes such as in retinoblastoma and Li–Fraumeni syndrome tend to be inherited dominantly. This phenomenon, in which a single functioning allele is lost, is called "loss of heterozygosity" (LOH).

Features suggestive of inherited cancer susceptibility in a family

These are:
- Several close (first- or second-degree) relatives with a common cancer.
- Several close relatives with genetically associated cancers (e.g., breast and ovary, or bowel and endometrial).
- Two family members with the same rare cancer.
- An unusually early age of onset.
- Bilateral tumors in paired organs.
- Synchronous or successive tumors.
- Primary tumors in two different organ systems in one individual.

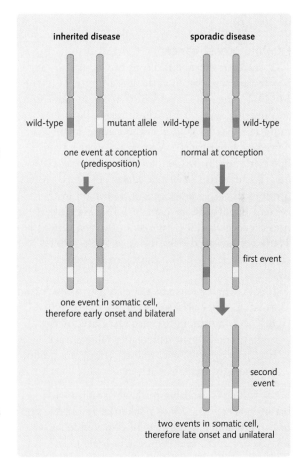

Fig. 7.37 Knudson's "two-hit" hypothesis. Note that two events must occur to lose tumor repressor function.

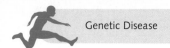

Examples of genetic cancer syndromes
Ataxia telangiectasia
This is an autosomal recessive disorder that affects 1 in 50,000. The *ATM* gene involved has been mapped to 11q23. It is thought to be involved in *p53*-mediated cell cycle arrest and apoptosis—that is, loss of function of the gene results in:
- Loss of cell cycle arrest.
- Loss of programmed cell death in response to DNA damage.

The onset is usually in childhood with progressive cerebellar ataxia, recurrent infections, and oculocutaneous telangiectasias. It is caused by a DNA repair defect and involves failure to excise nucleotide bases damaged by γ-radiation. These children have a raised serum α-fetoprotein, and they have nonrandom chromosome rearrangements. Approximately 30% die of myeloproliferative disease before 9 years of age.

Familial breast cancer
This accounts for about 5% of breast cancer, and it often presents at an early age. Mutations in the *BRCA-1* gene on 17q and *BRCA-2* gene on 13q account for over 50% of these cases. Both mutations have highly penetrant autosomal dominant inheritance. Women who have a germ-line mutation in *BRCA-1* or *BRCA-2* have a 40–85% lifetime risk of breast cancer and a 10–40% lifetime risk of ovarian cancer. (Women in the general population have an 11% lifetime risk of breast cancer and a 1.5% risk of ovarian cancer.) There are elevated risks for developing other cancers when these mutations are present as well:
- *BRCA-1* mutations are associated with increased prostate cancer risks in men.
- *BRCA-2* mutations are also associated with endometrial, renal, pancreatic, biliary tract, bladder, laryngeal carcinomas, lymphomas, and, occasionally, male breast cancer.

DNA testing is available for large families with breast cancer (e.g., 2% of Ashkenazi Jews have one of three founder mutations: BRCA$_1$ 185delAG, BRCA$_1$ 5382insC and BRCA$_2$ 6174delT).

Prophylactic bilateral mastectomies are sometimes considered following DNA analysis for women with a very strong family history.

Familial adenomatous polyposis coli
This is a rare autosomal dominant condition caused by a deletion in 5q21 resulting in a loss of function of the tumor suppressor gene, *APC*. This leads to the development of multiple benign adenomatous polyps of the large bowel (Fig. 7.38). A somatic mutation can result in the development of adenocarcinoma due to LOH (see above).

The diagnosis is based on:
- Family history.
- The presence of multiple intestinal polyps from childhood.
- Characteristic retinal changes in 80% of families.

There is a 90% risk of malignancy, and prophylactic whole-colon resection is often considered.

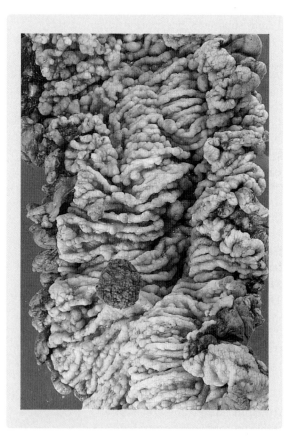

Fig. 7.38 Polyposis coli in large bowel. The multiple adenomatous polyps are clearly visible. (Courtesy of Dr. A. Stevens and Professor J. Lowe.)

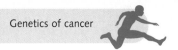

Fanconi syndrome

Fanconi syndrome is inherited as an autosomal recessive trait with an incidence of 1 in 350,000. More than one gene is associated with the syndrome. There is a DNA repair defect resulting in sensitivity to agents causing interstrand cross-links (e.g., alkylating agents). The clinical features include:

- Pancytopenia.
- Skin pigmentation.
- Congenital malformations, including abnormal hip joints and short or absent radii.

Acute nonlymphocytic leukemia develops in 5–10% of cases. Hepatocellular carcinoma and squamous cell carcinoma are also associated.

Li–Fraumeni syndrome

This is a rare autosomal dominant trait and is often due to mutation in the *p53* gene on 17p. It is commonly characterized by childhood cancers such as:

- Soft tissue sarcomas.
- Adrenal carcinomas.
- Brain tumors.

Later there is a high frequency of very early onset breast cancer, astrocytoma, and lung cancer. Direct mutation analysis is often possible, but of little benefit. The prognosis depends upon the number and sites of tumors.

Hereditary nonpolyposis colon cancer (HNPCC)

This is an autosomal dominant trait in which there is familial clustering of early-onset colon cancer (70% proximal) together with an increased risk of endometrial, ovarian, and renal tract tumors. Tumors are more frequently located in the proximal (right side) of the colon. The condition is associated with germ-line mutations in the DNA mismatch repair family of genes. Mutations in five genes—*hMSH2*, *hMLH1*, *hPMS1*, *hMSH6*, and *hPMS2*—have been identified so far. Mutations in *hMLH1* and *hMSH2* are by far the most common causes of HNPCC. Relatives are recommended to have yearly colonoscopy from 20–25 years of age.

Multiple endocrine neoplasias (MEN)

These are subdivided into MEN I, IIa, and IIb. They are rare autosomal dominant conditions:

- MEN I has been associated with the loss of a tumor suppressor gene mapped to 11q13.
- MEN IIa and IIb are caused by mutations in the *RET* oncogene on chromosome 10.

The clinical features are as follows (Fig. 7.39):

- MEN I is characterized by pituitary adenoma, hyperparathyroidism, and pancreatic adenomas (often gastrinomas, accounting for 50% of patients with Zollinger–Ellison syndrome).
- MEN IIa is characterized by pheochromocytoma, medullary thyroid carcinoma, and hyperparathyroidism.
- MEN IIb is characterized by neuromas of the mucous membranes, pheochromocytoma, megacolon, and medullary thyroid carcinoma.

Prenatal diagnosis is now possible by direct mutation analysis and MEN IIa and IIb are monitored by yearly calcitonin assays from 5–30 years of age for early detection of medullary thyroid carcinoma.

Neurofibromatosis type I (von Recklinghausen disease)

This has an incidence of 1 in 3000. It is an autosomal dominant condition in which there is a mutation in the tumor suppressor gene *NF1* on 17q. *NF1* is thought to be responsible for catalyzing the hydrolysis of Ras–GTP, an activated intracellular protein complex that brings about cell cycle progression. Loss of *NF1* causes accumulation of Ras–GTP resulting in an increased rate of cell turnover.

The condition has variable expression and is characterized by:

- Café-au-lait patches.
- Skin neurofibromas.
- Axillary freckling.
- Iris hamartomas.
- Spinal and autonomic neuromas.
- Pheochromocytoma.

Complications include scoliosis, learning difficulties, and seizures. Approximately 4% of cases develop central nervous system (CNS) tumors and 3% develop other tumors.

Neurofibromatosis type II

This is also autosomal dominant. It has an incidence of 1 in 35,000 due to a variety of mutations in the tumor suppressor gene *NF2* on chromosome 22q. It is characterized by:

- Bilateral vestibular schwannomas.
- Intracranial meningiomas.

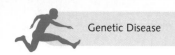

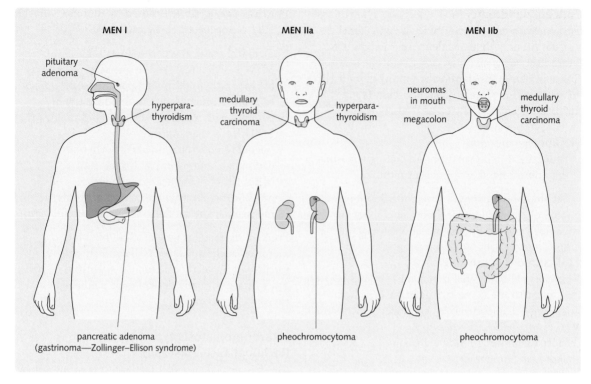

Fig. 7.39 Summary of features associated with multiple endocrine neoplasia (MEN).

- Café-au-lait patches.
- Lens opacities.
- CNS tumors.

Prenatal diagnosis is possible by direct and indirect DNA analysis, and carriers can be offered screening with magnetic resonance imaging (MRI) scans and audiology.

Tuberous sclerosis

This is an autosomal dominant trait with loci on 9q (*TSC1*) and 16p (*TSC2*). It has an incidence of 1 in 10,000 and there are characteristic skin changes in early childhood, including:
- White patches seen under ultraviolet light (Wood's lamp).
- A fibroangiomatous (facial) rash.

Intracranial calcification and periventricular hamartomas are seen on computerized tomography (CT); 90% of cases develop epilepsy, and 60% of cases are associated with mental retardation.

Retinoblastoma

Bilateral cases and 15% of unilateral cases of this childhood tumor of the eye are inherited as an autosomal dominant trait due to a mutation in the *Rb* gene on chromosome 13q14. There is an incidence of 1 in 18,000. The onset:
- Is usually in the first 2 years.
- Is first detected by a white light reflex or a squint.

Some cases are detected by neonatal screening for a red reflex. Survivors have an increased risk of adult tumors in various organs. The majority of retinoblastomas (60%) are sporadic and result in only one tumor in one eye. These are not hereditary, but are due to two inactivating mutations that have occurred somatically in the same retinoblast.

Wilms tumor

This renal tumor is mostly sporadic; however, 1% are inherited as an autosomal dominant trait.

Diagnosis is based on the presence of a renal mass with characteristic histology. Some cases are associated with a microdeletion syndrome at 11p13 in which there is aniridia, genitourinary abnormalities, and mental and growth retardation (WAGR). There is an increased risk of Wilms' tumor in Beckwith–Wiedemann syndrome.

Xeroderma pigmentosum

This has an incidence of 1 in 70,000. There are at least nine subgroups, and these are characterized by:
- Defective DNA excision repair.
- Extreme ultraviolet light sensitivity.

Clinical features of xeroderma pigmentosum are:
- Progressive corneal and skin scarring on exposure to sunlight.
- Multiple skin cancers by 20 years of age.

von Hippel–Lindau disease

This is a rare condition mapped to 3p25–26. Affected individuals characteristically have multiple renal cysts and early onset of bilateral, multifocal renal carcinoma (clear cell carcinoma). CNS tumors are also associated. These tend to be hemangioblastomas, which are benign but associated with high morbidity.

Cowden syndrome

This is an autosomal dominant multiple hamartomatous syndrome. There is progressive macrocephaly in childhood with mild to moderate delay in psychomotor development. Adults develop multiple hamartomas. There is a high risk of thyroid, gastrointestinal, breast, and ovarian cancers (which often develop in harmartomas). The gene is PTEN, on chromosome 10.

Gorlin syndrome

This is also known as nevoid basal cell carcinoma syndrome. This is an autosomal dominant condition causing a predisposition to basal cell carcinoma of the skin, medulloblastoma, and ovarian fibromas. There are associated congenital malformations including dental malformations, cleft palate, and bifid ribs. The gene is PTCH, on chromosome 9.

Peutz–Jeghers syndrome

This is an autosomal dominant condition causing multiple hamartomatous polyps in the gastrointestinal tract (GIT) and mucocutaneous pigmented lesions in the lips, face, and oral mucosa. There is a 2–3% risk of adenocarcinoma of the GIT. The responsible gene has been mapped to the short arm of chromosome 19.

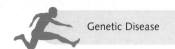

- Define genotype, phenotype, homozygote, heterozygote, and compound heterozygote.
- What is a triplet repeat expansion? Outline the salient features of three diseases in which this type of mutation is thought to be important, and discuss the molecular basis for anticipation.
- What is the difference between a loss of function mutation and a gain of function mutation?
- Describe the patterns of autosomal dominant, autosomal recessive, X-linked recessive, and X-linked dominant.
- List two autosomal dominant, two autosomal recessive, and two X-linked recessive disorders, and describe their salient features.
- What is the difference between allelic and locus heterogeneity in a single gene disorder?
- Define penetrance and variable expressivity.
- Explain why Angelman syndrome and Prader–Willi syndrome can result from both uniparental disomy and microdeletion.
- What is mosaicism, and how might it explain the presence of an X-linked recessive phenotype in a carrier female?
- Define aneuploidy, triploidy, trisomy, and monosomy.
- Discuss the role of nondisjunction and anaphase lag in monosomy.
- Describe the salient features of Down, Turner, and Klinefelter syndromes.
- What is a balanced translocation?
- What is an isochromosome?
- Name a syndrome that results from a structural chromosome abnormality, and discuss its salient features.
- What is the difference between polygenic and multifactorial inheritance?
- Describe the threshold model of multifactorial inheritance.
- Explain the concept of heritability in the context of multifactorial disorders.
- List four multifactorial disorders.
- Describe the multistage process of carcinogenesis with reference to colorectal cancer.
- List five differences between tumor suppressor genes and oncogenes.
- Explain Knudson's two hit hypothesis with reference to retinoblastoma.
- What features in a pedigree would lead you to suspect a familial cancer syndrome?
- List three examples of genetic cancer syndromes, and discuss their salient features.

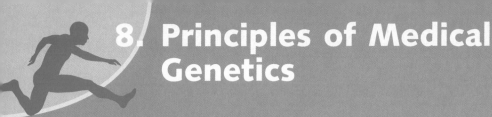

8. Principles of Medical Genetics

Population genetics and screening

Terminology

Allele

An allele is one of a series of possible alternative forms of a given gene or DNA sequence at a given locus.

Mutation

A mutation is a permanent heritable change in the sequence of DNA.

Polymorphism

Polymorphism is the occurrence in a population of two or more alternative genotypes, each at a frequency greater than that which could be maintained by recurrent mutation alone. A locus is arbitrarily considered to be polymorphic if the rarer allele has a frequency of at least 0.01. Any allele rarer than this is a "rare variant."

Introduction

It is estimated that between 2 and 5% of all newborns have congenital malformations or genetic disorders, accounting for one-third of pediatric hospital admissions. Moreover, many of the common causes of morbidity and mortality in later life—such as coronary heart disease, diabetes, and cancer—have a significant genetic component. Clinical genetics services extend beyond the person that presents with a genetic disease to their whole family. The clinical geneticist has many roles to play in the management of individuals and families affected by a genetic disease, including:

- Establishing an accurate diagnosis.
- Providing information about prognosis.
- Calculating the risks of developing or transmitting the disorder.
- Exploring with the patient ways in which the development or transmission of the disorder may be modified.

With a few exceptions, most genetic disorders are at present incurable. Therefore, the emphasis is placed on identifying individuals who are at risk of having an affected child so that they can make informed reproductive choices. Such individuals may be identified:

- In specific families where a genetic disorder has already arisen.
- In certain groups at an increased risk of genetic disease (e.g., Tay–Sachs disease in Ashkenazi Jews, Down syndrome in pregnant women over the age of 35 years).

Information on the diagnosis, management, and counseling of specific genetic disorders can be found on http://www.genetests.org/

Population genetics

Population genetics is the study of the genetic composition of populations. Allele frequencies, and, therefore, the frequency of disease-causing mutations, vary between populations. Different allele frequencies are characteristic of distinct populations, reflecting their specific geographical and genetic origins. Thus, some diseases may be much more common in some groups than others (Fig. 8.1).

If clinical geneticists are to offer an accurate assessment of risk of a genetic disease, they must know how common the disease-causing mutation is in the relevant population. This is particularly important in recessive disorders, where unaffected heterozygotes are carriers of the disease-causing gene. One way of determining the carrier frequency would be to sample a large number of people and use molecular genetic techniques such as polymerase chain reaction (PCR) to identify mutant alleles. However, this would be arduous and not all disease-causing mutations have been cloned. The Hardy–Weinberg principle enables the frequency of a disease-causing allele in a

Selected examples of disease alleles with different frequencies in different populations	
Allele/disease	**Population variation**
β^S allele of β-globin gene (sickle-cell anemia)	Higher in Africa, less common elsewhere. Allele frequency 1/20 among African Americans; <1/200 among Hispanic Americans
β^C allele of β-globin gene	High in West Africa (specifically Ghana and Burkina Faso) where allele frequency is 1/6. Allele frequency 1/100 among African Americans
Cystic fibrosis (all disease alleles)	High in European and US Caucasian populations (allele frequency 1/40–1/50); low in Finnish, Asian, and African populations
Phenylketonuria (all disease alleles)	Higher among Europeans of Celtic and Northern European background (allele frequency 1/67–1/90). Allele frequency 1/125 in Switzerland and Italy, 1/223 among African Americans, 1/330 in Japan. 1/500 in Finland
Tay–Sachs disease	High frequency in Ashkenazi Jews (allele frequency 1/60); hundredfold lower in other groups
Familial hypercholesterolemia	High in certain regions of Quebec (allele frequency 1/244) and in Afrikaners in South Africa (allele frequency 1/140). Allele frequency 1/1000 in Europe and United States
Myotonic dystrophy	Allele frequency 1/50,000 in Europe and nonexistent in sub-Saharan Africa. Allele frequency 1/950 in certain regions of Quebec

Fig. 8.1 Selected examples of disease alleles with different frequencies in different populations. (Adapted from Nussbaum, McInnes, and Willard, 2001.)

Fig. 8.2 The Hardy–Weinberg equation. Consider if two heterozygotes mate, Aa × Aa. The distribution of AA, Aa, and aa genotypes in the population correspond to p^2, 2pq, and q^2, respectively. If A and a are the only alternative alleles for the same gene locus, then, p^2 + 2pq + q^2 = 1. (a, recessive allele; A, dominant allele; p, frequency of A; q, frequency of a.)

population to be calculated from the disease incidence (provided that the population is in Hardy–Weinberg equilibrium).

Hardy–Weinberg principle

The Hardy–Weinberg law is a mathematical equation that forms the basis of population genetics. It states that allele frequencies within a population tend to remain constant from one generation to the next, provided that:

- The population is large.
- There is random mating.
- The mutation rate remains constant.
- Alleles are not selected for (i.e., they confer no survival or reproductive advantage).
- There is no migration into or out of the population.

A population with constant gene and genotype frequencies is said to be in Hardy–Weinberg equilibrium.

The Hardy–Weinberg equation is derived by considering a population carrying an autosomal gene with two alleles A and a. The frequency of the dominant allele A in gametes is represented by p, and the frequency of the recessive allele a in gametes is represented by q (Fig. 8.2). Since there are only two alleles, p + q = 1 and q = 1 − p

In the combination of alleles that forms the next generation:
- The chance that both male and female gametes will carry the A allele is p × p = p^2.
- The chance that the gametes will produce a heterozygote is (p × q) + (p × q) = 2pq.
- The chance that both male and female gametes will carry the a allele is q × q = q^2.

These are the only possibilities; therefore:

$$p^2 + 2pq + q^2 = 1$$

This equation can be used to calculate the allele frequency and the heterozygote frequency in a population if disease occurrence is known, provided that the population is in Hardy–Weinberg equilibrium.

For autosomal recessive (AR) conditions, disease incidence = q^2; gene frequency = q; heterozygote frequency (i.e., frequency of carriers of AR condition) = $2pq$. For example, an AR disorder occurs with a frequency of 1 in 1600 liveborn births:

- Incidence, $q^2 = 1/1600$.
- Gene frequency (a), $q = 1/40$; dominant allele A has gene frequency $p = 39/40$.
- Heterozygote frequency, $2pq$ is $2 \times 39/40 \times 1/40$, which is approximately 1/20.

For autosomal dominant (AD) conditions:

- Nearly all affected are heterozygotes, so q^2 is approximately 0.
- If the condition is rare, p^2 is approximately 1.
- Disease gene frequency (A) is approximately $2pq$, which is approximately $2q$.

The assumptions underlying Hardy–Weinberg equilibrium are not always found in a natural population. However, an understanding of the Hardy–Weinberg model provides a method to test when a population is *not* in equilibrium, and allows us to identify factors that have upset this theoretical balance.

Factors that disturb Hardy–Weinberg equilibrium

A population is not in Hardy–Weinberg equilibrium if the genotype frequencies do not arise in the proportions predicted by the Hardy–Weinberg law (Fig. 8.3). This may arise as a result of a number of mechanisms, discussed below.

Nonrandom mating

Random mating refers to the selection of a partner regardless of that partner's genotype. The tendency of individuals to select partners who share certain characteristics (e.g., height) is called assortive mating, which is a form of nonrandom mating. Nonrandom mating may also result from

A	Allele frequencies determined from genotype frequencies			
	Genotype			
	TT	Tt	tt	Total
No. of individuals	40	40	20	100
No. of T alleles	80	40	0	120
No. of t alleles	0	40	40	80

Total number of alleles = 120 + 80 = 200

Frequency of T = p = 120/200 = 0.6

Frequency of t = q = 80/200 = 0.4

B	Using χ^2 test to determine whether a population is in Hardy–Weinberg equilibrium		
	Genotype		
	TT	Tt	tt
Observed (O)	40	40	20
Expected (E)	$p^2 \times 100 = 36$	$2pq \times 100 = 48$	$q^2 \times 100 = 16$
O – E	4	–8	4
$(O – E)^2/E$	16/36 = 0.44	64/48 = 1.33	16/16 = 1

$\chi^2 = \Sigma(O – E)^2/E = 0.44 + 1.33 + 1 = 2.77$

Fig. 8.3 Determining whether a population is in Hardy–Weinberg equilibrium given the genotype frequencies. (A) The genotype frequencies are used to determine the allele frequencies. (B) Chi squared (χ^2) tests are used to determine whether the population differs significantly from one in Hardy–Weinberg equilibrium. The observed (O) genotype frequencies are those seen in the population. The expected (E) genotype frequencies are those predicted if the population is in Hardy–Weinberg equilibrium, using the allele frequencies calculated in A. From χ^2 tables (with one degree of freedom and 95% confidence intervals), a population does not differ significantly from one in Hardy–Weinberg equilibrium if χ^2 is less than 3.84.

consanguinity (i.e., mating of individuals who are genetically closely related to each other).

Mutation

If a locus has a high mutation rate, theoretically there will be an increase in the number of mutant alleles in the population. In practice, this does not occur for populations that are in Hardy–Weinberg equilibrium because the mutation rate is balanced against a reduction in reproductive fitness in affected individuals.

Selection

The reduced reproductive fitness of affected individuals acts as a negative selection, which leads to a gradual reduction in the frequency of the mutated gene and disturbance of the Hardy–Weinberg equilibrium. In practice, this is balanced by the mutation rate for populations that are in equilibrium.

In some cases, selection may increase fitness and for some autosomal recessive disorders heterozygotes show an increase in fitness relative to unaffected homozygotes. For example, carriers of sickle-cell anemia are comparatively resistant to malaria, which is thought to explain the high incidence of the sickle-cell trait in West Africa. This phenomenon is called heterozygote advantage.

It is thought that the high frequency of cystic fibrosis (CF) mutations in Caucasians (carrier frequency 1/20) can be explained by heterozygous advantage. It is proposed heterozygotes are resistant to the effects of gastrointestinal infection with cholera and dysentery compared with unaffected homozygotes. Conversely, in tropical regions CF is virtually unknown. The higher sweat sodium content in heterozygotes may be a disadvantage in these areas where water is in short supply.

Genetic drift

In small populations, one allele may be transmitted to a high proportion of offspring by chance, resulting in marked changes in allele frequency between the two generations and a disturbance in Hardy–Weinberg equilibrium. This phenomenon may contribute to the "founder effect" (see below).

Migration

The introduction into the population of new alleles as a result of migration and subsequent intermarriage will result in a change in the relevant allele frequencies, and thus a disturbance to Hardy–Weinberg equilibrium.

Founder effect

Founder effects arise in small isolated populations that breed amongst themselves. If, by chance, one of the small group of original founders had a certain disease gene, this will remain overrepresented in successive generations as the population expands. For example, several rare autosomal recessive disorders occur at a relatively high frequency amongst the Old Order Amish (an isolated religious group that tend to intermarry).

 The expression of genes and their frequency is undoubtedly influenced by the environment. However, it can be argued that genes may themselves influence the environment, at least socially and politically. For example, Queen Victoria was a carrier of hemophilia A, and two of her great grandsons who were heirs to the thrones of Russia (Tsarevich Alexis) and Spain (Crown Prince Alfonso) inherited this X-linked recessive trait. Tsarevich Alexis' hemophiliac status led to his mother's involvement with the deeply unpopular Rasputin, who claimed to be able to control his bleeding. This in turn resulted in the abdication of the tsar and, indirectly, to the success of the Bolshevik revolution. When the Spanish Royal family were already facing overthrow, the death of Crown Prince Alfonso from blood loss following a car accident triggered an attempted revolution in Spain, which ultimately resulted in the Spanish civil war.

Population screening and carrier detection

Population screening is the screening of all members of a population regardless of their family history. It is used to identify carriers of recessive traits and to detect presymptomatic individuals. Presymptomatic testing is sometimes called predictive testing.

The aim of carrier detection is usually to identify asymptomatic heterozygotes for AR traits, although it is sometimes used to detect carriers of AD disorders that have limited penetrance or late onset. If two partners are identified as being heterozygotes for a mutation at the same locus, genetic counseling can be offered before conception and prenatal tests offered as appropriate. Carrier detection tends to be confined to small ethnic populations in which there is an anomalously high incidence of a particular disease due to either the founder effect or heterozygous advantage.

Prenatal diagnosis concerns the use of tests in pregnancy to determine whether an unborn child is affected with a particular disorder. Figure 8.4 describes some of the tests available in prenatal diagnosis and their relative risk to the pregnancy.

Criteria for a screening program

A genetic disease is suitable for screening if it fulfills the following criteria:
- Clearly defined disorder.
- Appreciable frequency.
- Advantage to early diagnosis or carrier detection.
- Few false positives (test specificity).
- Few false negatives (test sensitivity).
- Benefits outweigh the costs.

Methods used for carrier detection and presymptomatic diagnosis
Direct mutation detection

If the mutation (or mutations) that causes a specific disease has been defined, carriers or presymptomatic individuals can be identified by direct mutation analysis using DNA techniques such as PCR, Southern blotting or fluorescence *in situ* hybridization (FISH) (see Chapter 6). For example, individuals carrying Huntington, cystic fibrosis (the most common mutations), and myotonic dystrophy mutations may be identified in this manner.

Linkage to polymorphic marker

Genetic linkage is the tendency for alleles close together on the same chromosome to be transmitted together through meiosis (see Chapter 6). It allows disease genes for which the causal mutation is unknown to be followed through generations, using a linked polymorphic marker that lies sufficiently near the disease gene for recombination to be unlikely. The marker is often a microsatellite (Fig. 8.5). Linkage analysis allows the detection of disease in families where the causative gene is known but an unidentified mutation is segregating in this gene for a given family.

Biochemical tests

Biochemical tests form an important part of prenatal and presymptomatic diagnosis. Over 100 inborn errors of metabolism can be detected by fetal enzyme assays using cultured amniocytes or chorionic villus samples. Newborn babies can be screened for errors of metabolism by simple biochemical tests on a blood sample.

Phenylketonuria (PKU) is routinely screened for in all newborn babies. A sample of blood is taken from a heel prick from all newborn babies. The blood is placed on a Guthrie card and used to detect PKU, congenital hypothyroidism, and galactosemia. Following the detection of PKU, the amino acid phenylalanine is excluded from the diet, and this prevents the development of symptoms.

Newborn screening

Newborn genetic screening identifies treatable genetic disorders (such as phenylketonuria, galactosemia, maple syrup urine disease, and congenital adrenal hyperplasia) in newborn infants. Early intervention to treat these disorders (usually through dietary management) can eliminate or modify clinical symptoms that would otherwise lead to severe disability, mental impairment, or death. In the United States, the screening programs are administered by the individual states. Each state determines which disorder will be screened and how to cover the costs associated with the screening, follow-up, and diagnosis. Prevalence and severity of a condition as well as the availability and effectiveness of a treatment often are factors in determining whether a state will screen for that condition. The development of

Tests used for prenatal diagnosis

Test	Gestation	Procedure	Abnormalities detected	Risk of procedure
Amniocentesis	16–18 weeks (routinely) 14–32 weeks is possible	Amniotic fluid is removed via a long needle inserted transabdominally. Cells are cultured for up to 2 weeks	Fetal sexing, karyotyping, and enzyme assay	Miscarriage rate estimated at 0.5–1% above the normal rate at 16 weeks
Chorionic villus sampling	10–12 weeks	Biopsy usually taken transabdominally or transvaginally	Fetal sexing, fetal karyotyping, biochemical studies, DNA analysis (cell culture not necessary)	Miscarriage rate estimated at 0.5–1% above average at 10 weeks
Cordocentesis	18 weeks+	Fetal blood sample obtained by inserting a fine needle into fetal umbilical cord	Suspected fetal infection or mosaicism, unexplained hydrops, single gene disorders, fragile X, blood disorders	Procedure-related loss approximately 1–2%; risk of rhesus isoimmunization
Ultrasound	Routine scan performed at any time in pregnancy (often scheduled at 16–18 weeks)	Visualization of fetus by transabdominal ultrasound probe	Over 280 congenital malformations	Non-invasive test with low associated risk
Maternal serum screening; infectious screen (TORCH screen), triple test (serum AFP, HCG, and estradiol)	16–18 weeks	Sample of maternal blood collected	Detection of infections that may cause congenital malformations (see Chapter 8); triple test estimates relative risk of NTDs and Down syndrome based on serum levels of HCG, AFP, and estradiol	Very low

Fig. 8.4 Some of the tests available in prenatal diagnosis. (AFP, α-fetoprotein; HCG, human chorionic gonadotrophin; NTDs, neural tube defects; TORCH, toxoplasmosis, other agents, rubella, cytomegalovirus, herpes simplex.) Associated risk refers to the risk that the test may damage the fetus.

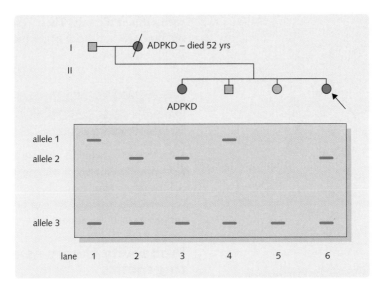

Fig. 8.5 Detection of autosomal dominant polycystic kidney disease (ADPKD) using microsatellite linkage. Using a PCR microsatellite site known to be linked to the disease gene locus, three alleles (each corresponding to a different repeat element) are detected. The affected mother has passed the disease gene and allele 2 to the affected daughter (lane 3) and her normal gene and allele 3 to each unaffected child (lanes 4 and 5). This could be a scenario where the mother and daughter have already both developed ADPKD and the test shows that the youngest daughter (lane 6) also has the disease gene so is at high risk of developing the disease. She should, therefore, have genetic counseling and regular kidney scans to detect disease-causing cysts early.

tandem mass spectrometry has allowed for rapid testing for numerous genetic disorders, leading to calls for a uniform panel of screened conditions across all states.

Screening in "at risk" populations
Thalassemia
Carrier detection of β-thalassemia is undertaken for Mediterranean populations and populations of South East Asia by finding a microcytosis—mean corpuscular volume (MCV) less than 75 fL with a low mean corpuscular hemoglobin (MCH) less than 25 pg, and an increased hemoglobin A_2 concentration.

Tay–Sachs disease
Carriers are detected by measurement of serum β-N-acetylhexosaminidase, and the test is targeted at the Ashkenazi Jewish population.

Cystic fibrosis
Cystic fibrosis is the most common serious AR condition to affect Caucasians. Carrier detection is now routinely offered to all pregnant women, using a panel of approximately 20–25 of the most common *CFTR* mutations.

General population screening tests
These are usually quick and simple tests that can be used to assess a woman's relative risk of having an affected child. Maternal serum is used in many of these tests. At 16–18 weeks' gestation, women can be tested for maternal serum α-fetoprotein (MSAFP), human gonadotrophin (HCG), and estradiol. These variables can be used to assess the relative risk of a number of fetal conditions including neural tube defects (spina bifida) and trisomy 21 (Down syndrome). Additional testing approaches are under consideration for first trimester screening, and may soon become part of standard clinical care.

Trisomy 21 and other chromosomal abnormalities
The detection of Down syndrome combines the biochemical serum marker results with maternal age to form a combined risk (Fig. 8.6). MSAFP and HCG are also disturbed in other chromosomal abnormalities:
- MSAFP is low in trisomies 21, 18, and 13, and normal in X chromosomal abnormalities.
- HCG is high in trisomy 21, low in trisomy 18, and normal in trisomy 13 and chromosome X abnormalities.

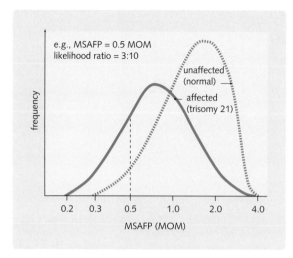

e.g., MSAFP = 0.5 MOM
likelihood ratio = 3:10

unaffected
(normal)

affected
(trisomy 21)

frequency

0.2   0.3   0.5   1.0   2.0   4.0

MSAFP (MOM)

Fig. 8.6 Screening for trisomy 21. Maternal serum α-fetoprotein (MSAFP) levels are used to generate likelihood ratios, which are derived from overlapping distribution of affected and unaffected pregnancies. Likelihood ratio and maternal age are used together to generate a combined risk. If there is a high combined risk, refer for amniocentesis. If there is a low combined risk, provide reassurance. (MOM, multiples of the median.)

Neural tube defects

Neural tube defects are associated with a high MSAFP because more of the fetal protein leaks into the amniotic fluid as a result of the malformation. As part of the routine 16–18-week check, pregnant women are referred for a detailed ultrasound scan if the MSAFP is on the 95th centile or above. Other conditions associated with a high MSAFP at 16–18 weeks are:

- Missed abortion.
- Esophageal atresia.
- Exomphalos.
- Sacrococcygeal teratoma.
- Bladder neck obstruction.
- Fetal–maternal hemorrhage.

Cascade screening

Cascade screening is the identification within a family of carriers for an autosomal recessive disorder or persons with an autosomal dominant gene following ascertainment of an index case. Once an individual has been diagnosed with a condition, family members at high risk are offered testing. If more people within the family are identified with the gene, the results may be used to identify further family members at risk, who are then offered the test. These results, in turn, redefine risk status for other members of the family—and so on.

Risk assessment and genetic counseling

For families in which a disease is showing a recognizable pattern of Mendelian inheritance the risk to other family members of developing or transmitting the disorder can be calculated by simple probability theory.

Probability theory as applied to genetics

The probability of a single event occurring can be expressed as a fraction:

$$p = \frac{\text{number ways events can happen}}{\text{total number of possibilities}}$$

Probability is a useful way of demonstrating the risk of specific genetic event(s) occurring.

Laws of addition and multiplication of probability
The law of addition

If two events could not happen at the same time, they are said to be mutually exclusive. The probability that either event will occur is equal to the sum of their probabilities. The law of addition is:

$$p = p_1 + p_2$$

The law of addition is sometimes called the "or" law because it is the probability that one event or another event will occur.

The law of multiplication

An independent event is one that has no effect on subsequent events. The outcome of the first event has no effect on subsequent events. The probability that all the events will occur is equal to the product of the individual probabilities. The law of multiplication is:

$$p = p_1 \times p_2$$

The law of multiplication is sometimes called the "and" law because it is the probability that one event and another event will occur.

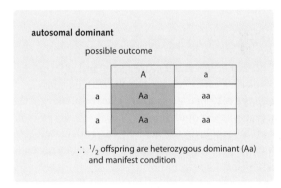

Fig. 8.7 Mendelian inheritance and risk calculation I. The condition manifests itself only when it is homozygous. If both parents are carriers of the allele, the risk of developing the condition is one-quarter. (a, mutant allele; A, normal allele.)

Calculating risks from pedigree information
Autosomal recessive conditions
Autosomal recessive disorders are only manifested if two mutant copies of the gene are inherited (Fig. 8.7). Therefore, for a child to have a recessive disorder the mother must be a carrier AND the father must be a carrier AND the child must inherit both mutant genes. Expressing this statement mathematically gives:

p(child has a recessive disorder
= p(mother is a carrier) × p(father is a carrier)
× p(child inherits both genes)

p(mother is a carrier) and p(father is a carrier) can be calculated from the pedigree information or from the frequency of carriers in the population.
p(child inherits both genes) = 1/4 (calculated from a knowledge of Mendelian inheritance; see Fig. 8.7).

Fig. 8.8 Mendelian inheritance and risk calculation II. Only one copy of mutant allele is needed to manifest symptoms. If one parent is affected, the risk of having an affected child is one-half. (a, recessive nonmutant allele; A, dominant mutant allele.)

Autosomal dominant conditions
Autosomal dominant conditions are manifested if one mutant gene is inherited (Fig. 8.8). Therefore, for a child to have a dominant disorder either the mother has the disease gene AND the child inherits it OR the father has the disease gene AND the child inherits it. Expressing this statement mathematically gives:

p(child has a dominant disorder)
= p(mother has the disease gene) × p(child inherits the disease gene) × p(father has the disease gene) × p(child inherits the disease gene)

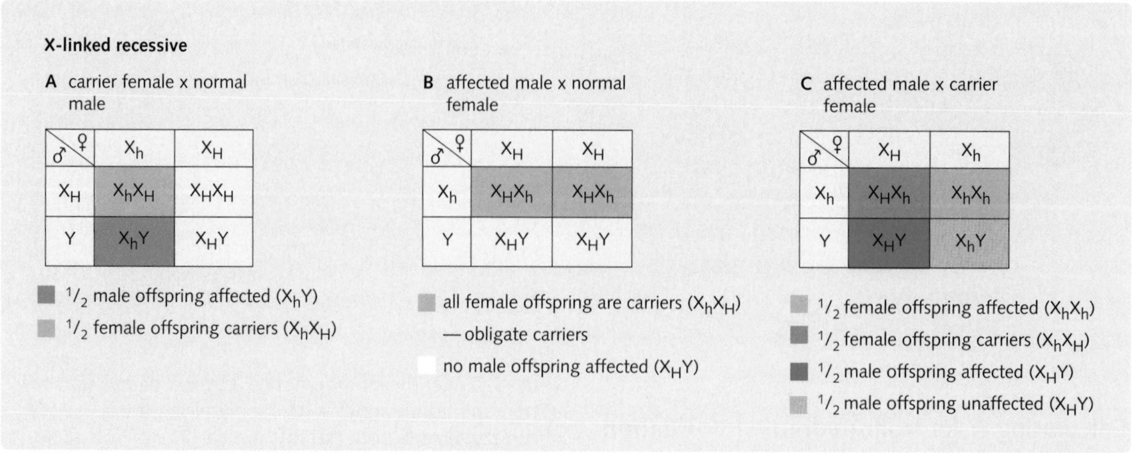

X-linked recessive

A carrier female x normal male

♂ \ ♀	X_h	X_H
X_H	X_hX_H	X_HX_H
Y	X_hY	X_HY

■ $^1/_2$ male offspring affected (X_hY)

■ $^1/_2$ female offspring carriers (X_hX_H)

B affected male x normal female

♂ \ ♀	X_H	X_H
X_h	X_HX_h	X_HX_h
Y	X_HY	X_HY

■ all female offspring are carriers (X_hX_H)

— obligate carriers

□ no male offspring affected (X_HY)

C affected male x carrier female

♂ \ ♀	X_H	X_h
X_h	X_HX_h	X_hX_h
Y	X_HY	X_hY

■ $^1/_2$ female offspring affected (X_hX_h)

■ $^1/_2$ female offspring carriers (X_hX_H)

■ $^1/_2$ male offspring affected (X_HY)

■ $^1/_2$ male offspring unaffected (X_HY)

Fig. 8.9 Mendelian inheritance and risk calculation III. The mutant allele is expressed in all males who inherit it since only one copy of X-linked alleles is carried. Affected male passes allele on to all female offspring and no male offspring, e.g., hemophilia A. (X_h, mutant allele; X_H, normal allele.)

p(mother has the disease gene) and p(father has the disease gene) can be calculated from the pedigree information or from the frequency of the disease in the population.

p(child inherits the gene) = 1/2 (calculated from a knowledge of Mendelian inheritance; see Fig. 8.8).

X-linked recessive conditions

The situation is more complicated with X-linked recessive disorders because the situation varies according to whether the child is a girl or a boy (Fig. 8.9).

Bayes' theorem

Additional information may be used to modify the risk calculated from the pedigree data in order to obtain a more accurate value. For example, given that Huntington disease generally manifests in middle age, a suspected carrier who has not yet developed the disease at age 30 years is still likely to have the mutation. However, if they have not developed the disease by age 60 years, given that the condition would have been expected to manifest by this age, it is less likely that they carry the mutation. Bayesian analysis is a method for taking such considerations into account by determining the relative probabilities of two alternative outcomes:

- The "prior" probability is based on classical Mendelian inheritance.
- The "conditional" probability is based on observations that modify the prior probability, such as existing unaffected offspring, results of screening tests, or the age of the offspring.

A "joint" probability is calculated as the product of the prior and the conditional probability. A final "relative" probability is the proportional risk of one alternative with respect to the other (Figs 8.10 and 8.11).

Aspects of genetic counseling
Establishing the diagnosis

Genetic counseling is the provision of information to affected individuals or family members at risk of a disorder that may be genetic. The consultands (individuals attending counseling) are informed of:

- The consequences of the disorder.
- The probability of developing or transmitting it.
- Ways in which it may be prevented or ameliorated.

An accurate diagnosis is essential to genetic counseling so that the correct advice can be given. A medical history of all affected family individuals is needed and a pedigree constructed. Miscarriages,

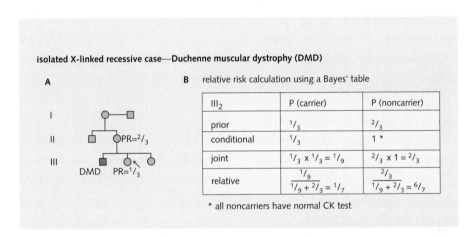

Fig. 8.10 Estimation of carrier risks using Bayes' theorem I. (A) Mother (I₂) is an obligate carrier as she has an affected brother and son. Daughter (II₂) has already had three unaffected sons. What is the risk that she is a carrier? (B) The relative risk calculated can be displayed on a Bayes' table.

Fig. 8.11 Estimation of carrier risks using Bayes' theorem II. (A) Isolated case of DMD in III₁; assess carrier risk in his sister, III₂. Approximately one-third of cases arise from new mutations—neither mother nor sister would have the mutation. If mutation was inherited from the mother, the carrier risk for the sister would be halved. Now assume the daughter has a normal creatine kinase (CK) test. In general, two-thirds of carriers have raised CK and one-third have normal CK. (B) The relative risk calculated can be displayed on a Bayes' table.

unexplained mental handicap, or malformed children, and parental consanguinity should be asked about specifically.

Investigations may involve chromosomal or DNA analysis or specific biochemical tests related to the disease being screened for.

Presenting the risks in context

Once the diagnosis and mode of inheritance have been established, carrier risk and recurrence risk for the consultands can be estimated, based on Mendelian rules and Bayes' theorem.

Discussing options, communication, and support

The counselor must aim to be nonjudgmental and nondirective toward the consultands when discussing their future options. At best, the counselor can give the consultand reassurance that the recurrence risk is no greater than the population risk. If the recurrence risk is high, the counselor must explore the feelings of the consultand towards the disease in terms of the emotional, physical, and financial implications. With these in mind the counselor can provide information about the options open to them such as:

- No further pregnancies—advice about reliable forms of contraception should be given.
- Prenatal diagnosis—selective termination of affected fetuses.
- Artificial insemination of donor sperm (AID)— if the male has an AD condition or both partners are carriers for an AR condition.
- In vitro fertilization (IVF) with preimplantation genetic diagnosis.
- Ignoring the risk and coping if an affected child is born.

Follow-up sessions should be offered and, with informed consent, the consultands should be kept on a register so they can be recalled if new prenatal or carrier tests are developed.

Ethical considerations in genetic counseling
Consanguinity and incest
Incest is the mating of first-degree relatives. It has been outlawed in most human societies because of its risk of serious genetic disease (AR disorders). In the US, first cousins are the closest relatives allowed to marry. The risk of disease or serious congenital malformation in a child born to first cousins is 1 in 20. This rises to 1 in 11 in a highly inbred family. Therefore, a detailed anomalies scan is indicated during the pregnancy as well as careful monitoring during and after the pregnancy.

Disputed paternity
Paternity testing uses modern DNA fingerprinting techniques. It is based on the detection of microsatellites in genomic DNA. These are a series of allelic polymorphisms created by tandem arrangements of multiple copies of short (2–6 nucleotide) DNA repeats. There are multiple microsatellite sequences scattered throughout the genome. PCR based methods of DNA fingerprinting produce an allele specific pattern that is unique for each individual and the probability that two unrelated people have the same fragment pattern is less than 3×10^{-11} when a particular set of microsatellite markers is used.

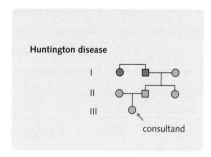

Fig. 8.12 Huntington disease. The grandfather and his sister both died of Huntington disease. The father is now in his late thirties and is still unaffected. The daughter (consultand) is now 18 years old and wants to know if she is affected.

Since humans are diploid, cells contain two copies of each microsatellite. Parents transmit one of their two alleles to their offspring, so allele patterns that arise in the child's DNA fingerprint will be identifiable in the fingerprint of the biologic father.

Confidentiality and conflicts of interest
The laws of patient confidentiality must be observed. This can sometimes be a problem if a family has a disease with a very clear pattern of inheritance and only some members of the family want to know their risks of being affected. Figure 8.12 shows an example of a conflict of interest.

There are DNA tests available that detect the presence of the trinucleotide repeat expansion that gives rise to Huntington disease. However, if the DNA test shows the granddaughter is positive for the repeat expansion, it would imply that her father is also positive and is likely to develop the disease before she does. If he does not want to know this, her attendance at counseling may create severe family tension.

Genetic consultation and history taking

Structure of the genetic consultation
Some important points
An accurate diagnosis is essential if relevant genetic advice is to be given. Some disorders that are superficially similar may have totally different

etiologies and modes of inheritance (e.g., dwarfism). Incorrect assumptions about the underlying diagnosis may, therefore, lead to totally misleading risk calculations. It is important that information is given in a way that the consultands (people receiving the advice) can understand. It is useful to ask them what they understand about genetics before attempting to explain the nature of the disease.

Counseling should be nonjudgmental and nondirective. The counselor should aim to make the consultands aware of the risk of having an affected child, the possible means of prevention including prenatal diagnosis and carrier detection, and treatment of the disease.

 In a genetic history, the family is of paramount importance and may be discussed first.

Outline of the interview

Presenting complaint
Are the symptoms felt by the patient or noticed by the parents?

History of the presenting complaint
Allow the patient (or more often the parents) to talk about what they perceive to be the problem; find out what they expect from the consultation and their concerns. Ask about:
- The nature of the complaint.
- Extent of any deficit.
- The onset and time course of the complaint.
- The pattern: constant or intermittent, frequency, duration.
- Precipitating and relieving factors.
- Other relevant symptoms.
- Any previous treatment or investigations for this complaint.

Family history
Particular attention should be given to relatives with relevant disorders. A family tree should be constructed to show how the condition has been passed on through the family. A standardized set of symbols is used, as described in Fig. 7.1. The male line is conventionally placed on the left and members of the same generation are placed on the same horizontal level. An arrow is used to indicate the proband (affected individual whose diagnosis caused the consultands to seek advice).

Inquire specifically about:
- Infant deaths, stillbirths, and abortions as this may alter recurrence risks (e.g., spina bifida is associated with an increased risk of neural tube defect in subsequent children).
- Consanguinity.
- Illegitimacy (discreetly!), as this may explain unexpected disease incidences.

An accurate family tree should reveal the mode of inheritance of the genetic disease and its penetrance and possibly where it originated from in the first place. In this way, realistic risk calculations can be made for the family with regard to future pregnancies.

Social history
The social history may have relevance to the consultand's reproductive choices. Relevant details include marital status, children, religious beliefs, education level, occupational history, accommodation, diet, exercise, and risk behaviors such as smoking and alcohol consumption.

Past medical history
Previous medical conditions should be enquired about where appropriate. Past medical history should also include obstetric history (e.g., maternal health, teratogen exposure, viral infections).

Drug history
Details of all prescription and over-the-counter drugs, any known allergies, and exposure to toxins such as alcohol, tobacco, or industrial toxins should be obtained.

Review of the systems
There should be an emphasis on finding any conditions that may have a genetic component or be suggestive of a syndrome or an association (Fig. 8.13).

Summary
Give a full summary when presenting the case.

189

Systems review	
System	**Things to ask about**
Cardiovascular	Congenital heart disease, hypertension, hyperlipidemia, vessel disease, heart attacks, strokes
Respiratory	Recurrent lung infections, asthma, bronchitis
Gastrointestinal	Atresia (at any level), fistulas (e.g., tracheoesophageal), recurrent diarrhea, chronic constipation
Genitourinary	Ambiguous genitalia, abnormal renal function
Musculoskeletal	Muscle wasting or weakness
Neurological	Developmental milestones, hearing, vision, coordination, fits

Fig. 8.13 Systems review in genetic history taking.

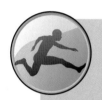

Red flags, although not 100% sensitive or specific, should prompt the clinician to consider a genetic cause or contribution to a patient's condition and to act accordingly (e.g., testing, intervention, counseling, follow-up, or referral to a medical geneticist). Common red flags are summarized in the mnemonic Family **GENES**:

Family—**F**amily history. Multiple affected siblings or individuals in multiple generations. Don't forget that lack of a family history does not rule out genetic causes.

G—**G**roups of congenital anomalies. Two or more anomalies are much more likely to indicate the presence of a syndrome with genetic implications.

E—**E**xtreme or exceptional presentation of common conditions. Early onset of disease or unusually severe reaction to infectious or metabolic stress, for example.

N—**N**eurodevelopmental delay or degeneration. Developmental delay, developmental regression in children, or early onset neurologic deterioration in adults, for example.

E—**E**xtreme or exceptional pathology. Rare tumors or other pathology or multiple primary cancers in one or different tissues, for example.

S—**S**urprising laboratory values. Abnormal laboratory values in an otherwise healthy individual; extreme laboratory values for a typical clinical situation.

Common presentations of genetic disease

Most syndromes and disorders mentioned in this section are discussed in Chapter 7.

Development

There are eight areas of childhood development:

- Hearing.
- Vision.
- Gross motor skills.
- Fine motor skills.
- Language comprehension.
- Expressive language.
- Behavior and emotional development.
- Social skills.

These areas are interconnected, and they affect each other (e.g., difficulty in vision affecting fine motor skills).

In assessment, observation is divided into:

- Development rate (check whether within normal range).

- Pattern of development (qualitative rather than quantitative milestones observed).
- Final level of attainment (e.g., adult IQ level).

Deviations in development

Deviations can be the result of abnormalities in any of the areas listed above.

Hearing loss

Hearing loss can be conductive or sensorineural. Conductive deafness in childhood is rarely directly genetic. Sensorineural deafness is uncommon, and it is not always genetic.

Vision

In 50% of cases, visual impairment has genetic causes.

Gross motor skills

Conditions that affect muscle tone or nerve supply will impair gross motor skills. The quality of the movement can be affected, the child may fall over, or there may be a regression of motor skills.

Fine motor skills

These are also affected by neuromuscular problems, but it should be remembered that vision has a large impact on this developmental category.

Behavior development and social skills

There are specific genetic syndromes that have characteristic behavior patterns. For example:
- Gregarious personality—Williams syndrome.
- Inappropriate laughter with absent speech—Angelman syndrome.
- Motor and vocal tics—Gilles de la Tourette syndrome.

Many genetic conditions have an effect on behavioral development due to the complicated impact of factors including hospitalization, decreased IQ, illness behavior, stigmatization, and coping with a chronic illness.

Language is affected by all the above areas of development, and it is assessed in the two areas of:
- Speech (vocal sounds made).
- Language (comprehension and expression).

An example of the effect that a genetic disease can have on language development is Down syndrome where:
- Low IQ affects language comprehension.
- Conductive deafness due to secretory otitis media affects speech and language.
- Macroglossia affects sound production.

Failure to thrive

Failure to thrive is defined as suboptimal growth and weight gain in infants and toddlers. It is usually detected when values plotted on a centile chart begin to cross centile lines. Many childhood conditions are first diagnosed when the child presents with failure to thrive. Causes can be divided into organic and non-organic (environment deprivation).

Genetic causes of organic failure to thrive are:
- Decreased food intake. This can be primary (e.g., inability to feed due to cleft palate) or secondary to chronic illness (e.g., cystic fibrosis).
- Decreased food absorption (e.g., due to cystic fibrosis causing pancreatic insufficiency).
- Increased energy requirements (e.g., due to cystic fibrosis).
- Metabolic disorders (e.g., mucopolysaccharidoses).
- Miscellaneous causes, including chromosomal disorders and syndromes.

Oral and facial deformities

Abnormal facies are common in genetic conditions so it is important to make accurate measurements of the facial landmarks if an abnormality is suspected (e.g., interpupillary distance). Craniofacial syndromes can be described using the terms:
- Hypertelorism—increased interpupillary distance.
- Hypotelorism—decreased interpupillary distance.
- Low-set ears—upper border of ear attachment is below level of inner corner of the eye (inner canthus).
- Upslanting palpebral fissures—inner canthi are below outer canthi.
- Downslanting palpebral fissures—outer canthi below inner canthi.
- Epicanthic folds—skin folds over inner canthi.
- Brachycephaly—short anteroposterior skull length.

Examples of craniofacial malformations include:
- Cleft lip and palate—seen in many syndromes of Mendelian inheritance (e.g., chondrodysplasia punctata), chromosomal disorders (e.g., trisomy 13), and non-Mendelian syndromes (e.g., Pierre Robin syndrome—cleft palate with mandibular hypoplasia).

- Craniosynostosis—premature fusion of sutures can be due to genetic syndromes (e.g., Crouzon syndrome).
- Treacher Collins syndrome—hypoplasia of the mandible, with downslanting palpebral fissures, deformed ears in 80%, and deafness in 40%.
- Sturge–Weber syndrome—hemangiomatous facial lesion (port wine stain) in ophthalmic division of trigeminal nerve distribution. Hemangiomatous extension into the brain may cause epilepsy, learning difficulties, and paralysis. It is almost always sporadic.

Although not a malformation, it should be noted that abnormal head circumference is associated with some genetic conditions. For example:

- Microcephaly reflects decreased brain growth as seen in cases of severe learning difficulties.
- Macrocephaly is seen in central nervous system (CNS) storage disorders (e.g., mucopolysaccharidoses) and Cowden syndrome.

Eye disorders
Choroidoretinal degenerations
These include:

- Retinitis pigmentosa—autosomal recessive in 80%, autosomal dominant in 15%, and X-linked in 5% (but 50% of males). It is normally isolated, but it can be part of a syndrome. Many distinct genes have been implicated in this disorder.
- Night blindness—usually autosomal dominant and isolated.

Nystagmus
Causes of nystagmus may be primary ocular disease or nystagmus may be secondary to neurologic or vestibular disorders. Ocular albinism is an example and is X-linked recessive.

Other eye disorders
These include:

- Disorders of color vision—all are X-linked recessive, and they occur in 8% of males. Because of the high frequency of these mutant alleles in the population about 1 in 150 women are also colorblind (both parents had the mutant allele on the X chromosome).
- Leber's optic atrophy—discussed under mitochondrial inheritance (see Chapter 7).

- Corneal dystrophies—require specialist opthalmological referral (e.g., clouding seen in mucopolysaccharidosis).
- Retinal detachment—commonly associated with high myopia. Genetic syndromes associated include Stickler syndrome.
- Retinoblastoma—(see Chapter 7).
- Cataracts—congenital cataracts can be associated with syndromes (e.g., Down syndrome) and genetic metabolic disorders (e.g., mucopolysaccharidosis). Some genetic disorders can cause cataracts in later life (e.g., myotonic dystrophy, which is Mendelian, and diabetes mellitus, which is polygenic).
- Kayser–Fleischer rings—due to copper accumulation in the cornea and seen in Wilson disease.
- Glaucoma—congenital glaucoma can be primary following AR inheritance or associated with other syndromes (e.g., retinoblastoma, Sturge–Weber syndrome).
- Refractive errors—can be associated with syndromes (e.g., myopia and Marfan syndrome).
- Cyclops—all are lethal and sporadic.
- Microphthalmos and anophthalmos—both these abnomalities can be features of many chromosomal disorders (e.g., trisomy 13).
- Aniridia—may be associated with Wilms tumor.
- Ptosis—may be isolated as an autosomal dominant disorder, or it may have a neuromuscular cause (e.g., myotonic dystrophy).

Ear disorders
Severe congenital sensorineural deafness
First exclude external factors such as rubella and cytomegalovirus infection. About 40–50% of genetic causes are due to AR inheritance and 10% are due to AD inheritance; X-linked inheritance is rare.

Partial nerve deafness
Some forms are present at birth while others are progressive. More than 10% have AD inheritance, for example, otosclerosis, which is a mixed conductive, and neural deafness, which has a progressive course and incomplete penetrance.

Syndromes associated with deafness
Waardenburg syndrome is associated with deafness and it is autosomal dominant. The characteristics are a white forelock and decreased IQ. Two

distinct forms are recognized, attributable to mutations in *MITF* (chromosome 7) and *PAX* 3 (chromosome 2). Alport syndrome is also associated with deafness (see Chapter 7, Fig. 7.16).

External ear malformations

These can be related to syndromes (e.g., fragile X is associated with very large ears, Treacher Collins with small deformed ears).

Skin disorders

These include:
- Ichthyoses—can be associated with syndromes (e.g., chondrodysplasia punctata—Conradi syndrome).
- Epidermolysis bullosa—a heterogeneous group of disorders that can be AD or AR.
- Nevi—can be isolated AD or associated with syndromes (e.g., Turner syndrome). They must be distinguished from the lesions of tuberous sclerosis and neurofibromatosis, and pigmented lesions over spina bifida.
- Cavernous hemangiomas—usually sporadic (e.g., Sturge–Weber syndrome).
- Albinism—autosomal recessive. There are two main types, attributable to mutations in different genes, which vary in their severity.
- Vitiligo—usually AD.
- Acanthosis nigricans—primary acanthosis nigricans is AD, but acanthosis nigricans can also be secondary to other disorders, and it may be acquired as a result of visceral malignancy.

Skin tumors

There are a number of very rare Mendelian inherited skin tumors. Skin tumors may also result from genetic DNA repair disorders, for example, xeroderma pigmentosum (see Chapters 5 and 7). Kaposi sarcoma has an inherited form. Most cases of malignant melanoma are nongenetic, but an AD predisposition has been described. Basal cell nevus (Gorlin) syndrome predisposes to basal cell carcinoma (see Chapter 7).

Bone and connective tissue disorders

The following syndromes are discussed in Chapter 7:
- Achondroplasia.
- Marfan syndrome.

- Ehlers–Danlos syndrome.
- Mucopolysaccharidoses.
- Congenital dislocation of the hip.
- Talipes.

Other bone and connective tissue disorders are:
- Chondrodysplasia punctata—there is a characteristic facies with a saddle nose (nasal hypoplasia), frontal bossing, and a short stature. This syndrome is also characterized by cataracts, mental retardation, and ichthyoses.
- Lethal dysplasias—e.g., thanatophoric dwarfism.
- Osteopetrosis—characterized by hard, dense, and brittle bones, described as "marble bone" disease. Decreased marrow may result in anemia and thrombocytopenia, and compression of cranial nerves may result in optic atrophy and deafness. The mild form is AR; the severe form is AD.
- Polydactyly (extra digits)—this can be isolated as an AD condition or form part of a syndrome (e.g., trisomy 13; Ellis–van Creveld syndrome).
- Brachydactyly (short fingers)—generally this is AD and associated with syndromes such as Turner syndrome.
- Rockerbottom feet—a fat pad is increased on the sole. It is associated with trisomy 18.
- Limb reductions—these are associated with vertebral, anal, tracheoesophageal, and renal (VATER) anomalies, and other syndromes.
- Osteogenesis imperfecta—brittle bone disease caused by a collagen defect: type 1 causes blue sclera and deafness; type 2 is lethal; type 3 is characterized by fractures at birth with increasing deformity; type 4 is characterized by fragile bones and blue sclera.

Neuromuscular disorders
Muscular dystrophies

There are many types of muscular dystrophy, the most important being X-linked Duchenne and Becker muscular dystrophies (see Fig. 7.15). Muscular dystrophies present with muscular weakness and often progressive loss of motor milestones.

Spinal muscular atrophies

These are disorders of the anterior horn cell, and they present with weakness, wasting, and loss of reflexes. Most are AR.

Hereditary motor sensory neuropathies

These present with progressive distal muscle wasting. They are usually of AD inheritance (e.g., type I Charcot–Marie–Tooth disease; see Fig. 7.16).

Other neuromuscular disorders

These include:
- Myotonic disorders—present with delayed muscle relaxation (e.g., myotonic dystrophy, see Fig. 7.5).
- Metabolic myopathies—present with floppiness, weakness, or cramps (e.g., glycogen storage disorders and mitochondrial cytopathies).

Central nervous system and psychiatric disorders

Central nervous system disorders include:
- Rett syndrome—presents with deterioration in cognition, autistic behavior, and stereotyped hand movement.
- Gilles de la Tourette syndrome—presents with tics.
- Ataxia—many syndromes present with ataxia, some of which are inherited, the most common being Friedreich ataxia (see Fig. 7.5) and ataxia telangiectasia (see Chapter 7).
- Neural tube defects.
- Huntington disease (see Chapter 7).

Dementia

Dementia presents with a global impairment of higher cognitive function. Presenile dementia occurs before 65 years of age. Early onset is often caused by Alzheimer disease that has an inherited component, sometimes behaving as an AD disorder. It is also a feature of Down syndrome.

Neurocutaneous syndromes

These are neurofibromatosis, tuberous sclerosis, and von Hippel–Lindau disease (see Chapter 7).

Mental retardation

This is seen in a wide variety of genetic diseases and disorders frequently associated with mental retardation can be:
- Autosomal dominant (e.g., Huntington disease, tuberous sclerosis).
- Autosomal recessive (e.g., ataxia telangiectasia, mucopolysaccharidoses, phenylketonuria).

- X-linked (e.g., fragile X syndrome).
- Chromosomal (e.g., Down syndrome, Klinefelter syndrome, Turner syndrome, Prader–Willi syndrome).
- Metabolic (e.g., Wilson disease).

Schizophrenia

This is a multifactorial disorder with a genetic element (see Chapter 7).

Affective psychoses

These have multifactorial causation.

Behavioral disorders

Most behaviors are a combination of genetic and environmental factors, but some syndromes are associated with consistent behaviors (e.g., XYY syndrome with antisocial outbursts).

Disorders of thoracic development

Disorders of thoracic development include:
- Pectus excavatum—seen in Noonan syndrome.
- Wide nipples and shield-like chest—seen in Turner syndrome.
- Gynecomastia—seen in Klinefelter syndrome.
- Kyphoscoliosis (anterior chest wall deformity)—seen in Marfan syndrome.
- Chest infection—seen in cystic fibrosis and α_1-antitrypsin deficiency.

Congenital heart disease

Examples of congenital heart disease include:
- Pulmonary stenosis and atrial septal defects in Noonan syndrome.
- Aortic stenosis and pulmonary stenosis in Williams syndrome.
- Ventricular septal defect and patent ductus arteriosus in Edwards syndrome or Patau syndrome.
- Coarctation of the aorta in Turner syndrome.
- Truncus arteriosus and pulmonary atresia in DiGeorge syndrome.
- Aortic incompetence and dissecting aortic aneurysm in Marfan syndrome.
- A cardiovascular abnormality (e.g., atrioventricular septal defects, patent ductus arteriosus, tetralogy of Fallot) in 40% of cases of Down syndrome.
- Ellis–van Creveld syndrome (polydactyly and CHD).

Other heart disorders

These include:

- Cardiomyopathies—may be seen in muscular dystrophies and Friedreich ataxia.
- Coronary artery disease—familial hypercholesterolemia accounts for 10% of early coronary artery disease.
- Hypertension—this is multifactorial.
- Dextrocardia and bronchiectasis—seen in Kartagener syndrome, which is characterized by defective ciliary function and is AR with 50% penetrance.

Gastrointestinal disorders

These include:

- Infantile pyloric stenosis—shows polygenic inheritance.
- Exomphalos and gastroschisis—exomphalos can be associated with Beckwith syndrome, in which there is also macroglossia and hypoglycemia. Exomphalos is associated with major congenital abnormalities, while gastroschisis is not.
- Umbilical hernia—seen in Wilms tumor.
- Bowel atresia—meconium ileus is seen in cystic fibrosis (not true atresia) and duodenal atresia is seen with increased frequency in Down syndrome. Hirschsprung disease results from aganglionic segments of large bowel (not true atresia)—familial cases show mutations in *RET*.
- Peptic ulcer—has a multifactorial inheritance.
- Celiac disease—associated with HLA-DR3 and HLA-B8. It is also seen in families transmitting other autoimmune disorders.
- Intestinal polyposis—see Chapter 7.
- Imperforate anus—associated with VATER syndrome.
- Pancreatitis—this can be hereditary, and it is also seen in cystic fibrosis, both causing malabsorption and recurrent abdominal pain.

Liver disease

Metabolic liver disease presenting with cirrhosis, acute hepatitis, or portal hypertension is seen in Wilson disease, where there is aberrant copper deposition in the liver, brain, and cornea; it is inherited as an autosomal recessive disorder. Other liver disorders include:

- Hemochromatosis—see Fig. 7.13.
- α_1-antitrypsin deficiency—an important cause of neonatal hepatitis and cirrhosis, with some adults developing emphysema. It is AR.

- Hyperbilirubinemias—present with jaundice and tend to result from enzyme deficiencies. An example of this is Gilbert syndrome, which is often completely benign.
- Biliary atresia—presents in the infant with persistent jaundice and pale stools. Occasionally associated with chromosomal trisomies.
- Polycystic disease of the liver—isolated cases are AR, but adult polycystic kidney disease (which is AD) can be associated with a few hepatic cysts.

Genitourinary tract disorders

Genitourinary tract disorders include:

- Polycystic kidney disease—this commonly presents with deteriorating renal function, or the infantile form may be detected on routine antenatal ultrasound scan. There is an adult form (AD) and a more severe infantile form (AR). It can also be associated with trisomy 13, trisomy 18, tuberous sclerosis, and Meckel syndrome.
- Alport syndrome—presents with microscopic hematuria and sensorineural deafness (see Fig. 7.16).
- Fabry disease—this X-linked disorder presents with angiokeratomas of the skin, numerous cardiac signs, and hematuria (see Fig. 7.15).
- Urinary malformation—this can be detected on antenatal ultrasound, and it causes obstruction or recurrent urinary tract infections.
- Renal stones—present with renal colic (excruciating intermittent back pain). Hematuria may be present. Most are not usually due to single gene disorders, although there may be a genetic component. They are common in some rare inherited metabolic disorders (e.g., cystinuria), and they can occur more frequently in syndromes such as Lesch–Nyhan syndrome.
- Renal tumors—these present with hematuria, obstruction, or general ill health (cachexia and loss of appetite). Two important genetic renal tumors are Wilms tumor and renal carcinoma associated with von Hippel–Lindau syndrome.
- Hypogonadism—this presents with infertility in either sex or reduced testicular volume in males. It may be isolated or part of a syndrome (Fig. 8.14).
- Macroorchidism—greater than normal testicular volume and characteristic of fragile X syndrome (see Fig. 7.5).

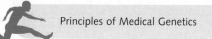

Hypogonadism as part of a syndrome	
Male	**Female**
Klinefelter syndrome (XXY)—usually sporadic	Turner syndrome (45,X)—usually sporadic
Kallmann syndrome (hypogonadotrophic hypogonadism with anosmia)—X-linked recessive	XX gonadal dysgenesis—autosomal recessive (sex limited)
Reifenstein syndrome (hypogonadism with hypospadias)—X-linked recessive mutation of androgen receptor	XY gonadal dysgenesis—X-linked recessive
Prader–Willi (hypogonadism with obesity, hypotonia, small hands and feet)—usually sporadic (risk to siblings 1–2%)	Testicular feminization (complete and incomplete)—X-linked recessive

Fig. 8.14 Hypogonadism as part of a syndrome.

• Virilized external genitalia (girls) or precocious puberty (boys)—these are the presentations of some forms of congenital adrenal hyperplasia, which occasionally presents as an emergency with a salt-losing crisis (see Fig. 7.13).

Recurrent abortions

These may result from parental or fetal factors. There may be an AR lethal disorder (increased risk with consanguinity), an X-linked lethal disorder in the male, or a cytogenetic abnormality in the germ line (e.g., translocation). Fetal causes include a major abnormality such as neural tube defects or chromosomal disorders.

Inborn errors of metabolism

Inborn errors of metabolism may present with metabolic acidosis, unusual body odors, hypoglycemia, respiratory distress, jaundice, urea and electrolyte imbalance, diarrhea, failure to thrive, lethargy, fits, and coma. Most are Mendelian (AR). Examples include porphyrias, mucopolysaccharidoses, phenylketonuria, Tay–Sachs disease, Gaucher disease, and aminoacidurias.

Blood disorders

Blood disorders include:

• Sickle-cell disease—may present with failure to thrive, neonatal jaundice, or crises (see Fig. 7.13). It can be detected by prenatal diagnosis or screening.
• Thalassemia—may present with anemia, neonatal jaundice, or stillbirth (see Fig. 7.13). It may be detected by prenatal diagnosis or screening.
• Glucose-6-phosphate deficiency—may present with neonatal jaundice or hemolysis precipitated by drugs or fava beans (see Fig. 7.15).
• Fanconi syndrome—may present with a pancytopenia.
• Immunodeficiencies—may present with recurrent infections; for example, X-linked Bruton agammaglobulinemia or, less commonly, severe combined immunodeficiency (SCID) (see Fig. 7.16) and ataxia telangiectasia (see Chapter 7).
• Coagulation disorders—may present with bleeding (e.g., hemophilia A and B (see Fig. 7.15) and von Willebrand disease (see Fig. 7.10)).

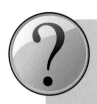

- Define allele, mutation, and polymorphism.
- List five factors that disturb Hardy–Weinberg equilibrium.
- What is the founder effect?
- What is the purpose of carrier detection? Give an example of its use.
- Describe cascade screening.
- Write formulas to express the laws of addition and multiplication.
- If both parents are carriers of an autosomal recessive disease, what is the probability their child will be affected? What is the probability that a parent with an autosomal dominant condition will transmit the disease to their child (assume their partner is unaffected)?
- How is Bayes' theorem used in genetic counseling?
- List three aims of genetic counseling.
- Describe the technique used to resolve disputed paternity.
- Outline the structure of the genetic consultation.
- What should be discussed in the systems review in a genetic consultation?
- What are the important aspects of the social history in a genetic consultation?
- What are the eight areas of childhood development?
- List two genetic disorders of each of the following: eye, ear, bone and connective tissue, central nervous system, gastrointestinal tract, genitourinary tract, and blood.

A

AAUAAA sequence, 97
ABO blood groups, 65
abortion
  recurrent, 196
acanthosis nigricans, 193
achondroplasia, 147, 149
acid phosphatase, 58
actin, 53
  function, 53–54
actin-binding proteins, 54
actin filaments, 53, 54
action potential, 44
active chromatin, 84
active transporter, 40
acute intermittent porphyria, 147, 149
AD see Alzheimer disease (AD)
adenomatous polyposis coli (*APC*) gene, 172
adenosine monophosphate (AMP), 81
adenosine triphosphate (ATP), 38, 40, 55, 56, 58
adenylate cyclase pathway, 49
adhesion molecules, 65–69
ADPKD see autosomal dominant polycystic kidney disease (ADPKD)
adrenoleucodystrophy, 153, 154
affective psychoses, 194
agglutination
  in blood transfusion, 65
alanine, 15
albinism, 193
alleleic heterogeneity, 153
alleles, 177, 178
Alport syndrome, 141, 156, 195
Alzheimer disease (AD), 168
amino acid
  as buffers, 17
  classification by side-group type, 15–16
  condensation into protein, 14
  covalent modification, 14
  cross-linkage, 14
  D and L isomers, 13
  essential, 13
  ionization properties, 14
  nonessential, 13
  properties, 13
  solubility, 14
  structure, 13
AMP see adenosine monophosphate (AMP)
amyloid precursor protein (APP) gene, 168
anaphase, 77, 79
anchoring junctions, 61–63, 63
aneuploidy, 159
Angelman syndrome, 157, 158, 165, 191
aniridia, 192
ankyrin, 34
annealing temperature, 127
antibiotics
  mitochondria, 104
  protein synthesis, 104
  transcription, 98–99
  translation inhibiting, 104
anticipation, 157
antimicrobial agents, 110
α_1-antitrypsin deficiency, 195
aortic incompetence, 194
aortic stenosis, 194
APC gene, 172
APP see amyloid precursor protein (APP) gene
AR see autosomal recessive (AR)
arginine, 16
aryl sulfatase, 58
Ashkenazi Jews, 60
asparagine, 16
aspartic acid, 15
asthma, 168
ataxia, 194
atherosclerosis, 168
ATP see adenosine triphosphate (ATP)
atrial septal defects, 194
attachment proteins, 54
autocrine signaling, 45
autophagy, 58
autoradiographs, 133
autosomal disorders, 146, 149, 161
  conditions, 179, 185
  examples, 146, 150
  inheritance, 146
autosomal dominant polycystic kidney disease (ADPKD), 183

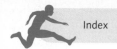

autosomal inheritance, 139
autosomal recessive (AR)
  conditions, 179, 185
  disorders, 147
    examples, 148, 151–152
    genes, 147
    inheritance, 147, 149
autosomes, 139
axonal transport, 57
axoplasmic flow, 58
azidothymidine (AZT), 29, 116
AZT *see* azidothymidine (AZT)

B
bacterial genetics, 110
bacterial toxins, 103
basement membrane, 69
Bayes' theorem, 186, 187
Becker muscular dystrophy, 153, 154
Beckwith–Wiedemann syndrome, 158, 175, 195
behavioral disorders, 194
behavior development, 191
benzylpenicillin, 111
biliary atresia, 195
biochemical tests, 181
blood disorders, 196
blood transfusion
  agglutination in, 65
bone disorders, 193
bowel atresia, 195
BRAC1, 76
  mutations, 172
BRAC2, 76
  mutations, 172
breast cancer, 76, 172
bronchiectasis, 195
buffer, 127

C
cadherins, 34, 66–67
  classes, 67
calcium channels, 48
calmodulin, 56
cAMP *see* cyclic AMP (cAMP)
cancer, 76
  genetics, 168–175
  genetic syndromes, 172
  pathways to malignancy, 169
  susceptibility in a family, 171
candidate gene approach, 136

carbohydrate degradation enzymes (e.g. galactosidase, glucosidase), 58
carcinogenesis
  multistage process, 169
carcinoma
  development, 170
cardiomyopathies, 194
carrier detection, 181
carrier proteins, 39
cascade screening, 184
catalysts, 25
cataract, 192
cathepsins, 58
cavernous hemangiomas, 193
CDH *see* congenital dislocation of the hip (CDH)
CDK *see* cyclin-dependent kinases (CDKs)
ceftizidime, 111–112
cefuroxime, 111
celiac disease, 195
cell
  adhesion, 61–71
  definition, 3
  differentiation, 10
  eukaryotic, 53
  labeling, 65
  motility, 53
  prokaryotic, 3–4
  shape, 53
  specialization, 10
  staging and prognosis, 11
  surface, 61–71
    receptors, 45
  wall synthesis
    inhibitors of, 110
cell–cell contact, 61, 62
cell–cell interactions, 61, 68, 76
cell cycle
  concept, 74
  extracellular regulation, 76
  regulation, 74
cell division
  overview, 77
cell junction
  types, 61
cell–matrix junctions, 62
cell membrane *see* membrane
cellular interaction, 61, 68, 76
central nervous system disorders, 194
centrioles, 9
cephalosporins, 111

CF *see* cystic fibrosis (CF)
CFTR *see* cystic fibrosis transmembrane regulator (CFTR)
Charcot–Marie–Tooth syndrome, 156
cholesterol, 32
   structure, 34
cholinesterase, 29
chondroitin sulfate, 69
chorioretinal degenerations, 192
Christmas disease, 153, 154
chromatids, 77, 78
chromatin, 73, 84
   fiber organization, 85
   inactive, 84, 85
chromosomal abnormalities, 183
chromosomal disorders, 159–165
   nomenclature, 160
   numerical, 160, 161
   overview, 160
   sex, 163
   structural, 160, 162–165, 165
   structure activity relationships, 166
   terminology, 159–160
   XX male, 161
   XXX, 161
   XYY, 161
chromosome condensation, 75
chromosome nomenclature (ISCN), 160
chromosomes, 7, 12, 77, 78, 80, 86
   anatomy, 86
   establishing linkage, 133–134
chronic progressive external ophthalmoplegia (CPEO), 159
cilia, 9, 56
cleft lip and palate, 168, 191
coagulation disorders, 196
coarctation of the aorta, 194
collagen, 70, 148
   fibrillar, 70
   structure, 70
   type IV, 71
collagenase, 58
colorectal cancer, 170
color vision disorders, 192
competitive antagonists, 49
complementation, 147, 150
complete mole, 157
compound heterozygote, 139
concordance
   in dizygotic twins, 167
   in monozygotic twins, 167

congenital adrenal hyperplasia, 148, 152
congenital dislocation of the hip (CDH), 167
congenital heart disease, 194
congenital malformations, 165, 177
conjugation, 112
connective tissue
   cell specialization, 11
connective tissue disorders, 193
connexin, 63
connexon, 63
Conradi syndrome, 193
consanguinity, 188
corneal dystrophies, 192
coronary artery disease, 165, 195
Corynebacterium diphtheriae, 103
Cowden syndrome, 175, 192
CPEO *see* chronic progressive external ophthalmoplegia (CPEO)
CpG dinucleotide, 85–86
craniosynostosis, 192
Cri du chat syndrome, 166
Crouzon syndrome, 192
cyclic AMP (cAMP), 48
cyclin-dependent kinases (CDKs), 74–76, 75
cyclins, 74–76
cyclops, 192
cysteine, 16
cystic fibrosis (CF), 39, 148, 152, 183
   gene therapy, 138
   mutations, 180
cystic fibrosis transmembrane regulator (CFTR), 34, 39
cytogenetic techniques, 128, 136
cytokinesis, 77
cytoskeleton, 9, 53
   components, 53–56
   functions, 53, 56

D
deafness, 159
   syndromes associated with, 192
deletion, 140, 165
dementia, 194
denaturing temperature, 127
dentatorubral-pallidoluysian atrophy (DRPLA), 145
deoxynucleotide triphosphates (dNTPs), 126
deoxyribonucleotides, 81
dermatan sulfate, 69
desmin, 55
desmosomes, 62
   structure, 63

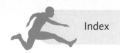

development areas, 190
development deviations, 191
dextrocardia, 195
diabetes mellitus, 165
   type 1 (insulin-dependent), 168
diakinesis, 78
dicer, 106
didanosine, 116
diffusion
   facilitated, 37, 38
   passive, 37
DiGeorge syndrome, 194
digestion of human DNA, 122
diplotene, 78
dissecting aortic aneurysm, 194
dizygotic twins
   concordance, 167
DMD see Duchenne muscular dystrophy (DMD)
DNA, 73, 80, 81
   electrophoresis, 122
   information carrier, 82
DNA damage, 76, 86–87, 139
DNA diagnostics, 136
DNA digestion, 121
DNA double helix, 81–82, 82
DNA fingerprinting, 188
DNA gyrase
   inhibitors, 110
DNA packaging, 84
DNA polymerases, 88–89
   eukaryotic, 89
   prokaryotic, 88
DNA polymorphisms, 132
DNA repair, 87
DNA repair mechanisms, 87
DNA repair systems, 164
DNA replication, 6, 80, 87–94, 139
   elongation, 92
   Escherichia coli, 91
   eukaryotic, 90, 92, 93
   prokaryotic, 90, 91
   termination, 92
DNA replication fork, 89
DNA sequence analysis, 129
DNA techniques, 181
DNA viruses, 113, 114
dNTPs see deoxynucleotide triphosphates
   (dNTPs)
dominant inheritance
   molecular basis, 146
dominant negative effect, 148

double-stranded RNA, 106
Down syndrome, 162, 194, 195
DRPLA see dentatorubral-pallidoluysian atrophy
   (DRPLA)
drug history, 189
drugs
   receptors, 48–50
Duchenne muscular dystrophy (DMD), 141,
   153, 154
duplication, 165
dynein, 57, 58
dystrophin gene 155

E
ear disorders, 192
ear malformation
   external, 193
ECM see extracellular matrix (ECM)
Edwards syndrome, 194
EFs see elongation factors (EFs)
EGF see epidermal growth factor (EGF) receptor
Ehlers–Danlos syndrome, 156
E-LAM, 68
elastin, 71
electrochemical gradient, 37
electrochemical potential difference of ions, 41
electrophoresis of digested human DNA, 122
electrophoresis of digested plasmid DNA, 122
Ellis–van Creveld syndrome, 194
elongation factors (EFs), 103
endocrine signaling, 45
endocytosis, 5, 58, 59
   receptor-mediated, 58
endomitosis, 80
endoplasmic reticulum (ER), 73, 103, 108
endotoxin, 67
environmental factors
   multifactorial disorders, 167–168
enzyme
   active sites, 25
   competitive inhibition, 29
   constitutive, 104
   genetic variation of function, 29
   induced fit hypothesis, 25
   inducible, 104
   inhibitors, 28–29
   kinetics, 27
   lysosomal, 58
   mechanisms of action, 25
   reaction rates, 27–28
   regulation of activity, 26

repressible, 104
specificity, 25
structure, 26
epidermal growth factor (EGF) receptor, 46
epidermolysis bullosa, 193
epigenetic mechanisms, 107
epilepsy, 168
epithelial tissue
  cell specialization, 11
ER *see* endoplasmic reticulum (ER)
erythrocyte cytoskeleton, 56
erythromycin, 112
Escherichia coli, 90
  DNA replication, 91
  prokaryotic polymerization, 92
  RNA polymerase (RNAP), 94
E-selectin, 67, 68
essential hypertension, 168
euchromatin, 12, 73
eukaryotes, 3–5, 82
  gene expression in multicellular, 10
  protein synthesis, 103
  transcriptional regulation, 105
eukaryotic cell, 4–5, 73
eukaryotic DNA polymerases, 89
eukaryotic DNA replication, 90, 92, 93
eukaryotic genes, 109
  structure and evolution, 109–110
eukaryotic organelles, 5
eukaryotic ribosome, 84
eukaryotic RNA polymerase, 95
eukaryotic transcription
  elongation, 97
  initiation, 95–97
  vs. prokaryotic transcription, 98, 103
  termination, 97
exocytosis, 59
exomphalos, 195
extension temperature, 127
extracellular matrix (ECM), 61, 62, 69, 71
eye disorders, 192

F
FA *see* Friedreich ataxia (FA)
Fabry disease, 153, 154, 195
facial deformities, 191–192
failure to thrive, 191
familial hypercholesterolemia, 147, 149, 195
family history, 189
family selection, 133
Fanconi syndrome, 173, 196

Faraday's number, 41
α-fetoprotein, 172
FGF *see* fibroblast growth factor (FGF) receptor
fibrillin, 71
fibrils, 70
fibroblast growth factor (FGF) receptor, 46
fibroblasts, 71
fibronectin, 71
filaments, 53
fine motor skills, 191
FISH *see* fluorescence *in situ* hybridization
    (FISH)
flagella, 9
fluid mosaic model, 31
fluorescence *in situ* hybridization (FISH), 128,
    129, 165, 181
founder effect, 180
F plasmids, 112
fragile X syndrome, 85, 142, 195
Friedreich ataxia (FA), 144, 148, 152, 195
fructose-6-phosphate, 30
functional cloning, 135

G
G-actin, 53
GAGs *see* glycosaminoglycans (GAGs)
galactosidase, 58
gamete, 77
gametogenesis, 79–80
gap junctions, 63–65
gastrointestinal disorders, 195
gastroschisis, 195
Gaucher disease, 60–61, 148, 151
G-banding, 128
gel electrophoresis, 121–122
gels, 133
gene cloning and characterizing, 132–136
gene duplication, 110
gene expression
  gene frequency, 180
gene expression control, 104–107
gene expression in multicellular eukaryotes, 10
gene inheritance
  X-linked, 146
GENES
  mnemonic, 190
genes
  structure, 109–110
gene splicing, 97
gene therapy (GT), 113, 136
  germ line, 136

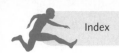
gene therapy (GT) (*Continued*)
  somatic cell, 136
  trials, 136
genetic code, 99–100
genetic counseling, 184–188, 185
  confidentiality and conflicts of interest, 188
  diagnosis, 186
  discussing options, communication, and
      support, 187
  ethical considerations, 188
  interview outline, 189
  presenting the risks in context, 187
  structure, 188
genetic disease, 139–175
  common presentations, 190–195
genetic disorders, 166, 177
  website, 177
genetic diversity, 79–80
genetic drift, 180
genetic heterogeneity, 153
genetic history *see* history taking
genetic linkage, 181
genetic linkage analysis, 132–133
genetic maps, 130–131
  fine, 134
genetic markers to cloned gene, 134
genetic material
  transfer mechanisms, 112
genetics
  molecular
    applied to medicine, 121–138
    basic techniques, 121–130
    basis of, 71–117
  principles of, 177–197
genitourinary tract disorders, 195–196
genome, 77
genome sequencing, 131
genomic DNA, 123
genotype, 139
genotype frequencies, 179
GFAP *see* glial fibrillary acidic protein (GFAP)
Gibbs–Donnan equilibrium, 42–43
Gilbert syndrome, 195
gilia, 9
Gilles de la Tourette syndrome, 147, 149, 191,
    194
glaucoma, 192
glial fibrillary acidic protein (GFAP), 55
glucose-6-phosphate dehydrogenase (G6PD),
    29
  deficiency, 153, 154, 196

glucose transporter, 40
glucosidase, 58
glucuronidase, 58
glutamine, 16
glycine, 15
  titration, 17
glycocalyx, 6
glycoproteins, 65, 70
glycosaminoglycans (GAGs), 69
glycosidases (e.g. glucuronidase, hyaluronidase),
    58
GMP *see* guanosine monophosphate (GMP)
Golgi apparatus, 7
Golgi complex, 58
Gorlin syndrome, 175
G6PD *see* glucose-6-phosphate dehydrogenase
    (G6PD)
G-proteins, 48, 49
Gram-negative bacteria, 110
gross motor skills, 191
growth factors, 76
GT *see* gene therapy (GT)
guanosine monophosphate (GMP), 81
guanosine monophosphate (GMP)-140, 68
gynecomastia, 194

H
HAART *see* highly active antiretroviral therapy
    (HAART)
haplotype genes, 111
Hardy–Weinberg equation, 178, 179–181
Hardy–Weinberg equilibrium, 133
Hardy–Weinberg principle, 178
HCG, 183
HDL *see* high-density lipoprotein (HDL)
hearing loss, 191
hemochromatosis, 147, 148, 151, 195
hemophilia A, 153, 154, 180
hemophilia B (Christmas disease), 153, 154
Henderson–Hasselbalch equation, 14
heparin-binding EGF, 46
heparin sulfate, 69
hereditary motor sensory neuropathies, 194
hereditary nonpolyposis colon cancer (HNPCC),
    173
heritability, 167
heterochromatin, 12, 73
heteronuclear RNA (hnRNA), 83, 97
heterophagy, 58
high-density lipoprotein (HDL), 168
highly active antiretroviral therapy (HAART), 116

Hirschsprung disease, 195
histidine, 16
histones, 73, 85
history taking, 188–189
  systems review, 190
HIV-1, 29, 113
HIV-2, 113
HIV/AIDS, 116
HLA *see* human leucocyte antigen (HLA)
HNPCC *see* hereditary nonpolyposis colon
        cancer (HNPCC)
hnRNA *see* heteronuclear RNA (hnRNA)
homozygote, 139
hormones, 76
  definition, 45
Human Genome Project, 10, 130–132
human leucocyte antigen (HLA), 111
  complex, 110
Huntington disease, 140, 142–143, 157, 188
hyaluronidase, 58
hybridization, 123
hydrolases, 58
hydrophilic interactions, 31
hydrophobic interactions, 31
hydroxylation, 107
hyperbilirubinemia, 195
hypertension, 195
hypoglycemia, 195
hypogonadism, 195, 196

I
ICAM, 67, 69
ICF *see* immunodeficiency, centromeric
        instability and facial anomalies (ICF)
        syndrome
ichthyoses, 193
Ig *see* immunoglobulin (Ig) family
IGF *see* insulin growth factor (IGF) receptor
IL-1 *see* interleukin-1 (IL-1)
immunodeficiencies, 196
immunodeficiency, centromeric instability and
        facial anomalies (ICF) syndrome, 85
immunoglobulin (Ig) family, 67
imperforate anus, 195
imprinting, 157
incest, 188
infantile pyloric stenosis, 195
inheritance patterns, 139
inositol lipid pathways, 48
inositol phospholipid signaling pathway, 50
insertion, 140

insulin-dependent diabetes mellitus, 168
insulin growth factor (IGF) receptor, 46
integrins, 68
integrins binding, 68
interleukin-1 (IL-1), 67
intermediate filaments, 53, 54–55
interphase, 74
intestinal epithelium, 57
introns
  structure and evolution, 109–110
inversion, 145, 164
ion channels, 39
ions
  distribution across cell membrane, 37
  electrochemical potential difference, 41
ISCN *see* chromosome nomenclature (ISCN)
isochromosome, 165
isoleucine, 15

K
kanamycin, 112
Kartagener syndrome, 9, 195
karyotype, 77, 159
Kayser–Fleischer rings, 192
Kearns–Sayre syndrome (KSS), 159
Kennedy disease, 140, 144
α-keratin, 21
kinesins, 57, 58
Klinefelter syndrome, 163, 194
Knudson's "two-hit" hypothesis, 171
KSS *see* Kearns–Sayre syndrome (KSS)
kyphoscoliosis, 194

L
lac operator, 106
lac operon, 106
lac repressor, 106
lactam, 110
lactate dehydrogenase
  structure, 27
laminin, 71
lamins, 73
law of addition, 184
law of multiplication, 184
LDL *see* low-density lipoprotein (LDL)
Leber's hereditary optic neuropathy, 159
Leber's optic atrophy, 192
Leigh disease, 159
leptotene, 78
Lesch–Nyhan syndrome, 153, 154
leucine, 15

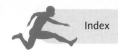

leucocyte function-associated (LFA1), 68
LFA1 *see* leucocyte function-associated (LFA1)
Li–Fraumeni syndrome, 171, 173
ligand
    definition, 45
Lineweaver–Burk plot, 29
linkage analysis, 132–133
lipases, 58
lipids, 31–32
liver disease, 195
locus heterogeneity, 153
LOD score, 133
loop formation, 84
low-density lipoprotein (LDL), 147, 168
    receptors, 60
lysine, 16
lysosomal storage
    diseases, 59
lysosomes, 7
    definition, 58
    functions, 58

M
macroglossia, 195
macroorchidism, 195
major histocompatibility complex (MHC), 65
malignancy, 76
MAP kinase, 47
MAPs *see* microtubule-associated proteins
        (MAPs)
Marfan syndrome, 147, 149, 194
maternal serum α-fetoprotein (MSAFP), 183, 184
maturation-promoting factor (MPF), 75
Meckel syndrome, 195
medical history, 189
meiosis, 134, 160, 161
    definition, 77
    phases, 78–79
meitoic recombination, 164
MELAS, 159
membrane
    biologic, 31–32
    cell, 31–51
        transport across, 36–41
    fluidity, 35
    mobility components, 36
    permeability, 36
    proteins, 32
    semipermeable, 37
    solute movement across, 38

structure, 31
    transition from gel to liquid crystal, 35
membrane potential, 41–44
    definition, 41
    maintenance, 41
    resting, 43
membrane recycling, 59
MEN *see* multiple endocrine neoplasia (MEN)
Mendelian characteristic, 132
Mendelian disorders
    heterogeneity in, 153
Mendelian inheritance, 185, 186
Mendelian inheritance of gene disorders, 145
Mendelian inheritance of single gene disorders,
        145–146
Mendelian inheritance *vs.* multifactorial
        inheritance, 166–167
mental retardation, 194
MERRF, 159
messenger RNA (mRNA), 7, 82
metabolic myopathies, 194
metabolism
    inborn errors, 196
metaphase, 77, 78
methionine, 16
methylation, 85–86
MHC *see* major histocompatibility complex
        (MHC)
Michaelis constant, 28
Michaelis–Menten equation, 27
Michaelis–Menten graph, 27
Michaelis–Menten kinetics, 37
microarray resequencing chips, 129–130
microcephaly, 192
micro RNAs (miRNAs), 105, 106
microsatellite linkage, 183
microsatellite markers, 132
microtubule, 53, 55–56
    formation, 56
    structure, 56
microtubule-associated proteins (MAPs), 55
microtubule organizing center (MTOC), 86
microvillus, 9
    structure, 57
migration, 180
miRNAs *see* micro RNAs (miRNAs)
mitochondria, 7
mitochondrial disorders
    examples, 159
mitochondrial DNA (mtDNA), 100, 158

mitochondrial inheritance, 158
mitosis, 74, 75
 definition, 77
 phases, 77
mitotic spindle, 58
monosomy, 159, 160–161
monozygotic twins
 concordance, 167
mosaicism, 158–159
MPF see maturation-promoting factor (MPF)
mRNA see messenger RNA (mRNA)
MSAFP see maternal serum α-fetoprotein
 (MSAFP)
mtDNA see mitochondrial DNA (mtDNA)
MTOC see microtubule organizing center
 (MTOC)
mucopoly-saccharidoses, 156
multifactorial disorders, 165–168, 166–167
 examples, 168
 overview, 165–168
 risk to relatives, 168
 threshold model, 167
multifactorial inheritance vs. Mendelian
 inheritance, 166–167
multiple endocrine neoplasia (MEN), 173
muscle contraction, 57
muscle tissue
 cell specialization, 11
muscular dystrophies, 193, 195
mutation, 76, 139, 177, 180
 effects on protein products, 141
 functional effects on protein, 145
 gain of function, 145
 loss of function, 145
 main classes, groups and types, 141
 mechanisms, 139
mutation analysis, 136
mutation detection, 181
myoglobin, 21
myosin, 56
 structure, 56
myosin II, 56
myosin proteins, 54
myotonic disorders, 194
myotonic dystrophy, 143

N
NADH, 26
NA⁺/K⁺ ATPase, 40
NARP, 159

N-CAM, 67
Nernst equation, 41–42
 derivation, 42
nervous tissue
 cell specialization, 11
neural tube defects, 168, 184
neurocutaneous syndromes, 194
neurofibromatosis type I (von Recklinghausen
 disease), 173
neurofibromatosis type II, 173–174
neurological disorders, 140
neuromuscular disorders, 193
nevi, 193
newborn screening, 181
nicotinic acetylcholine receptor, 46
nocodazole, 56
nonhistones, 73
non-Mendelian inheritance
 mechanisms, 157
nonrandom mating, 179–186
Noonan syndrome, 194
Northern blotting, 124
nuclear envelope, 73
nuclear matrix, 73
nuclear pores, 73, 74
nucleases (e.g. acid RNase, acid DNase),
 58
nucleic acids, 80–84
 isolation, 121
 production, 81
 structure, 80
nucleic acid synthesis
 inhibitors of, 110
nucleoli, 73
nucleoplasm, 73
nucleoproteins, 73
nucleosides, 80, 81
nucleosomes, 84
nucleotide cofactor binding domain, 28
nucleotides, 80, 81
nucleus, 6
 organization, 73–74
 structures, 73, 74
nystagmus, 192

O
occludin, 62
Okasaki fragments, 93
OMIN see Online Mendelian Inheritance in
 Man (OMIM)

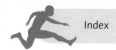

oncogenes, 169
  transduction position, 170
oncogenesis, 76
oncogenes *vs.* tumor suppressor genes,
  169
Online Mendelian Inheritance in Man (OMIM),
  153
oogenesis, 80
oral deformities, 191–192
organelles
  membranous, 5
  nonmembranous, 9
  specialized, 9
organism
  definition, 3
  multicellular, 10
osteogenesis imperfecta, 70

P
p53, 76–77
  major roles, 77
pachytene, 78
pancreatitis, 195
paracrine signaling, 45
partial mole, 157
partial nerve deafness, 192
Patau syndrome, 194
patent ductus arteriosus, 194
paternity testing, 188
PCR *see* polymerase chain reaction (PCR)
Pearson syndrome, 159
PECAM, 67
pectus excavatum, 194
pedigree analysis, 133
pedigree charts, 139, 140
penetrance, 153
penicillins, 110, 111
pentose sugars, 81
peptic ulcers, 165, 168, 195
peroxisomes, 7
Peutz–Jeghers syndrome, 175
PFK I *see* phosphofructokinase I (PFK I)
pH, 14
phagocytes
  motility, 57
phenocopy, 165
phenotype, 139
phenylalanine, 15
phenylketonuria, 148
phenylketonuria (PKU), 151, 181
phosphatases (e.g. acid phosphatase), 58

phosphatidylcholine, 32, 33
phosphatidylethanolamine, 32, 33
phosphatidylsenine, 32, 33
phosphofructokinase I (PFK I), 29, 30
phospholipids, 31, 32, 33
  mobility, 36
  packing, 34
phosphorylation, 107
physical maps, 131
PKU *see* phenylketonuria (PKU)
plasma membrane, 5
plasmid DNA, 123
ploidy, 77
point mutations, 139, 140
polycystic disease of the liver, 195
polycystic kidney disease, 156, 195
polygenic inheritance, 165
polymerase chain reaction (PCR), 89, 126, 181,
  183
  based techniques, 136
  controls, 127
  mechanism of action, 127
  negative control, 127–128
  reverse transcriptase, 128
  vs. Southern hybridization, 128
  visualizing the products, 127
polymorphic marker, 132
  linkage, 181
polymorphism, 177
polyploidy, 159, 160
polyposis coli, 172
population genetics, 177
population screening, 181
  tests, 183
positional candidate gene approach, 135
positional cloning, 132, 135
posttranslational modification
  disorders, 109
  proteins, 107–109
potassium, 39–40
potassium in cell membrane potential, 43
Prader–Willi syndrome (PWS), 157, 158, 165
prenatal diagnosis, 181, 182
presymptomatic diagnosis, 181
primary lysosomes, 58
primers, 126, 133
probability theory, 184
prokaryotes, 3–5
  protein synthesis, 100–103
  transcriptional regulation, 105
prokaryotic DNA polymerases, 88

prokaryotic DNA replication, 90, 91
prokaryotic polymerization
    Escherichia coli, 92
prokaryotic posttranscriptional modification, 94–5
    addition of 5′ cap, 97
prokaryotic replication, 90
prokaryotic transcription, 94
    vs. eukaryotic transcription, 98, 103
proline, 15
prophase, 77, 78
protease inhibitors, 116
proteases (e.g. cathepsins, collagenase), 58
protein expression control, 104–107
proteins
    actin-binding, 54
    biologic, 32
    carrier, 39
    glycosylation, 107
    integral, 31, 32
    membrane, 32, 35
    mobility, 36
    peripheral, 31
    posttranslational modification, 107–109
protein synthesis, 99–104
    antibiotics, 104
    eukaryotes, 103
    factors affecting, 103–104
    inhibitors, 112
    prokaryotes, 100–103
proteoglycans, 69, 70
proteome, 131
P-selectin, 67, 68
Pseudomonas aeruginosa, 112
psychiatric disorders, 194
ptosis, 192
pulmonary arteriosus, 194
pulmonary stenosis, 194
pump, 37, 58
purines, 80–81
    biosynthesis, 80–81
PWS *see* Prader–Willi syndrome (PWS)
pyrimidine, 80–81
    biosynthesis, 80–81
    synthesis, 81

Q
quinolones, 110

R
Ras, 34, 47
receptor, 45–50

cell surface, 45
    drugs, 48–50
    metabotropic, 48
    steroid, 48, 50
receptor-mediated endocytosis, 58
recessive inheritance, 153
    molecular basis, 147
reciprocal translocation, 164
recombination, 133
recombination fraction (RF), 133
refractive errors, 192
renal stones, 195
renal tumors, 195
replication bubble, 90
RER *see* rough endoplasmic reticulum (RER)
restriction endonucleases, 122
restriction enzymes, 121
restriction enzymes, fragment size produced and
        cuffing frequency, 122
restriction fragment length polymorphisms
        (RFLPs), 132
restriction maps, 122, 125
retinal detachment, 192
retinitis pigmentosa, 156
retinoblastoma, 174, 192
retroviruses, 113, 116
    replication, 115
retrovirus genome, 115
Rett syndrome, 85, 194
reverse transcriptase
    PCR, 128
reversible antagonists, 49
RF *see* recombination fraction (RF)
RFLPs *see* restriction fragment length
        polymorphisms (RFLPs)
ribonucleosides, 81
ribosomal RNA (rRNA), 7, 83
ribosome clusters, 7
ring chromosomes, 165
RISC *see* RNA-induced silencing complex (RISC)
risk assessment, 184–188
risk calculation, 185, 186
RNA, 80, 81
    synthesis, 82
RNA chain elongation, 95
RNA-induced silencing complex (RISC), 106
RNA interference (RNAi), 105, 106
RNAP *see* RNA polymerase (RNAP)
RNA polymerase (RNAP)
    Escherichia coli, 94
    eukaryotic, 95

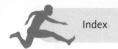

RNA replication, 6
RNA splicing, 98
RNA synthesis, 93–99
RNA viruses, 113, 115
Robertsonian translocation, 164
rough endoplasmic reticulum (RER), 7, 58, 103
rRNA *see* ribosomal RNA (rRNA)

S
sarcomeres, 57
SBMA *see* spinobulbar muscular atrophy (SBMA)
schizophrenia, 165, 168, 194
screening
 "at risk" populations, 183
screening program criteria, 181
secondary lysosomes, 58
second division, 79
second-messenger system, 45
selectins, 67
selection, 180
SER *see* smooth endoplasmic reticulum (SER)
serine, 16
severe combined immuno-deficiency, 156
severe congenital sensorineural deafness, 192
sex chromosome disorders, 161, 163
SH2 binding domain, 46, 47
Sherman's paradox, 142
sickle-cell disease, 148, 151, 196
signal peptide, 107
single gene disorders, 139
 autosomal dominant, 146
 autosomal recessive, 146
 causes, 139
 Mendelian inheritance of, 145–146
 Mendelian patterns of inheritance, 139
 non-Mendelian inheritance, 153
 terminology, 139
single gene disorders with more than one mode of inheritance
 example, 156
single gene inheritance
 X-linked recessive, 146
single nucleotide polymorphisms (SNPs), 132
siRNA *see* small interfering RNA (siRNA)
skin disorders, 193
skin tumors, 193
slicer, 106
small interfering RNA (siRNA), 105
smooth endoplasmic reticulum (SER), 7, 103
smooth muscle cells, 11

SNPs *see* single nucleotide polymorphisms (SNPs)
snRNPs, 98
social history, 189
social skills, 191
sodium pump, 40
Southern analysis, 123
Southern blotting, 124, 125, 136
Southern hybridization, 126
 vs. polymerase chain reaction (PCR), 128
spectrin, 57
spermatogenesis, 80
S phase, 78
sphingomyelin, 32, 33
spinal muscular atrophies, 193
spinobulbar muscular atrophy (SBMA), 144
spinocerebellar ataxia, 145
Staphylococcus aureus, 111–112
Stickler syndrome, 192
storage diseases
 lysosomal, 59
Sturge–Weber syndrome, 192, 193
substitution, 139
sulfatases (e.g. aryl sulfatase), 58
sulfation, 107
sulfonamides, 110

T
Taq polymerase, 126
taxol, 56
Tay–Sachs disease, 61, 148, 151, 183
telomerase, 93–94
telophase, 77, 79
tenascin, 71
tetracycline, 112
TGF-α *see* transforming growth factor-α (TGF-α)
thalassemia, 183, 196
α-thalassemia, 148, 151
β-thalassemia, 148, 151
thermocycling, 127
thoracic development disorders, 194
threonine, 16
tight junctions, 61, 62
TK *see* tyrosine kinase (TK)
TNF *see* tumor necrosis factor (TNF)
transcription
 antibiotics, 98–99
 definition, 94
 elongation, 94
 initiation, 94

prokaryotic, 94
    termination, 94–95
transcriptional regulation, 104
    eukaryotes, 105
    prokaryotes, 105
transfer RNA (tRNA), 82–83
    secondary structure, 83
transformation, 112
transforming growth factor-α (TGF-α), 46
transition, 139
translation
    definition, 99
    elongation, 101–103
    initiation, 101
    termination, 103
translocation, 159, 162–163
transmembrane proteoglycans, 68
transmembrane signaling, 45
transport
    active, 38
    axonal, 57
    mechanisms, 39–41
    primary active, 38
    secondary active, 38–39
    summary of types, 39
transporter
    active, 40–41
    glucose, 40
transporter molecule
    summary of types, 41
transversion, 139
Treacher Collins syndrome, 192
trimethoprim, 110
trinucleotide repeat disorders
    genetics, 145
triplet repeat expansions, 140
    diseases caused by, 142–145
triploidy, 159
trisomies, 160
trisomy 13, 162
trisomy 18, 162
trisomy 21, 183, 184
tRNA *see* transfer RNA (tRNA)
troponin, 56
truncus arteriosus, 194
tryptophan, 15
tuberous sclerosis, 157, 174
tubulin, 53, 55, 56
tumor necrosis factor (TNF), 67
tumor suppressor genes, 76, 169–171
    examples, 171

    in inherited cancers, 171
    vs. oncogenes, 169
Turner syndrome, 163, 193, 194
type 1 (insulin-dependent) diabetes mellitus,
    168
tyrosine, 15, 46
tyrosine kinase (TK)
    receptors, 46, 47
    signal transduction, 47

U
UBE3A gene, 157
umbilical hernia, 195
uniparental disomy, 157
urinary malformation, 195

V
valine, 15
van der Waals forces, 32
variable expressivity, 157
variable number tandem repeat (VNTR), 132
VATER syndrome, 195
VCAM, 67
vector systems, 136–137
ventricular septal defect, 194
vimentin, 55
vinblastine, 56
viral genetics, 113
virus
    life cycle, 114
visual impairment, 191
vitamin D, 165
vitiligo, 193
VNTR *see* variable number tandem repeat
    (VNTR)
von Hippel–Lindau disease, 175, 195
von Recklinghausen disease, 173
von Willebrand disease, 147, 149, 196

W
Waardenburg syndrome, 192
Western blotting, 124
Williams syndrome, 191, 194
Wilms tumor, 174–175, 195
Wolf–Hirschhorn syndrome, 166

X
X chromosomes, 150, 161
xeroderma pigmentosum, 175
X-linked disorders, 148
X-linked dominant inheritance, 150

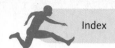

X-linked genes, 150
X-linked inheritance
  molecular basis, 150
X-linked recessive conditions, 186
X-linked recessive disorders
  examples, 150–152, 155
X-linked recessive inheritance, 148, 153

Y
Y chromosome, 161

Z
zidovudine, 116
zygotene, 78